Cleft Palate
and Communication

Contributors to This Volume

JAMES F. CURTIS

LEONARD D. GOODSTEIN

ELISE HAHN

DOROTHY A. HUNTINGTON

C. M. KOS

KENNETH L. MOLL

HUGHLETT L. MORRIS

WILLIAM F. PRATHER

RALPH L. SHELTON, Jr.

D. C. SPRIESTERSBACH

CLEFT PALATE
AND COMMUNICATION

EDITED BY

D. C. SPRIESTERSBACH

DEPARTMENT OF SPEECH PATHOLOGY AND AUDIOLOGY
AND
DEPARTMENT OF OTOLARYNGOLOGY AND MAXILLOFACIAL SURGERY
UNIVERSITY OF IOWA
IOWA CITY, IOWA

AND

DOROTHY SHERMAN

DEPARTMENT OF SPEECH PATHOLOGY AND AUDIOLOGY
UNIVERSITY OF IOWA
IOWA CITY, IOWA

ACADEMIC PRESS   New York and London   1968

ACADEMIC PRESS INC.
111 Fifth Avenue, New York, New York 10003

United Kingdom Edition published by
ACADEMIC PRESS INC. (LONDON) LTD.
Berkeley Square House, London W.1

LIBRARY OF CONGRESS CATALOG CARD NUMBER: 68-18682

PRINTED IN THE UNITED STATES OF AMERICA

FH

To Wendell Johnson

The editors dedicate this book to one who was not only their colleague, but also their teacher, mentor, and good friend, and whose influence upon their attitudes and thinking has been immeasurable. He was teacher, mentor, and good friend to countless other persons throughout the world. His greatness is to be found in the impact that he had on people. He argued consistently for the philosophy that knowledge could not be packaged and claimed by narrowly defined professions. He startled many by questioning arbitrary academic units which tended to inhibit the solution of problems because they fostered a kind of academic provincialism.

The results of his life's work are a matter of record which reveals a man who had imagination, idealism, and optimism, a record to which many men aspire but few achieve.

List of Contributors

Numbers in parentheses indicate the pages on which the authors' contributions begin.

JAMES F. CURTIS (27), *Department of Speech Pathology and Audiology, University of Iowa, Iowa City, Iowa*

LEONARD D. GOODSTEIN (201), *Department of Psychology, University of Cincinnati, Cincinnati, Ohio*

ELISE HAHN (225), *California State College at Los Angeles, Los Angeles, California*

DOROTHY A. HUNTINGTON (1), *Division of Speech Pathology and Audiology, Stanford University School of Medicine, Palo Alto, California*

C. M. KOS (169), *Iowa Clinic of Otology, Iowa City, Iowa*

KENNETH L. MOLL (61), *Department of Speech Pathology and Audiology, University of Iowa, Iowa City, Iowa*

HUGHLETT L. MORRIS (119, 225), *Department of Speech Pathology and Audiology, and Department of Otolaryngology and Maxillofacial Surgery, University of Iowa, Iowa City, Iowa*

WILLIAM F. PRATHER (169), *Veterans Administration Hospital, and Speech Department, University of Washington, Seattle, Washington*

RALPH L. SHELTON, JR. (225), *University of Kansas School of Medicine, Kansas City, Kansas*

D. C. SPRIESTERSBACH (269), *Department of Speech Pathology and Audiology, and Department of Otolaryngology and Maxillofacial Surgery, University of Iowa, Iowa City, Iowa*

Preface

During the 25 years following the organization of the American Cleft Palate Association (originally the American Academy of Cleft Palate Prosthesis) an increasing interest in the problems of persons with cleft lip and palate has resulted in a greater number of studies of various facets of these problems by investigators in many professions. Since the primary purpose of much of the physical management of the cleft is to provide a structure which functions adequately as part of the speech mechanism, many of the investigators, particularly the speech pathologists, have studied the relationships between the clefts and the communication abilities of the persons with the clefts. The results of these studies have been published largely in scholarly journals in fields such as surgery, dentistry, and speech pathology. The results of some of the studies have been and are now being reported in textbooks, but not in a systematic way. The purpose of this book is to present a systematic review devoted solely to the work which has been done to date on the communication problems of individuals with cleft lip and palate. It is our hope that this review will establish new, or at least more available, bases for our understanding of the communication problems of the persons with clefts, that it will identify the gaps in our understanding and the reasons for them, and that it will stimulate further research, both basic and applied, which will help to close these gaps. We assume that other reviews such as this one will be needed periodically in the future.

This book has been written primarily for those professional persons who have specialized in the communication problems of persons with clefts. The authors have assumed that the reader will have a considerable amount of sophistication about the "cleft palate problem," including familiarity with the relevant literature and with the research techniques which have been employed. Thus, this book has not been written to provide an effective introduction to the problem. On the contrary, we feel that it will be helpful for advanced courses and seminars, and as a resource book for investigators in any of the fields concerned with cleft lip and palate, and most particularly, for advanced students and researchers concerned with the communication problems.

We have attempted to organize the material in the book in a logical fashion. The first two chapters deal with the normal processes of speech production. Chapter III deals with the work which has been done to describe the nature of the communication problems associated with cleft lip and palate. Chapter IV reviews the work which has been done in an attempt to account for these problems. Chapters V and VI proceed to describe the work which has been done on the psychological and audiological aspects of these problems. Chapter VII draws upon all of these chapters and upon additional work to review the state of our knowledge concerning the diagnostic and therapeutic techniques for evaluating the communication problems of persons with clefts. Finally, Chapter VIII includes some commentary on the attitudes and motivations which have provided the impetus for the investigations which have been made to date and suggests some possible directions for the development of professional activities in the future.

As attested by the material in this book, we are aware that the communication skills of persons with cleft lip and palate are highly dependent on the physical status of the speech mechanism. We join many other specialists, however, in the conviction that there may be other important bases for the communication problems. Because we consider that the central and major core of the behavioral aspects of the problem is related to the audiological and psychological areas, we have confined our discussion to these two areas but without any intention of implying that we have rejected other behavioral aspects in specific instances. We have chosen not to consider issues related to physical management in this text, first, because a great deal has already been published in this area and, second, because review of that work here would necessarily have limited the depth with which we would have been able to explore the communication problems.

Many persons have had a hand in assisting with the development of this material. These have included administrators, colleagues, graduate students, and members of the office staffs of our several institutions. We are grateful indeed for their help and their support, and we extend our sincere thanks to them. We are especially indebted to Lucy Eggert who has typed the manuscript (some of it several times as the final version was developed), who has checked out endless details, and who has reminded us in her gentle but effective way that time was moving on. Finally, we are all greatly indebted to Hughlett L. Morris, whose interest and counsel during the final stages of the preparation of the manscript were crucial to its completion.

Grateful acknowledgment is also made of the support which has come from several agencies which made it possible for us to carry on our own investigations. The work at the University of Iowa has been supported over the years by grants M-1158 (National Institute of Mental Health) and D-00853 (National Institute of Dental Research), Public Health Service. The work at the University of Kansas has been supported by grants DE-02004 (National Institute of Dental Research), Public Health Service and by a grant from the Easter Seal Research Foundation.

December, 1967   D. C. SPRIESTERSBACH
DOROTHY SHERMAN

Contents

LIST OF CONTRIBUTORS   vii

PREFACE   ix

Chapter I. **Anatomical and Physiological Bases for Speech**   1

   Dorothy A. Huntington

    I.   Introduction   1
   II. Speech Production   2
       References   22

Chapter II. **Acoustics of Speech Production and Nasalization**   27

   James F. Curtis

    I.   Fundamental Acoustic Properties of Speech Signals   28
   II. Acoustic Theory   30
  III. Nasalization of Speech   45
  IV. Source Functions   53
   V. The Respiratory System   58
       References   60

Chapter III. **Speech Characteristics of Individuals with Cleft Lip
and Palate**   61

   Kenneth L. Moll

    I.   General Incidence of Speech Problems   63
   II. Speech Sound Articulation and Intelligibility   68
  III. Nasal Voice Quality   95
  IV. Language Development   108
   V. Other Speech Dimensions   110
  VI. Summary   112
       References   113

Chapter IV. **Etiological Bases for Speech Problems** 119
Hughlett L. Morris

   I. Articulation Disorders 121
  II. Voice Disorders 149
 III. Language Development 153
 IV. Discussion 156
  V. Summary 165
     References 165

Chapter V. **Audiological and Otological Considerations** 169
William F. Prather and C. M. Kos

   I. Introduction 169
  II. Incidence of Hearing Loss and Aural Pathology 170
 III. Incidence of Hearing Loss and of Aural Pathology in Relationship to
     Other Variables 174
 IV. Discussion and Implications for Management 194
     References 198

Chapter VI. **Psychosocial Aspects of Cleft Palate** 201
Leonard D. Goodstein

   I. Introduction 201
  II. The Parents of a Child with a Cleft Lip or Palate 203
 III. The Psychosocial Development of the Child with Cleft Palate 209
 IV. The Personality and Adjustment of the Child with Cleft Palate 213
  V. The Psychosocial Problems of the Adolescent and Adult with Cleft Palate . 217
 VI. Some Methodological Considerations in Cleft Palate Research 218
 VII. Recapitulation 220
     References 222

Chapter VII. **Diagnosis and Therapy** 225
Ralph L. Shelton, Jr., Elise Hahn, and Hughlett L. Morris

Part One: DIAGNOSIS 226
   I. Velopharyngeal Competence 227
  II. Speech Problems 237
 III. Oral-Facial Structures 239
 IV. Neural Function 241
  V. Hearing Acuity and Auditory Perception 244
 VI. Psychosocial Adjustment 245
 VII. Language Maturity 246
 VIII. Concluding Statement 248

Part Two: THERAPY 249
   I. Procedures for Articulation Therapy 251
  II. Therapeutic Exercise and Motor Learning 253
 III. Procedures for Voice Therapy. 257
 IV. Procedures for Language Development and the Improvement of
      Communication 259
  V. Concluding Statement 261
     References 261

Chapter VIII. Some Professional Implications. 269

D. C. Spriestersbach

   I. "Professions" 269
  II. The Team 273
 III. The Speech Pathologist 275
 IV. Summary 278
     References 279

AUTHOR INDEX 281
SUBJECT INDEX 288

Cleft Palate
and Communication

CHAPTER

I

Anatomical and Physiological Bases for Speech

Dorothy A. Huntington

I. Introduction 1
II. Speech Production 2
   A. Respiration in Speech 2
   B. Vocal Fold Vibration 4
   C. Articulation 6
   References 22

I. Introduction

An understanding of normal speech, and also of any speech which deviates from normal, includes a knowledge of three different and complexly interrelated aspects of the speech process: the production of speech, the acoustic characteristics of the speech signal, and speech perception. Much remains to be learned not only about their interrelationships but also about each of these aspects of normal speech. Fortunately, the refinement of traditional techniques of investigation and the development of a variety of new techniques have gradually yielded new information and have made possible new insights into the speech processes.

In terms of its production, speech is a learned process which makes use of portions of the tracts and certain of the structures involved in the primary life processes of respiration and deglutition. The use made of these tracts and structures for producing speech, however, involves activities and adjustments which in many ways differ substantially from those involved in respiration and deglutition. For this reason, a description of the function of the various structures which concerns itself largely with their vegetative functions may be somewhat misleading when applied to an understanding of the processes involved in connected discourse. Certain important

1

differences have already been specified, and future systematic analyses of speech production may reveal many others not presently recognized.

The present chapter will be concerned with certain aspects of normal speech production. Discussion of the acoustic attributes of the sounds of speech and of some of their implications for speech perception are presented in Chapter II.

II. Speech Production

A. RESPIRATION IN SPEECH

In general, speech may be considered to be the product of the selective modification and control of an outgoing airstream. Researchers making use of measures of respiratory volumes and of relative air pressures to study the nature of the expiratory air flow have contributed a certain amount of information concerning the relationship of respiration to speech production. Anatomical inference, observations of body-wall movement, and x-ray and electromyographic techniques have provided some indication of which structures, and sometimes which particular muscles, may be involved in the respiratory process.

In quiet connected discourse, both the volumes of air and the air pressures involved are only slightly greater than those required for normal vegatative breathing. It is obvious, however, that the particular demands of speech will substantially alter certain relationships. The most essential difference, in terms of respiration, is in the control of expiration, a control which is manifested in the temporal ratio of the inhalation-exhalation phases within the respiratory cycle. In quiet breathing, these phases are of about equal duration and the air flow is regular. In speaking, the inhalation phase is markedly shortened, the exhalation phase is protracted, and the outgoing air flow is conspicuously irregular. The prolongation of the exhalation phase for speech involves the control of those forces which reduce the size of the thoracic cavity (and hence increase the pressure of the contained air) and also involves the control of the amount of resistance which certain of the structures along the respiratory tract present to the outflow of air.

1. *Inspiration*

Air moves into and out of the lungs as a consequence of disparities between intrapulmonary and atmospheric air pressures. Intrapulmonary pressure is decreased as the muscles used for inspiration, in contracting, increase the size of the thoracic cavity in its several dimensions.

The lungs increase in capacity by following the outward movements of the thoracic walls largely because of the pressure differential between the atmosphere and the pleural spaces. The inflation of the lungs is opposed by the elasticity and stiffness of the pulmonary structures and the resistance of the respiratory tract to air flow.

2. *Expiration*

Exhalation depends upon decreasing the volume of the respiratory system. This decrease can be accomplished by a variety of movements which depend, in part, on which structures were moved and which muscles were contracted during inspiration. The extent of their specific contributions will be influenced by posture. A number of nonmuscular forces of importance in expiration, particularly in the early stages, include gravity, the untorquing of the costal cartilages with the accompanying inward movement of the ribs, and the elastic recoil of the structures compressed, stretched, or displaced during inhalation. These structures commonly include not only the alveoli, bronchioles, and other thoracic tissues but also the muscles and other tissues of the abdominal wall and also the abdominal viscera. As the diaphragm gradually relaxes, it is aided in its ascent by the recoil of the displaced and compressed abdominal viscera and the elastic recoil of the abdominal wall.

All of these nonmuscular forces exert their maximal effect when the volume of the lungs is greatest at the start of expiration. Research findings indicate that these forces are balanced or checked by the activity of certain of the muscles used in inspiration which may gradually cease their activity after the onset of expiration (Murphy *et al.*, 1959; Ladefoged, 1962).

In expiration which is greater in volume than is the expiration of vegative breathing, the active contraction of the abdominal muscles is commonly involved, especially that of the lateral abdominals which compress the viscera. Campbell (1958) has emphasized the importance of the abdominal muscles to expiration in man.

Air begins to flow outward from the lungs as the intrapulmonary pressure is elevated above atmospheric pressure sufficiently to overcome the resistance which the respiratory tract offers both to turbulent and to laminar air flow. With increasing rate of air flow, a disproportinate increase in the pressure gradient results from increasing resistance which accompanies the increasing turbulent component. The diameter and length of the air passageways are related to lung volume; thus air flow resistance also is related to lung volume.

In general, current views hold that expiration provides a mean subglottal breath pressure which is maintained throughout a given utterance in a relatively stable fashion by a balance of opposing respiratory forces. Superimposed upon this mean pressure level are characteristic fluctuations thought to be systematically related, in ways not yet specified, to the production of syllables, the variations in stress patterns, and the effects of articulatory closures. During phonation there are, of course, rapid periodic pressure fluctuations associated with the vibratory cycle of the vocal folds.

B. VOCAL FOLD VIBRATION

During expiration the vocal folds are a source of potential turbulence in the airstream. When partially or completely adducted, they reduce or arrest the flow of air. In the presence of continued expiratory pressure they may be set into vibration, and when they are, phonation results.

Because of the problems involved in observing rapidly vibrating structures in a relatively hidden location, the factors governing the vibration of the vocal folds have been the subject of repeated controversy. Many of the disagreements have arisen aş direct consequences of limitations in the instrumentation employed and have been resolved only by the development of new or improved equipment. Bell Telephone Laboratories (Farnsworth, 1940) pioneered in high-speed motion picture photography of normal vocal fold action. Subsequently, notable contributions based upon the use of this technique have been made by several investigators, including Moore and von Leden (1958), Timcke et al. (1958, 1959), Rubin (1960), and van den Berg (1960). These films have served to resolve questions concerning the synchronization of the vibratory movement of the folds as well as to provide other new information concerning vocal fold action.

Phonation during speech involves the approximation of the vocal folds. The vibratory rate of the folds will be determined by their effective length, elasticity, and vibrating mass as well as by the subglottal breath pressure. When they are elongated, that is, placed under longitudinal tension, their margins are quite thin and the vibrating mass is small. The length of the folds is primarily a function of the opposition between the thyroarytenoid and the cricothyroid muscles, with approximation for phonation and length adjustment further controlled by the lateral portions of the thyroarytenoid and the lateral cricoarytenoids. The effective length is further determined by the medial compression which these latter muscles supply (van den Berg, 1960). It is apparent that the term "vocal fold tension" is ambiguous if it is taken to refer to the entire fold. The longitudinal tension of the ligament will be least when the thyroarytenoid portion of the vocal fold is shortest. While the muscle may be made somewhat "tense" by stretching, the amount of this tensing will be limited by the relative inelasticity of the vocal ligament. The muscle may contract actively ("tense") and shorten itself by varying amounts, depending on the opposition of the cricothyroids and certain extrinsics. This action will decrease the tension of the ligament.

In the production of low pitched sounds, the vocal folds vibrate relatively slowly, are comparatively thick and flaccid, and are comparatively short as contrasted with the folds in the production of higher pitches. When the folds are relatively thick, the upper and lower portions of their medial margins display somewhat different vibratory patterns. There is an apparent phase difference between the two, the lower margin leading the upper. This difference decreases with decreasing thickness of the folds and disappears when the folds are very thin.

At such low pitches there is also an increase in the relative duration of the closure portion of the cycle. This increase appears to be systematic. Sonesson (1960) has related this increased closure time to the increased thickness observed and to the increased phase difference between the upper and lower surfaces of the folds. Relative closure duration may be directly associated with the phase difference. Measurements of the relative closure duration of the folds at high pitches do not show a systematic relationship between relative closure duration and pitch. There appears to be considerable individual variability. More data are needed to establish this point and its relevance to the dependence of closure duration on vocal fold thickness and phase difference. The phase difference observed is related to the air pressure against surfaces of the folds and to the rate of air flow between them. Additional information concerning the relative rate of vocal fold movement to and away from the midline also appears to be needed. Apparently this rate of movement depends upon the factors governing intensity. At low intensity levels, the lateral movement is the more rapid while at high intensities the rate of medial movement is greater than the rate of lateral movement (Timcke et al., 1958). Lieberman (1963, 1967) has examined the perturbations of periodicity which typically occur in phonation and has associated them with changing subglottal breath pressures, alteration of the laryngeal mass, and changes in configuration of the vocal tract.

Hollien (1960) has found systematic relationships between vocal pitch and laryngeal size, higher pitch ranges being associated with smaller larynges. Hollien and Curtis (1960) also found that low-pitched voices were associated with greater vocal fold thickness and larger vocal fold areas than were high-pitched voices. These same investigators, in a subsequent study (1962), observed a consistent elevation and tilt of the vocal folds with increased vocal pitch.

Instrumental and methodological problems have hindered seriously the measurement of breath stream dynamics. Subglottal breath pressure measurement is a case in point. The general relationship of increased intensity as a concomitant of increased subglottic pressure, however, is well established. The effects of increased subglottal pressure on the fundamental frequency of the voice are not as well understood. Further, since most of the information thus far obtained applies to sustained sung vowels, it is probably not appropriate at present to apply the details of this information to connected speech. Analog studies of speech, however, do corroborate the main findings of the physiological investigations.

Air flow has been measured in a variety of ways. One of the chief difficulties in instrumentation for this purpose has been the slow response-time of the system. Smith (1960) and van den Berg (1962) have discussed some of the difficulties and have suggested specifications for appropriate instrumentation. Response times now available appear to be adequate for many kinds of mean air flow measurements.

C. ARTICULATION

The air emitted through the glottis enters that portion of the respiratory tract often called the vocal tract. For purposes of description, the vocal tract is conventionally divided into several regions, although it is increasingly apparent that functionally, at least in speech, the configurations of such regions are highly interrelated rather than discrete. In the tract above the glottis are the laryngeal ventricles, the aditus, the pharynx, the oral cavity, and the nasal cavities. Each of these is, for purposes of description, sometimes further subdivided. Certain constrictions of the tract serve as approximate boundaries for these regions. These include the epiglottis, the aryepiglottic folds, and the faucial pillars as well as the tongue and the velum together with the palatopharyngeal folds.

Whereas the air passageways below the level of the larynx may be modified slightly in diameter and length under various conditions of respiration, the amount of modification possible is comparatively slight and not a primary concern in differentiating the speech sounds from each other. (It is, however, increasingly apparent that the acoustic effects of modifying these cavities cannot be completely disregarded in a description of certain of the phenomena associated with speech.). In contrast to a relative lack of modifiability in the subglottal tract, the vocal tract, which extends upward from the level of the glottis, is highly modifiable and is readily changed both in size and shape. In the process of articulation, these supraglottal cavities are systematically changed in more or less patterned ways. Through the introduction of constrictions and the approximation of structures in various locations, cavity configurations are modified. These modifications interact throughout the vocal tract.

Vocal tract configurations have been studied in a variety of ways. These have included direct observation with the use of a small mirror or combination of mirrors. Contacts of the tongue with other oral structures have been recorded by both direct and indirect palatography for isolated utterance and for continuous speech. Externally observable events have been recorded by high-speed photography. Transducers of various sorts have been placed externally and internally both within the cavities and along their walls. Roentgenography, including lateral still film and lamino-graphy and also direct cineradiography and cinefluorography, has been employed. The precise recording of the continuously and rapidly changing relationships along the vocal tract continues to be a problem. Electrical stimulation and electromyography have been employed to ascertain the neuromuscular events responsible for the changes. Inferences concerning contacts and configurations have been drawn from acoustic analysis of the speech signal. Inferences have been drawn from measurements of the breath stream at various points along the tract and externally. Inferences deriving from many sources have been tested upon electrical models. It is apparent that no method alone is free from possible artifact of recording or error of interpretation and that many methods must be used to complement and supplement each other if the data derived are to be fully interpreted.

1. *Pharyngeal Configurations*

The larynx, pharynx, mandible, tongue, and velum are all complexly interconnected, largely by musculature attached to the hyoid bone, as are certain of the muscles which help to determine the positions of the cervical vertebrae and head. Bosma and Fletcher (1962) have emphasized the importance of these interrelationships. Any movement of one of these structures may result in movements of the others, or may impose constraints upon their movements. In addition, movements of the shoulder girdle and upper thorax may well result in changes in the relationships of the laryngeal cartilages and in the configurations of the vocal tract.

The larynx and hyoid bone are intimately associated with the inferior portion of the pharynx and help to stabilize it. While the larynx and hyoid do not execute extensive movements in speech as they typically do in yawning and swallowing, they are not stable in speech. Their movements, in addition to influencing the relative positions of the laryngeal cartilages, may affect the whole vocal tract to some extent.

The pharynx is supported superiorly by a complex musculature which, in part, helps to control palatal position and the size of the velopharyngeal port. Certain of these superior structures, consequently, are affected by the movements of the rest of the vocal tract. Thus, the inferior hyoid and laryngeal attachments together with the superior attachments determine the length of the pharynx. In addition, under certain circumstances, the nasal tract may be coupled to the pharyngeal tract by varying amounts of velopharyngeal opening and may serve as a superior extension of the vocal tract. The nasal tract extends from the nasopharynx to the nares, communicating there with the external air. The nasal cavities typically are not bilaterally symmetrical.

The muscles which help to determine the length of the vocal tract by controlling its inferior support do this in part by positioning the larynx. The whole group of extrinsic laryngeal muscles, therefore, may be involved indirectly or directly in controlling the vocal tract as well as the larynx. The inferior pharyngeal constrictor, by virtue of the attachment of the inferior portion of its fibers to the cricoid cartilage and the superior portion of its fibers to the thyroid, is potentially opposed to the hyoid group in the control of both laryngeal position and pharyngeal dimensions. Similarly, the hyoid muscle group is involved not only in determining laryngeal cartilage adjustment and laryngeal position but also in changing the configuration of the vocal tract. These interactions have been examined primarily in connection with swallowing and yawning, during which gross changes in the pharynx are apparent. Little attention has been paid to the contribution of these muscular interactions to normal speech, although "tenseness" in the anterior throat region has often been described in vocal disorders, and the "open throat" in singing has been much discussed. Sonninen (1956) has pointed out some of the implications of the effect of extrinsic laryngeal muscle contraction on pharyngeal configuration, particularly with reference to singing at very high pitches. Although comparatively small and rapid laryngeal movements are commonly observed in normal speech, this movement and the associated pharyngeal changes have not yet been adequately described with respect to the normal articulation of speech. Hudgins and Stetson (1935), however, did describe laryngeal depression in conjunction with the voicing of consonants.

Posteriorly, the pharynx is indirectly and loosely attached to the vertebral column, separated from direct contact with it by the prevertebral space. There apparently are few constraints on the vertical excursion of the pharynx. The presence of the vertebral column, however, limits its anteroposterior diameter and dictates, in conjunction with the diverse musculature centering upon the hyoid, the dependence of the pharynx upon the skull and vertebral column. Little information is available at present on changes in the transverse configurations and dimensions of the pharynx, although there is reason to believe that such changes may be significant.

It has been demonstrated conclusively that differential movements of the pharynx are associated with speech production (Holbrook and Carmody, 1937; Truby, 1962). Most of the evidence concerning these movements comes from information based upon x-ray films, largely from lateral exposures because of the technical difficulties involved in frontal plane representation.

The various techniques of radiological investigation with specific reference to speech have been explored and compared by several investigators, including Moll (1960), Subtelny and Subtelny (1962), Truby (1962), Björk (1961), Abramson and Cooper (1963), and Shelton et al. (1963). A number of limitations and complementary characteristics of these techniques have been evaluated. Because of the rapidity of articulatory movements, for example, very precise correlation of a particular exposure and the associated utterance is necessary in speech studies. There is danger, otherwise, of misinterpreting the film.

An associated difficulty in the interpretation of cinefilms, conventional or x-ray, involves the number of frames per second needed to resolve the motions being investigated. Very evidently this problem must be solved in different ways for different purposes.

2. Couplings and Configurations of the Upper Vocal Tract

The superior portion of the oropharynx is coupled to the oral cavity via the faucial isthmus and may be coupled to the nasopharynx and hence to the nasal tract. The anterior portions of the pharynx are, of course, intimately involved in the differential movements of the tongue, the mandible, and the floor of the mouth. The tongue extends from the hyoid into the oral cavity, its posterior surface acting as a highly mobile anterior wall of the pharynx. The movement of the mandible carries the tongue and the floor of the mouth with it. The palatoglossus, attached to the lateral margins of the tongue and extending above it to attach to the margins of the soft palate, forms the bulk of the anterior faucial arch. It is intimately associated not only with tongue position but also with velopharyngeal relationships. It may assist in the depression of the palate or in the elevation of the tongue. The posterior faucial arch consists primarily of the palatopharyngeus muscle. These muscles, which aid the convergence of the pharyngeal walls, may also assist in the elevation of the pharynx or the depression of the palate. Thus, the position of the velum is, to some extent, dependent upon the activity of the lingual, the mandibular, and the pharyngeal muscles.

These various muscles, tending directly and indirectly to lower the palate, are opposed by the superior support of the levator and also by the tensor muscles of the palate. The levator muscles serve to elevate and retract the velum. The tensor muscles, upon contraction, exert a lateral force on the velum, tending to stiffen and flatten it, thus opposing the action of the inferior muscles somewhat less directly than do the levators. Bosma and Fletcher (1961) point out the functional interrelationships of the palatal tensors and the external pterygoid muscles. These muscles help to control the anteroposterior diameter of the pharynx in deglutition and respiration. The external pterygoid muscles, by their anterior positioning of the mandible, tongue, hyoid, and larynx, help to determine the configuration of the middle and lower portions of the pharynx. The positions of these structures, as well as that of the velum, in respiration and in chewing, sucking, and swallowing may thus result in configurations antithetical to those required in the production of certain of the sounds of speech.

The palatal levators and tensors, acting in concert with the constriction of the superior pharynx, close the velopharyngeal port. The regulation of this opening must be coordinated to a certain extent with the activities of the other articulators in speech. Very evidently, the rapidity and extent of closure will not be independent of the size of the opening and the degree of stability provided by the support mechanisms. The level at which closure occurs will also be influenced by this balance.

The nature of the velopharyngeal closure in normal speech is not yet completely specified. The distinction between nasal and nonnasal sounds is widespread among languages, but the particular classes of sounds so distinguished vary somewhat from language to language. Obviously, the nasal and oral tracts must be coupled for the production of the nasal speech sounds. The aperture joining them must be smaller for nonnasal sounds than it is for the nasals. Apparently there is a rough progression in the size of the opening under different conditions. It is fairly large during quiet breathing, becoming successively smaller in the production of nasal consonants, nasal vowels, and the nonnasal sounds. It is possible that, for some individuals, small amounts of coupling may be characteristically associated with certain of the primarily oral sounds, especially with those demanding a low tongue position for their production. For many sounds, the amount of velopharyngeal opening is probably dialectally conditioned as well.

In spite of the variations noted, certain generalizations concerning the nature of the velopharyngeal closure in normal speech production may be made. In the most conspicuous movement of the closure, the velum is elevated so that it approximates the posterior pharyngeal wall, assuming a "shoe"- or "boot"-shaped configuration with the anterior portion of the soft palate more or less parallel to the hard palate and the posterior portion approximately parallel to the posterior pharyngeal wall. These two structures may fail to meet, or the contact may be sufficiently firm that the pharyngeal wall appears on the lateral radiograph to be somewhat dented. Anteroposterior pharyngeal wall movement has been reported to be slight by many investigators; for example, Hagerty et al. (1958). Because of technical difficulties, mesial movement along the major (transverse) axis has been much less thoroughly explored. Although this movement has been considered to be of importance, clinical findings have suggested that transverse movement may not be reliably predicted from indications of anteroposterior movement, that is, of the minor axis of the port.

Björk (1961) compared measures of area obtained from transverse tomography with measures of the anterioposterior distance obtained from conventional lateral views during the production of various sustained nonnasal and nasal vowels and nasal consonants as well as during quiet respiration. Since the area measurements he obtained were directly related to the measured anteroposterior distance, he concluded that velopharyngeal aperture area may be calculated from conventional lateral measures. These data, of course, derive from relatively long exposures during which articulatory change was minimized.

Moll (1962) indicated that although there was a tendency for a somewhat larger velopharyngeal opening on sustained vowels than on vowels produced during connected speech, measurements from sustained sounds were considered to be fairly accurate predictors of velopharyngeal opening for vowels in nonnasal context. It appears, then, that for normal speech, anteroposterior velopharyngeal measurements may provide a good estimate of the area of opening. The nature of the synchronization of velopharyngeal coupling and nasal sounds as they appear in connected speech is, of course, another matter.

In the production of normal speech, the primary coupling of the pharynx is to the oral cavity, a cavity which may be adjusted to a variety of configurations as a function of movements of the mandible, lips, and tongue. The oral cavity is separated from the nasal cavities by the hard and soft palates. This superior surface of the cavity is bounded by the alveolar ridge and teeth. The floor of the mouth, with is primarily muscular, is bounded by the mandible and lower teeth. Because of the nature of its articulation with the temporal bone and the complex of muscles which govern its position, the mandible is capable of a wide variety of movements. It may be raised, lowered, protruded, retracted, and moved laterally to a small degree. The first two of these movements are the most important in normal speech. The masseter, the temporalis, and the external and internal pterygoid muscles are the principal elevators. The depression of the mandible may be affected by a number of muscles including those in the suprahyoid group, especially the mylohyoid, a part of the digastric, and the geniohyoid.

Anteriorly, the oral cavity is bounded by the lips. The size of the lip opening is determined partly, but not entirely, by the position of the mandible. The lips may be protruded, retracted, raised, compressed, everted, and lowered. The primary muscles involved in lip movement during articulation are the orbicularis oris and those muscles intimately associated with it. These include the risorius, the zygomaticus, the quadratus labii (inferior and superior), the mentalis, and the buccinator, as well as other smaller muscles which also affect the position of the angle of the lips. Lip movement is necessary in the production of certain consonants and is a usual concomitant of some of the vowels. Again, information on specific muscle action in speech production is lacking, but these muscles are thought to effect the narrowing and spreading of the mouth aperture and the positioning of the lips.

When the teeth are together, the tongue, which is primarily composed of muscles and which is, consequently, highly mobile, almost completely fills the oral cavity. Its tip may be pointed or rounded, raised or lowered, and protruded or retracted; it may be retroflexed, that is, raised and bent back. The blade of the tongue may be flattened or rounded. The dorsal surface may be made convex or concave. The posterior portion may be depressed or elevated, moved anteriorly, or retracted. It is important to note that tomographic evidence (Truby, 1962) confirms that these diverse configurations are not related to each other in a simple fashion in the production of a given sound.

The tongue muscles are divided into the extrisic and intrinsic groups. There is a dearth of information concerning the specific actions of the muscles of both groups in the production of speech. The older view that the extrinsics govern tongue position and the intrinsics determine tongue configuration is apparently, however, an oversimplification (Heffner, 1950; Van Riper and Irwin, 1958). Abd-el-Malek (1939) and Strong (1956) have described the anatomy of the tongue in some detail. Strong, using palatograms, related the vectors of certain of the instrinsic muscle bundles to consonant production. MacNeilage and Sholes (1964), in accordance with results of an electromyographic investigation, have described certain lingual muscle functions during vowel production.

Both the extrinsic and intrinsic muscles perform actions which are important in articulation, not only in the movements for shaping the configurations for a given sound, but also, and even more importantly, in the movements necessary in progressing from one sound to another in connected speech. The extrinsic group of tongue muscles is composed of the genioglossus, hyoglossus, palatoglossus, and styloglossus muscles. In altering the position of the tongue, the genioglossus may pull the tongue forward and down; the hyoglossus may pull it backward and down; and the palatoglossus and the styloglossus may pull it backward and upward. In addition to changing tongue position, however, these actions may aid the intrisic muscles in determining tongue configuration. The intrinsic tongue muscle group consists of the superior and inferior longitudinal, the transverse and the vertical muscle groups. Both pairs of longitudinals, in addition to contracting the anteroposterior dimension of the tongue by acting together, may elevate or depress the tip or deflect it laterally by contracting differentially. The transverse muscle fibers may narrow the tongue and the vertical fibers may flatten it. In these actions, the intrinsic muscles may be aided by the synergic action of various extrinsic tongue muscles. Furthermore, it is apparent that these actions will not be independent of the actions of closely related muscles in the pharyngeal and velar regions.

It is clear that the intimate interrelationships of the cavities and couplings throughout the entire vocal tract from the vocal folds to the lips are such that the articulatory configurations for speech sounds involve the entire vocal tract. Furthermore, these complex configurations are in continuous change in the production of speech. Fortunately, while relatively little information is currently available concerning the specific actions of the muscles involved in articulatory movements, certain aspects of the changing configurations of the structures are fairly generally agreed upon.

3. *Articulatory Adjustment for the Sounds of Speech*

Each of the sounds of speech is characterized by more or less distinctive patterns of articulatory movement, configuration, or contact. Descriptions of speech sounds are, of course, bound to a given language and in some cases to a given dialect. The articulation patterns described here refer to General American English. Since English orthography does not unequivocally designate these sounds, it is necessary to employ a phonetic alphabet (Kenyon and Knott, 1944).

It is convenient for purposes of discussion to divide the speech sounds into two categories, vowels and consonants, even though such a division is somewhat arbitrary. Vowels are contrasted with consonants in that vowels do not require that the airstream be occluded or driven through an aperture with appreciable force, and hence are not dependent upon air flow or pressure patterns in any distinctive way for their differentiation. Further, vowels are considered to be capable of being sustained without articulatory movement. No vowel in General American English requires the coupling of the nasal and vocal tracts and none requires lateral as contrasted with frontal emission. All vowels require that the vocal folds furnish the acoustic signal, whether phonated or aspirated, and all require characteristic oral differentiation of the signal from that of any other vowel. Like consonants, vowels occur as features of syllables but, unlike consonants in English, a vowel may constitute an entire stressed syllable. Under some circumstances, however, certain consonants may perform the syllabic function of the vowel in unstressed syllables.

While all of the configurative aspects of the vocal tract have potential relevance in the specification of each of the speech sounds, certain traditional simplifications of the details of articulation have proved to be useful. The vowels, for example, have been classified according to a diagram displaying the position of the highest portion of the tongue with reference to both its anteroposterior and vertical locations. The condition of lip-rounding, or of lip-spreading, may or may not be indicated, since, in English, either is a concomitant of anteroposterior location. Similarly, incisor separation and the configuration of the pharynx, although known to be of importance in the determination of vowel character, have traditionally been assumed to vary consistently with the tongue position parameters. The patterned movement of vowel articulation is such, generally speaking, that the simple description provided by the vowel diagram has been demonstrated to be useful and to agree well with acoustic data.

Traditional consonant descriptions also represent a simplification. Consonants are typically classified in terms of the presence or absence of voicing, the manner of production (for example, plosive, nasal, fricative, lateral, glide), and the place of tongue contact with, or greatest proximity to, another articulator.

These traditional vowel and consonant specification systems represent "normalized" or generalized sound types and do not include the characteristic changes in articulatory position and durational relationships which occur typically in connected speech. These generalized articulatory descriptions hold under the assumption that the entire vocal tract is both structurally and functionally normal. Departures therefrom anywhere along the tract can be expected to disrupt the concomitant adjustments implicit in the simplified descriptions of these articulations whether or not they distort the speech sound. Compensatory articulations will alter the characteristic patterns of transitional movement as well.

The vowels are produced by a graduated series of modifications involving the configuration of much of the vocal tract. Each vowel may be produced in a sustained steady-state condition and in isolation. When this is done, certain more or less constant relationships may be described as typical for each vowel. Traditionally, the parameters of interest are indicated by the anteroposterior location of the high point of the tongue and the relative separation of this high point and the palate. While any precise measurement of the degree and location of tongue height will not be the same for different individuals, or for a given individual in different conditions of utterance, certain relational values can be reliably indicated. The vowel /i/ as in *heed* represents the highest and most anterior position of the tongue hump. The front vowel series /i/, /ɪ/ as in *hid*, /ɛ/ as in *head*, and /æ/ as in *had* represents a progressive lowering and retraction of this high point. Similarly, the back vowel series progresses downward from the highest back position from /u/ as in *who*, through /ʊ/ as in *hood*, /ɔ/ as in *hawed*, and /ɑ/ as in *hod*. The remaining ("central") vowels are produced with the high point in a more or less intermediate position with /ɝ/ as in *heard*, the highest, followed by /ʌ/ as in *hut* and the unstressed schwa, /ə/. While the several changes in the position of the tongue hump in these series are not necessarily equidistant, the relationships are preserved by normal speakers.

Certain of the General American syllabic nuclei have been classed as diphthongs. They are characterized by distinctive, as opposed to adventitious or assimilative, change in articulatory configuration during their production. While they may be prolonged, they cannot be sustained. Diphthongs are described as displaying certain of the characteristics of the simple vowels and are accordingly transcribed by a combination of symbols representing the two vowels which they most closely resemble at initiation and termination. Intermediate characteristics are ignored since they are considered to be dictated by the positions assumed at onset and termination. Variability in production and in perception has given rise to some discussion as to which of two adjacent vowels best represents each component of the diphthongs. Since, however, the elements of the diphthongs typically only approximate the simple vowels in terms of all the requisite features, arbitrary distinctions must inevitably be made in a generalized description. Close phonetic transcription of particular utterances is another matter. For present purposes, the General American diphthongs are considered to be /aɪ/ as in *high*, /aʊ/ as in *how*, and /ɔɪ/ as in *boy*. In addition, in this dialect, the mid-front vowel /e/ and the mid-back vowel /o/ are considered to be characteristically diphthongized, that is, /eɪ/ as in *bait* and /oʊ/ as in *boat*.

In addition to tongue position, certain other articulatory adjustments are characteristic, although not invariant, concomitants of a given vowel articulation. Movement of the mandible carries the base of the tongue upward for high vowels, downward for low, and, consequently, incisor separation is customarily least for /i/, greatest for /a/. Lip separation tends to be generally associated with incisor separation. In contrast to certain vowels in a number of other languages, marked differential lip configuration is not a necessary correlate of any General American vowel. It is apt to occur, however, as a concomitant variation in General American, particularly with the high vowels. Articulation of the high front vowels commonly includes a certain amount of lip spread, that is, retraction of the corners of the mouth with a more or less slitlike orifice. Articulation of the mid- and high-back vowels is usually accompanied by a certain amount of lip-rounding and protrusion.

As mentioned earlier, velar height and the degree of closure of the velopharyngeal port varies systematically with vowel articulation. In general, this appears to be associated with tongue position and pharyngeal configuration, that is, with the velum characteristically lower and the port more open for low vowels than for high vowels. (For normal vowels any opening is very slight.) In view of the anatomical relationships involved, this correspondence is to be expected, although it is not dictated. Although insufficient evidence is available to support the opinion, it is probably that conspicuous variations in these relationships might be found in studies involving cross-language and cross-dialect comparisons.

Traditional articulatory descriptions of the vowels have neglected pharyngeal modification as a factor in vowel differentiation. With few exceptions (for example, Heffner, 1950), phonetic texts containing diagrammatic representations of the vocal tract either show a pharynx of constant configuration or neglect it entirely, even texts in which considerable emphasis may be placed upon other details of vowel configurations. Initially, this neglect of the pharyngeal region probably reflected lack of information about systematic changes in the pharynx with vowel articulations. Its perpetuation suggests the tacit assumption that oral and pharyngeal configurations display invariant relationships. There is reason to believe that this is not necessarily the case. These relationships do not appear to obtain in all languages (Ladefoged, 1964), and in any given language they may well be more or less radically modified by compensatory articulations. Neglect of the pharynx in articulatory descriptions has resulted in the common misconception that the high point of the tongue represents the major constriction of the vocal tract during vowel production. This is not necessarily true, and the assumption is conspicuously misleading in the case of the low vowels, particularly /ɑ/, which is characterized by marked pharyngeal constriction and relatively slight tongue hump elevation (Parmenter and Bevans, 1933; Heffner, 1950; Truby, 1962; Abramson and Cooper, 1963).

As has been indicated previously, the consonants may be classified according to their manner of production, place of characteristic oral constriction, condition of voicing, and condition of nasalization. An additional category is necessary to include that group of sounds called the semivowel-glides which, as the name implies, share some of the distinguishing features of vowel-like sounds.

The consonants as a class are loosely distinguished from the vowels by several articulatory features. As has been pointed out, however, these differentiating features do not permit of a clear dichotomy between consonants and vowels on articulatory parameters and the labels are somewhat arbitrarily assigned. Even contextual criteria (for example, function within the syllable) will not unequivocally distinguish the traditional classes of vowels and consonants, since certain consonants may sometimes serve as the syllable nucleus, thus substituting for an unstressed vowel. In this case, one view holds that the sound actually belongs under the vowel classification (Pike, 1943). Generally speaking, however, a number of consonantal articulatory features contrast with those of the vowels. For example, consonants in certain of the classes cannot be sustained. Several classes of consonants make use of constrictions above the level of the glottis as sound sources, either solely or in conjunction with the primary sound source. Further, the consonants cannot be ranged along a graded positional continuum in the sense of that described for the vowels. This latter articulatory characteristic of consonants may be reflected in recent findings which suggest differential perceptual response functions for the two classes of sounds (Liberman *et al.* 1963).

All General American consonants can be assigned to one of four basic categories according to the manner of their production, that is, stop plosives, fricatives, nasals, and semivowel-glides. The stop plosives, /p/, /b/, /t/, /d/, /k/, and /g/, are all characterized by more or less complete oral and velopharyngeal occlusion, behind which a certain amount of air may be impounded under pressure. The fricatives, /f/, /v/, /θ/ as in *thing*, /ð/ as in *there*, /s/, /z/, /ʃ/ as in *shoe*, /ʒ/ as in *measure*, /hw/ as in *when*, and /h/, on the other hand, are characterized by a more or less narrow constriction through which the airstream is driven. They involve varied breath stream dynamics in their production. Thus both stop plosives and fricatives are characterized by constraints placed upon the airstream and on the consequent turbulent flow.

The consonants /tʃ/ as in *church*, and /dʒ/ as in *judge*, the so-called affricates, are commonly thought to combine distinguishing features from both the stop plosive and the fricative categories. The nasals, /m/, /n/, and /ŋ/ as in *think*, are characterized both by oral occlusion and by the opening of the velopharyngeal port. In contrast to the fricatives and to the plosives (which they otherwise closely resemble) the nasals do not require a conspicuous alteration in breath stream dynamics for their production. However, if sufficient air is admitted to the nasal cavities, the creation of turbulence there appears to be inevitable as a consequence of the complexity of the cavity configurations. The semivowel-glide class includes four sounds, /w/, /j/ as in *you*, /r/, /l/, which, while disparate in certain respects, are alike in all being nonnasal voiced continuent nonconstrictive consonants, as opposed to the voiced continuant fricatives, which require constriction. Several of these sounds are further distinguished from other consonants by certain time-bound changes in the articulatory configuration required for their production.

The description of place of articulation indicates not only the location of the characteristic articulatory constriction, but also specifies the articulators involved in creating it. The bilabials, which as the name implies require an approximation of the lips, include /p/, /b/, /m/, /w/, and /hw/. Of these, the first three require a close initial approximation. The labiodentals, /f/ and /v/, require a close approximation of the lower lip and the upper incisors. The lingua-dentals, /θ/ and /ð/ (the so-called voiceless and voiced *th*), require a close approximation of the anterior tongue and the upper incisors.

The alveolars, /t/, /d/, /n/, /s/, /z/, and /l/, involve a tongue-gum ridge constriction. The oral closure is complete for /t/, /d/, and /n/ and there is a close approximation for /s/, /z/, and /l/, with accompanying lateral emission of the airstream for /l/. The sounds /ʃ/ and /ʒ/ require a lingual-palatal constriction, and the sound /r/ a somewhat less close approximation of the tongue to the palate. Typically, for /r/ there is a certain degree of retroflexion of the tongue blade, often accompanied by movement of the lower lip as well. The linguavelars, /k/, /g/, and /ŋ/, require complete posterior oral closure. The affricates, /tʃ/ and /dʒ/, are complexly articulated and require combining the features of a stop and a fricative. The glide /j/ requires a rapid shift away from linguapalatal approximation. The voiceless glottal fricative /h/ requires that the vocal folds constrict the airstream only enough to provide a source of turbulence.

Generally speaking, all consonants have traditionally been dichotomized according to two remaining categories of classification, voiced-voiceless and nasal-nonnasal. The oppositions tense-lax and fortis-lenis have each been proposed as more distinctive in English than the voicing parameter. The experimental evidence presently available does not indicate the desirability of adopting either alternative terminology, however, and the traditional voiced-voiceless classifications are conventionally used.

Certain pairs of consonants are articulated in the same place and in the same manner, but differ in condition of voicing. These are the cognate stop plosives /p-b/, /t-d/, and /k-g/ and the cognate fricatives /f-v/, /θ-ð/, /s-z/, and /ʃ-ʒ/, and the affricates /tʃ-dʒ/. When the fricatives among these consonants are produced in isolation, the presence or absence of vocal fold vibration is their distinguishing characteristic. The same is true of the cognate plosives and affricates when they are articulated before a neutral vowel. In the production of the voiceless consonants, any air pressure differential across the glottis which may exist is probably not of distinctive significance. Presumably the respiratory tract is relatively unrestricted up to the level of the articulatory constriction. Production of the voiced member of each cognate pair, however, requires the restriction of the airstream at the glottis which is associated with the vibration of the vocal folds. Vibratory action of the folds necessitates a pressure differential across the glottis and also its periodic occlusion. The restrictions imposed on patterns of air flow by the vibration of the folds thus are such that air pressures at the level of articulatory occlusion or constriction for the voiceless consonants are potentially higher, and the volume of air involved is potentially greater, than for their voiced cognates. In general, it may be said that the voiceless sounds are at least potentially associated with a greater (or at least more uniform) intraoral pressure than are the voiced, and that the plosives and certain of the fricatives which depend upon a marked constriction in the tract tend to be associated with greater intraoral pressures than do the other classes of speech sounds (Stetson and Hudgins, 1930; Black, 1950; Malecot, 1955).

The three nasal sounds of English share the places of articulations of the three stop plosive voice-voiceless cognates: /m/ with /b/ and /p/, /n/ with /d/ and /t/, and /ŋ/ with /g/ and /k/. The members of these three groups of consonants share other sound production features as well. All members of all groups require complete oral occlusion. The primary distinguishing feature of the last member of each group which separates it from the other two is the absence of vocal fold vibration and associated air flow phenomena. The first member of each group differs from the other two primarily because of nasal coupling. The nonnasal members of each group may or may not, depending upon phonetic context and idiosyncracy, display a burst or some form of frication upon release. The nasals, in normal General American speech, do not. The nasals may be sustained, but typically are not. The nonnasal voiced cognates /b/, /d/, and /g/ may be prolonged only briefly since complete occlusion of the tract eliminates the pressure differential across the glottis needed to sustain vocal fold vibration. The nonasal voiceless cognates, /p/, /t/, and /k/ may also be prolonged during the occluded phase, but typically are not. Normally, the velopharyngeal closure is sufficiently complete during the articulation of nonnasal cognates to prevent the escape of an appreciable amount of air into the nasal cavities and to prevent acoustic coupling. Insufficient velopharyngeal closure may manifest itself in both measurable nasal escape of air and acoustic coupling.

These more or less traditional articulatory descriptions of consonant and vowel types, descriptions which attempt to specify the articulatory gestures which characterize and distinguish the speech sounds, are incomplete in many of their details. More elaborate treatments of certain of these descriptions are to be found in "The Principles of the International Phonetic Association" (1949) and in most phonetics texts. The system of categorization employed here is arbitrary in some of its aspects, as are all such systems. The application of any of these descriptions to the sounds which occur in speech is even more arbitrary, since certain articulatory features are inevitably not fully realized.

Classifications of this sort usually involve an implicit or explicit effort to minimize redundancy. The foregoing description, as is typical of all attempts at phonetic generalization independent of context, has largely ignored certain potentially distinctive articulatory characteristics. For example, the time parameter has been suggested only when articulatory change in time is categorically distinctive and not redundant. As a consequence, certain dichotomies—the voiced-voiceless distinction, for example—suggest that there is only one relevant variable, in this case the presence or absence of vocal fold vibration. Studies of connected speech, however, have indicated very clearly that more than the presence or absence of phonation is involved in this contrast. One of the distinctions between the so-called voiced and voiceless cognate pairs in speech is that of time. Voiced consonants are characteristically shorter than are their voiceless cognates in similar phonetic environments.

Not only is the discrete categorization of sounds necessarily arbitrary and oversimplified, but it perforce ignores the conspicuous effect of one sound upon another in speech. It is clear that sounds in speech are not produced as discrete entities, but rather are the product of continuously varying physiological adjustments. Thus it is that generalized articulatory configurations are rarely, if ever, realized, for each potential configuration is affected by those which precede and follow it rapidly in time.

The inevitability and the predictability of the influence of one articulatory gesture upon adjacent gestures raise the question of the discreteness of the speech sounds. Such articulatory interactions are the rule rather than the exception. Under these circumstances, the identity of a sound in speech clearly relies on its influence upon sounds adjacent to it as well as upon its own inherent distinctive articulatory attributes. Unfortunately, there is a dearth of physiological data on this aspect of speech. Most of the evidence concerning these interactions is either acoustic or perceptual (Harris, 1958). It is, however, consonant with theoretical descriptions of articulatory constraints. In the stream of speech, the articulators must move from one characteristic position (or its approximation) to another. Acoustic signals are generated during this transitional movement and hence reflect it.

The interdependence of sounds in connected speech is recognized in the phonetic construct of assimilation and in the linguistic construct of allophonic variation, both of which are concerned with the modification of a generalized "speech sound" by its phonetic environment. Other sources of departure from the abstraction are particularized and are concerned with both idiosyncratic and denotative circumstance of utterance. Phonetic assimilation involves the change of one or more of the primary or ancillary attributes of a segment of contextual utterance in predictable ways to the extent that it not only loses some of its conventionally distinctive attributes (reduction or "slighting"), but also incorporates some of the features of its environment. Such features may be irrelevant to, or even antithetical to, the generalized description of that speech sound as a postulated discrete entity.

Assimilative change can alter a specific sound token with respect to its sound type in a variety of ways and to a greater or lesser extent. Voiced sounds can be fully or partially devoiced, and the converse. Nonnasals can be nasalized. Place of articulation may be shifted in either the anteroposterior or the vertical direction or both. The degree of such shift may be sufficiently extensive to cause an identification of the sound not in correspondence with the intent of the talker (sound substitution). Articulatory context may also increase the probabilities of sound omission. Thus, the effects of phonetic context may cause the modification, reduction, substitution, or omission of specific speech sounds in lawful and predictable ways. Structural deficits may well disrupt these environmental interactions and result in defective connected speech.

The disparity in the constraints imposed upon the various adjustments along the length of the vocal tract in the production of the various sounds of speech means that certain articulators are free at any given moment to assume the configuration characteristic of the succeeding sound even as the sound preceding it is under production. For example, it has been demonstrated in a frame-by-frame analysis of high-speed cineradiography (Truby, 1959) that the tongue typically assumes the configuration for /l/ as in *play* even as the lips are occluded to build up intraoral breath pressure for the initial plosive. This natural process of coarticulation means, of course, that the articulatory configurations, as well as the acoustic signals they generate, will share some of the characteristics of both adjacent sounds rather than conform completely to the generalized description of either. Similar effects obtain from assimilative influences upon the functioning of the vocal folds and of the velopharyngeal closure as well.

Under these circumstances, it is understandable that the identification of discrete speech segments in connected utterance is not simple. It is apparent that, perceptually, each language with its dialects employs a limited set of "speech sounds" intuitively recognized by native speakers as entities. In all cases, however, these units which form the basic combinatory code are characterized by wide but predictable variances rather than by specific invariance. In addition to predictable variation, adventitious and idiosyncratic departures also occur. The articulatory and acoustic correlates of even the predictable variants are only partially understood.

It is apparent that progress is currently being made in the development of instrumentation suitable for continuous recording of articulatory data. One such system utilizing electromyographic techniques has been developed at Haskins Laboratories (Harris *et al.*, 1964). Kozhevnikov and Chistovich (1965), summarizing earlier descriptions of components, have described a multiple parameter system currently in use in Russia. Systems for the continuous recording of tongue-palate contacts (Kydd and Belt, 1964) and pressures (McGlone *et al.*, 1965) have been announced. Additional systems of various types are in the development stage. High-speed photography, stroboscopy, and roentgenography continue to be improved. Data reduction presents a particularly acute problem for these continuous recording systems, and is particularly intractable for the optical techniques.

Despite early and continuing instrumental limitations, certain aspects of the articulatory process have been described and certain theoretical constructs advanced. Chiba and Kajiyama published their classic researches in "The Vowel—Its Nature and Structure" in 1941. The summary of Stetson's long series of investigations, "Motor Phonetics" was published posthumously in 1951. No similarly comprehensive compilations of individual researches have appeared since, although the highly restricted field of static (as opposed to continuous) palatography has recently been surveyed in an historical review (Moses, 1964). Theoretical formulations of the probable functions of the articulatory muscles appear in the texts of Heffner (1950) and Van Riper and Irwin (1958). Strong (1956) and Ladefoged (1964) have postulated force vectors related to specific lingual muscles and muscle groups.

Certain of the dynamics of articulation have recently been examined with relatively new techniques. MacNeilage and Sholes (1964) mapped the surface of the tongue in an electromyographic (EMG) investigation of vowel articulation and suggested the muscle functions involved in the differential EMG patterns obtained. Kozhevnikov and Chistovich (1965), using data from contact electrodes, described lingual contacts as they vary in time. Fritzell (1963) obtained EMG evidence of velar muscular activity during nonnasal articulation as opposed to nasals, as did Harris et al. (1962). Harris et al. (1962, 1965) and Fromkin (1965) have described certain aspects of EMG patterns for bilabials, MacNeilage (1963) for a labiodental. Fujimura (1961) and Fromkin (1965) have measured lip opening in the production of labial consonants using photographic techniques, the latter author supplementing the photographs with plaster casts. Truby (1962), as previously mentioned, discussed a number of articulatory adjustments on the basis of cineradiographic and tomographic films. Radiographic techniques (Moll, 1960, 1965; Subtelny and Subtelny, 1962) have been used extensively, as indicated earlier, in investigations of the velar region and of articulatory adjustment for various speech sound combinations. When any of these techniques for obtaining continuous articulatory descriptions is combined with high quality tape recordings so that the synchronization of the two sets of data is exact, it is possible to describe certain of the acoustic correlates of the articulatory gestures.

REFERENCES

Abd-el-Malek, S. (1939). Observations on the morphology of the human tongue. *J. Anat.* **73**, 201–210.

Abramson, A., and Cooper, F. S. (1963). Slow motion X-ray pictures with stretched speech as a research tool. *J. Acoust. Soc. Am.* **35**, 1888A.

Björk, L. (1961). Velopharyngeal function in connected speech. *Acta Radiol. Suppl.* **202**, 1–94.

Black, J. W. (1950). The pressure component in the production of consonants. *J. Speech Hearing Disorders.* **15**, 207–210.

Bosma, J. F., and Fletcher, S. G. (1961). The upper pharynx. I. Embryology, anatomy. *Ann. Otol. Rhinol. Laryngol.* **70**, 953–973.

Bosma, J. F., and Fletcher, S. G. (1962). The upper pharynx. II. Physiology. *Ann. Otol. Rhinol. Laryngol.* **71**, 134–157.

Campbell, E. J. M. (1958). "The Respiratory Muscles and the Mechanics of Breathing." Year Book Publ., Chicago, Illinois.

Chiba, T., and Kajiyama, M. (1941). "The Vowel, Its Nature and Structure." Phonetic Soc. Japan, Tokyo.

Farnsworth, D. W. (1940). High speed motion pictures of the human vocal cords. *Bell Lab. Record* **18**, 203–208.

Fritzell, B. (1963). An electromyographic study of the movement of the soft palate in speech. *Folia Phoniat.* **15**, 307–311.

Fromkin, Victoria A. (1966). Neuro-muscular specification of linguistic units. *Lang. Speech* **9**, 170–199.

Fujimura, O. (1961). Bilabial stop and nasal consonants: a motion picture study and its acoustical implications. *J. Speech Hearing Res.* **4**, 233–247.

Hagerty, R. F., Hill, M. J., Pettit, H. S., and Kane, J. J. (1958). Posterior pharyngeal wall movement in normals. *J. Speech Hearing Res.* **1**, 203–210.

Harris, Katherine S. (1958). Cues for the discrimination of American English fricatives in spoken syllables. *Lang. Speech* **1**, 1–7.

Harris, Katherine S., Schvey, M. M., and Lysaught, G. F. (1962). Component gestures in the production of oral and nasal stops. *J. Acoust. Soc. Am.* **34**, 743A.

Harris, Katherine S., Rosov, R., Cooper, F. S., and Lysaught, G. F. (1964). A multiple suction electrode system. *Electroencephalog. Clin. Neurophysiol.* **17**, 698–700.

Harris, Katherine S., Lysaught, G. F., and Schvey, M. M. (1965). Some aspects of the production of oral and nasal labial stops. *Lang. Speech* **8**, 135–147.

Heffner, R.-M. S. (1950). "General Phonetics." Univ. of Wisconsin Press, Madison, Wisconsin.

Holbrook, R. T., and Carmody, F. J. (1937). X-ray studies of speech articulations. *Univ. Calif. Publ. Mod. Philol.* **20**, 187–238.

Hollien, H. (1960). Some laryngeal correlates of vocal pitch. *J. Speech Hearing Res.* **3**, 52–58.

Hollien, H., and Curtis, J. F. (1960). Laminagraphic study of vocal pitch. *J. Speech Hearing Res.* **3**, 361–371.

Hollien, H., and Curtis, J. F. (1962). Elevation and tilting of vocal folds as a function of vocal pitch. *Folia Phoniat.* **14**, 23–36.

Hudgins, C. V., and Stetson, R. H. (1935). Voicing of consonants by depression of the larynx. *Arch. Neerl. Phon. Exptl.* **11**, 1–28.

Kenyon, J. S., and Knott, T. A. (1944). "A Pronouncing Dictionary of American English." Merriam, Springfield, Massachusetts.

Kozhevnikov, V. A., and Chistovich, L. A. (1965). "Rech', Artikulvatsiva i Vosprivative." Moscow-Leningrad. English translation: "Speech Articulation and Perception." U. S. Dept. Comm., Clearinghouse for Fed. Sci. and Tech. Inform., Washington, D.C.

Kydd, W. L., and Belt, D. A. (1964). Continuous palatography. *J. Speech Hearing Disorders* **29**, 489–492.

Ladefoged, P. (1962). Subglottal activity during speech. *Proc. 4th Intern. Congr. Phon. Sci., Helsinki, 1961*, pp. 73–91. Mouton, The Hague.

Ladefoged, P. (1964). Some possibilities in speech synthesis. *Lang. Speech* **7**, 205–214.
Liberman, A. M., Cooper, F. S., Harris, Katherine S., and MacNeilage, P. F. (1963). A motor theory of speech perception. *Proc. Speech Commun. Seminar.* Roy. Inst. Technol., Stockholm, Sweden.
Lieberman, P. (1963). Some acoustic measures of the fundamental periodicity of normal and pathologic larynges. *J. Acoust. Soc. Am.* **35**, 344–353.
Lieberman, P. (1967). "Intonation, Perception, and Language." MIT Press, Cambridge, Massachusetts.
McGlone, R. E., Christiansen, R. L., and Proffitt, W. R. (1965). Lingual pressures during syllable production. *Asha* **7(A)**, 375.
MacNeilage, P. F. (1963). Electromyographic and acoustic study of the production of certain final clusters. *J. Acoust. Soc. Am.* **35**, 461–463.
MacNeilage, P. F., and Sholes, G. N. (1964). An electromyographic study of the tongue during vowel production. *J. Speech Hearing Res.* **7**, 209–232.
Malecot, A. (1955). An experimental study of force of articulation. *Studia Linguistica* **9**, 35–44.
Moll, K. L. (1960). Cinefluorographic techniques in speech research. *J. Speech Hearing Res.* **3**, 227–241.
Moll, K. L. (1962). Velopharyngeal closure on vowels. *J. Speech Hearing Res.* **5**, 30–37.
Moll, K. L. (1965). Photographic and radiographic procedures in speech research. *Asha Rept.* **1**, 129–139.
Moore, P., and von Leden, H. (1958). Dynamic variations of the vibratory pattern in the normal larynx. *Folia Phoniat.* **10**, 205–238.
Moses, E. R., Jr. (1964). "Phonetics: History and Interpretation," pp. 17-32. Prentice-Hall, Englewood Cliffs, New Jersey.
Murphy, A. J., Koepke, G. H., Smith, E. M., and Dickinson, D. G. (1959). Sequence of action of the diaphragm and intercostal muscles during respiration. II. Expiration. *Arch. Phys. Med. Rehabil.* **40**, 337–342.
Parmenter, C., and Bevans, C. (1933). Analysis of speech radiographs. *Am. Speech* **8**, 44–56.
Pike, K. L. (1943). "Phonetics." Univ. of Michigan Press, Ann Arbor, Michigan.
Rubin, H. J. (1960). The neurochronaxic theory of voice production—a refutation. *Arch. Otolaryngol.* **71**, 913–920.
Shelton, R. L., Jr., Brooks, Alta R., Youngstrom, K. A., Diedrich, W. M., and Brooks, R. S. (1963). Filming speed in cinefluorographic speech study. *J. Speech Hearing Res.* **6**, 19–25.
Smith, S. (1960). The electro aerometer. *Speech Pathol. Therapy* **3**, 27–29.
Sonesson, B. (1960). On the anatomy and vibratory pattern of the human vocal folds. *Acta Oto-Laryngol. Suppl.* **156**, 1–80.
Sonninen, A. A. (1956). The role of the external laryngeal muscles in length-adjustment of the vocal cords in singing. *Acta Oto-Laryngol. Suppl.* **130**, 1–102.
Stetson, R. H. (1951). "Motor Phonetics," Rev. ed. North-Holland Publ., Amsterdam.
Stetson, R. H., and Hudgins, C. V. (1930). Functions of the breathing movements in the mechanism of speech. *Arch. Neerl. Phon. Exptl.* **5**, 1–30.
Strong, L. H. (1956). Muscle fibers of the tongue functional in constant production. *Anat. Record.* **126**, 61–80.
Subtelny, Joanne D., and Subtelny, J. D. (1962). Roentgenographic techniques and phonetic research, *Proc. 4th Intern. Congr. Phon. Sci., Helsinki, 1961*, pp. 129–146. Mouton, The Hague.
"The Principles of the International Phonetic Association." (1949). Univ. College, London.

Timcke, R., von Leden, H., and Moore, P. (1958). Laryngeal vibrations: Measurements of the glottic wave. I. The normal vibratory cycle. *Arch. Otolaryngol.* **68**, 1–19.

Timcke, R., von Leden, H., and Moore, P. (1959). Laryngeal vibrations: Measurements of the glottic wave. II. The normal vibratory cycle. *Arch. Otolaryngol.* **69**, 438–444.

Truby, H. M. (1959). Acoustico-cineradiographic analysis considerations with especial reference to certain consonantal complexes. *Acta Radiol. Suppl.* **182**, 1–227.

Truby, H. M. (1962). Synchronized cineradiography and visual-acoustic analysis. *Proc. 4th Intern. Congr. Phon. Sci., Helsinki, 1961,* pp. 265–279. Mouton, The Hague.

van den Berg, Jw. (1960). "Voice Production: the Vibrating Larynx." Univ. of Groningen, Groningen, Netherlands.

van den Berg, Jw. (1962). Modern research in experimental phoniatrics. *Folia Phoniat.* **14**, 81–149.

Van Riper, C. G., and Irwin, J. V. (1958). "Voice and Articulation." Prentice-Hall, Englewood Cliffs, New Jersey.

Acoustics of Speech Production and Nasalization

James F. Curtis

I. Fundamental Acoustic Properties of Speech Signals 28
    A. Periodicity vs. Aperiodicity 28
    B. Duration 28
    C. Amplitude 29
    D. Spectral Composition 29
II. Acoustic Theory 30
III. Nasalization of Speech 45
IV. Source Functions 53
    A. The Larynx 53
    B. Frictional and Transient Sources 57
V. The Respiratory System 58
    References 60

Communication through speech may be broadly viewed as a chain consisting of three main parts: (a) the physiological processes of vocalization and articulation; (b) the acoustic signals that are produced by these physiological processes; and (c) the psychoacoustic events by means of which a listener converts the acoustic signals into a perceived message. Although all of these are important to an understanding of the speech communication process, in this chapter we shall be primarily concerned with the second of these main parts of the chain, viz., the acoustic signals. We shall by no means ignore the physiological processes of phonation and articulation since a reasonable understanding of the nature of the acoustic signals requires consideration of how they are generated. Moreover, many of the significant characteristics of the physiological processes of speech production may be deduced from information concerning the properties of the acoustic signals.

I. Fundamental Acoustic Properties of Speech Signals

A. PERIODICITY VS. APERIODICITY

The acoustic signals of speech may be conveniently divided into two broad classes: those which are relatively periodic in their vibratory character; and those which lack such periodicity. The regularity of vibratory pattern of the first class implies a sound-generating source having a motion that is correspondingly periodic in character. In the vocal apparatus such a source is provided by the larynx. All sounds which are vocalized thus belong to the first class. These include the vowel sounds and all voiced consonants.[1] Sounds which are relatively periodic in character are perceived as having a definite pitch, i.e., as being high or low in relation to the musical scale. Periodic sounds are usually called tones, in contrast to the nonmusical, aperiodic sounds to which the term noise is frequently applied.

Speech sounds belonging to the second class include the voiceless consonants, so-called because they are produced without laryngeal vibration. In English speech two types of noise-generating sources are utilized in the articulation of voiceless consonants: (1) air may be forced through a very narrow constriction, e.g., a constriction formed by the tongue and teeth, so that the airstream becomes turbulent; (2) air may be impounded behind a complete closure formed by the articulatory structures and then suddenly released as a sharp, explosive pulse. For both of these types of sound source the resulting vibratory motion in the air is aperiodic in character. Speech sounds generated by the first type of source are the fricative consonants. The second type of aperiodic source is required for stop plosive consonants. Some consonant sounds result from simultaneous excitation of the air in the vocal cavities by both periodic and aperiodic generating sources, since laryngeal vibration can occur at the same time that air is being forced through a narrow constriction or can be coincident with the release of impounded air in a short, transient pulse. Thus voiced fricative consonants and voiced stop plosives are possible.

B. DURATION

In addition to their characteristics as periodic or aperiodic sounds, the acoustic signals of speech have other properties that are significant in relation to the physiological events by which they are produced and which contribute to their perception. An obvious such dimension is duration. Vowels and many consonants, including fricatives, can be prolonged considerably.

---

[1] Whispered speech, which contains no periodic sounds, will be neglected in this discussion.

On the other hand, since they require pulse excitation, stop plosives are necessarily short, or transient, in character. Speech sounds may also be varied in duration as dictated by the requirements of speech rate, syllabic stress, etc.

C. AMPLITUDE

Speech sounds also vary characteristically with respect to their energy levels. For example, vowels have greater average sound energy levels than consonants, and some consonants characteristically have higher energy levels than others. Because the sound energy level is related to the amplitude of the vibratory disturbance that constitutes a sound wave, the term amplitude is often used to designate this dimension. Perceptible differences in sound amplitude are heard as differences in loudness. Thus, vowels are usually perceived as louder than consonants and when one speaks with an increase in sound energy level, he will be heard to speak more loudly. The variations in amplitude of speech signals depend both on the amplitude with which the air in the vocal cavities is excited by the source vibration (whether it is periodic motion generated by the larynx, a continuous noise, or a transient pulse) and on the transmission characteristics of the vocal cavities as the sound passes through them and is radiated to the air outside the speaker's mouth. Later discussion will consider the transmission characteristics of the vocal cavities in more detail.

D. SPECTRAL COMPOSITION

Thus far, three important acoustic dimensions of speech signals have been mentioned, viz., periodicity (or lack thereof), duration, and amplitude. However, to describe the acoustic properties of speech signals that enable us to make phonetic discriminations among various speech sounds, a fourth property, which may be termed spectral composition, must be specified. The spectral composition of speech signals is also important in relation to the perceptual aspect of speech which we refer to as voice quality. Since nasality, or nasal quality, is one such voice quality, and is a particularly significant aspect of the speech of many individuals with palatal clefts, spectral composition has special importance in the present context.

Spectral composition refers to the distribution of sound energy among the various frequency components which make up a complex sound. The reader is doubtless already familiar with the fact that, with the exception of special test tones generated in a laboratory, nearly all sounds are complex in the sense that the energy in the sound wave is not concentrated at a single frequency, but is distributed among a number of frequency components.

Both periodic tones and aperiodic noises are complex, but they differ characteristically with respect to the nature of their spectral compositions.

Although sounds which are truly periodic in nature may have a large number of frequency components, these can occur only at certain frequencies, viz., those frequencies which are integral multiples of the fundamental frequency of the sound wave. Such components are called harmonics, and the spectral composition of complex, periodic sounds is characterized by a distribution of energy among discrete harmonically related components. Although the sound waves of speech are never perfectly periodic, many speech signals approach periodicity closely enough so that all but a negligible part of the energy in these signals is distributed among harmonic components.

On the other hand, the spectral compositions of aperiodic sounds, such as those generated by creating turbulence in a jet of air, or by the sudden release of a transient pulse, may show energy at any frequency. The term *continuous spectrum noise*, sometimes used to refer to such aperiodic sounds, is appropriate because the energy may be continuously distributed along the frequency dimension. The phonetic differences among fricative and stop plosive consonants are perceived in part because they vary in their duration and overall intensity characteristics, but also, and very importantly, because of amplitude variations in the continuous distribution of energy with respect to frequency, i.e., because of differences in spectral composition.

II. Acoustic Theory

From what has already been said it follows that a very important part of the acoustic theory of speech is that which deals with the relationship between significant variations in spectral composition of speech signals and the physiological events in the vocal system which give rise to these spectral variations. Figure 1 illustrates in block diagram form most of the essential elements of the peripheral processes required for speech generation. The diagram indicates the functions that would need to be performed by an electrical device which would be capable of simulating the speech-generating processes for all of the various speech sounds. As a matter of fact, electrical speech synthesizers following the principles illustrated have been shown to be capable of generating speech sounds which are both natural in sound and readily recognized. The only element lacking in the diagram for the generation of very natural continuous speech is a programming system that would be capable of bringing about the rapid adjustments required for producing the highly complex dynamic variations in speech signals that are characteristic of continuous speech. The circuit represented in Fig. 1 has properties which are, in a number of respects, functionally analogous to

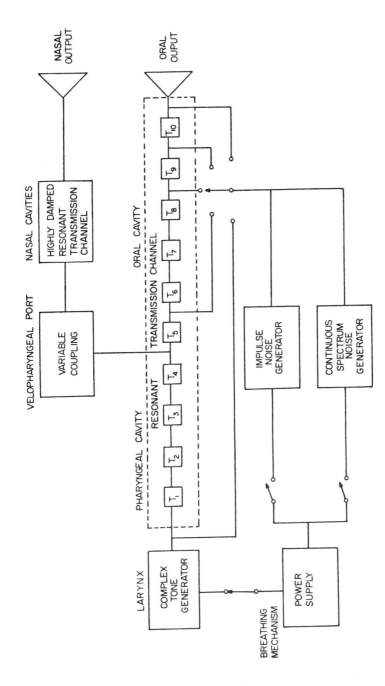

Fig. 1. Block diagram of a hypothetical electrical speech-synthesizing system which illustrates by analogy certain functional principles and relationships of the speech generation processes.

the properties of the vocal mechanism. As indicated in the diagram the block designated as the power supply can be thought of as analogous to the breathing mechanism. The function of the power supply is to furnish operating voltages to the electronic generators, which serve as the signal sources in the illustrated circuit. In a similar manner the breathing mechanism generates expiratory pressures from which the vibratory energy of the speech signals are generated. Three types of sources are shown in the diagram. The box designated as the complex tone generator represents the laryngeal vibrating source. It can be thought of as a relaxation oscillator which releases energy from the power supply in periodic pulses in much the same manner as the vibrating larynx releases air pressure from the lungs in relatively periodic pulses. A second source generates an aperiodic noise similar in character to the continuous spectrum noise which results from forcing the breath stream through a narrow constriction during fricative consonant articulation. The third source, designated as the transient noise source, generates an electrical input signal that is analogous to the acoustic transients produced by sudden release of stop consonant articulations.

In the diagram of Fig. 1 the vocal tract is represented by a series of blocks (designated T_1, T_2,..., T_{10}) rather than a single block. The purpose of this representation is to emphasize that the vocal tract does not act as a single simple resonator. Instead, it acts as a continuous, acoustic tube having a number of resonant modes. The shape of this acoustic tube can be varied considerably, of course, and for each variation in shape there will be a corresponding variation in the pattern of resonant modes. An approximate electrical analog for such a variable acoustical transmission line is a series of variable networks, each of which corresponds to a short section of tube having a fixed length but variable cross-sectional area. The complete vocal tract is then represented by the series connection of these networks.[2] Representation of the vocal tract as a series of blocks also provides the opportunity to indicate that the effective input from the continuous noise and transient sources may occur at various points along the transmission system representing the vocal tract. It should also be noted that the diagram includes a side branch corresponding to the nasal cavities and that the coupling between this side branch and the main tract can be varied, thus simulating the variable coupling of the nasal cavities to the oral tract which is governed by the velopharyngeal closure in the actual speech mechanism. The two loud speakers represent the radiation impendances through which the vibratory energy existing in the main vocal tract, or its side branch, may be radiated into the air.

[2] There is no intention to suggest that an electrical analog consisting of 10 sections can adequately simulate the articulatory shape variations of the vocal tract. Actual vocal tract analogs that have been built and operated successfully have consisted of 35 or more.

An alternate, and in some respects somewhat simpler, representation of the functions which are involved in the generation of any sound by the speech mechanism is expressed in the following symbolic equation:

$$| P(f) | = | S(f) | \cdot | H(f) | \cdot | R(f) |$$

This expression states that the sound pressure spectrum radiated from the vocal mechanism is equal to the product of three factors: the volume velocity spectrum generated by the source, $S(f)$, the transfer function of the vocal tract, $H(f)$, and the radiation characteristic, $R(f)$. Each of these is a complex function of frequency, as indicated by the notation, (f). The vertical bars indicate that we are concerned only with the magnitudes of these functions and not with their phase relations. Thus, each of them can be represented by a graph which shows how its magnitude varies as a function of frequency.

Of these three factors, the one that is most closely related to the spectral characteristics that cause us to hear phonetic differences among speech sounds is the transfer function of the vocal tract, $H(f)$. The radiation characteristic, $R(f)$, describes how the volume velocity spectrum at the lips or nares is radiated into the air as a sound pressure spectrum. $R(f)$ plays a very minor role in generating distinctive speech sound variations because it is primarily related to the shape of the speaker's face and head which does not change very greatly in relation to the sound being uttered. Measurements have shown that, despite the irregularities of facial features, the pattern of sound radiation in front of a speaker's lips is very similar to the pattern radiated from a sound source located on the surface of a spherical baffle. Hence, to a reasonable first approximation, a plot of $R(f)$ against frequency is a rising curve with a slope of 6 dB per octave, and this function may be considered to be a constant in the equation, irrespective of the particular sound that is being uttered.

It is also well known that the laryngeal spectrum can vary a great deal without appreciably altering those characteristics of the output sound spectrum that are significantly related to phonetic variations among vowels and various consonants. For example alterations of the laryngeal vibration may produce a high-pitched or a low-pitched voice, a loud voice or a soft voice, one that sounds harsh, or breathy, or artistically musical; but, because these alterations do not affect the transmission properties of the vocal cavity system, they do not change the phonetic perception of the vowel being phonated. It can also be shown that for voiced sounds there is negligible interaction between the source spectrum, $S(f)$, and the transmission properties of the vocal tract. That is to say, the spectrum which is generated by the laryngeal source is essentially independent of variations which may take place in the vocal tract. More concretely, if we are considering the glottal source during vowel phonation, the spectrum generated by the vocal fold vibration is essentially unaffected by the particular shaping of the oral and pharyngeal cavities that is required for a particular vowel. Thus, the laryngeal spectrum will be essentially the same for [i], [a] or [u], etc.

Since they are essentially independent factors in the speech generation process, we can appropriately consider the transmission properties of the vocal tract system and the sound-generating characteristics of the source separately. Because of their primary importance in relation to the formation of distinctive speech sounds, and in the control of nasalization of speech, first and most detailed consideration will be given in this chapter to the transmission properties of the vocal tract.

As previously mentioned, the factors which contribute to the spectral distribution of the output signal are complex functions of frequency that can be represented by graphs showing how the magnitudes of these functions vary as frequency is changed. In the case of the transfer function $H(f)$, which describes the transmission properties of the vocal tract, the graph is a plot for each frequency of the ratio formed by dividing the magnitude of the output signal by the magnitude of the input signal. If the transmission of the system at a particular frequency is large, this ratio will have a correspondingly large value. Conversely, if the system transmits little energy at some frequency, this ratio between output signal and input signal will be small. Thus, the transfer function curve represents the frequency-selective character of the vocal cavity transmission.

A particular mathematical theory has been developed for the analysis of such complex frequency functions. Although detailed consideration of the mathematics of complex frequency signals would be out of place in this chapter, consideration of a few of its implications will be useful to later discussion, since they are fundamental to the acoustic theory of speech production. This mathematical theory shows that graphs of complex frequency functions, such as $S(f)$ and $H(f)$, can be analyzed as compounds of sets of curves having somewhat simpler characteristics. Although these component curves may vary in certain respects, they all belong to a family having particular shape characteristics. This principle is illustrated in Fig. 2. In the upper graph of the figure, the four very similar solid-line curves are of the type that represent components of a complex frequency function. For mathematical reasons that need not concern us here, the functions represented by these curves are called *poles*. It is evident that each of these pole curves has a very similar shape. They differ, however, with respect to their location along the horizontal axis representing frequency. It is perhaps obvious that the frequency location of each can be specified by a single number, i.e., the frequency of the maximum, or peak, of the curve. The solid curve in the lower graph is the complex curve which is obtained if one sums algebraically the four component curves of the upper graph. Thus, the more complex curve of the lower graph may be considered a compound of the four simpler curves. The dashed curves in the upper and lower graphs show the effect of changing the frequency of the first, or lowest frequency, pole. The dashed curve in the lower graph is the algebraic sum of the dashed curve representing a lower frequency for pole 1 and the original curves for poles 2, 3, and 4. Note that changing the frequency of only one pole has altered the magnitudes at all frequencies of the composite curve. The two curves in the lower graph illustrate possible transfer function curves of a frequency-selective, that is, resonant, system, such as the vocal tract, and illustrate with a somewhat simplified example the principle that complex transfer functions can be analyzed into a set of component curves. Each

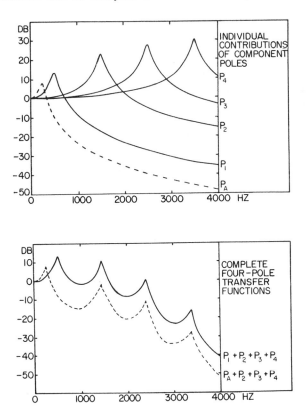

Fig. 2. Graphs illustrating the analysis of complete transfer functions into their component poles. The curves in the upper graph illustrate the individual contributions of poles having different frequencies, but equal bandwidths. The lower graph illustrates complete four-pole transfer function curves which may be derived by combining the contributions of individual poles from the upper graph. (Adapted from Fant, 1960.)

of the poles in this transfer function represents a resonant mode of the transmission system. These curves have the form of response curves of simple, single-tuned resonantors and each curve represents the contribution of the corresponding resonant mode to the frequency-selective character of the complete system, which, in turn, is represented by the composite graph derived by summing the individual pole curves.

In this somewhat idealized illustration, the poles differ in only one respect, viz., the pole frequencies. However, poles and their curves can also differ with respect to one other parameter, viz., bandwidth. Poles with small bandwidths are represented by curves having steep slopes in the region of maximum response and appear narrow and quite peaked. Those having large bandwidth values are represented by curves with less steep slopes which are wider and less sharply peaked in the region of their maxima. Thus, the complete curve of any pole is fully specified by stating only two numbers—one corresponding to the frequency of the pole and a second number giving its bandwidth. It follows that the composite curve which describes the complete frequency-selective character of a transmission system may be fully described by stating only the frequencies and bandwidths of the poles.

A further word needs to be said about bandwidth. The bandwidth of a pole corresponding to a resonant mode of a transmission system is related to a characteristic of the system that is called *damping*. The damping of a transmission system is related to the rate at which energy is absorbed by the system. Highly damped systems absorb energy rapidly, and conversely. Also, the greater the damping the wider will be the bandwidths of the poles, and vice versa. In an actual system the damping is seldom uniform for all resonant modes as shown by the graph of Fig. 2. Thus, the bandwidths of the poles of a particular system usually differ one from another.

One further point needs to be made before we leave this discussion of the mathematical theory of complex frequency signals. Thus far we have considered only systems whose transmission characteristics may be specified by taking account of their resonant modes. However, some systems have characteristic antiresonances as well as resonances; in fact, some may have only antiresonances. The mathematical theory takes this into account in a manner very similar to that covered in the previous discussion of poles. The contribution of antiresonances to the complete transfer function can be shown to correspond to curves which have the form of inverted pole curves. The functions defining these curves, which slope downward to minima instead of upward to maxima, are called *zeros*. The complete curve of a zero, like that of a pole, may be fully specified by two numbers—its frequency and its bandwidth. Finally, the complete transfer function of a frequency-selective transmission system which has both resonant and antiresonant modes may be described completely by an analysis into the poles and zeros which correspond, respectively, to these resonances and antiresonances and by determining their respective frequencies and bandwidths.

As previously stated, the pharyngeal-oral channel acts as a frequency-selective, or resonant, transmission line which modifies the spectrum of the acoustic input, whether this input is the more or less periodic oscillation produced by the vocal fold vibration, or whether it is either a continuous noise or impulse noise generated by the airstream interacting with a consonant constriction. The particular effect produced is described by the transfer function previously mentioned. A simplified illustration of this is shown in Fig. 3. The line spectrum at the left of the figure is a simplified representation of the volume velocity spectrum generated by the vocal folds. The curve in the middle part of the figure represents a simplified,

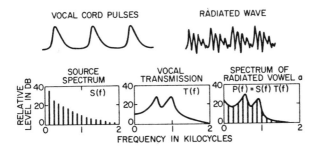

Fig. 3. Simplified decomposition of the spectrum of a two-resonance vowel sound. The output of the vocal system is the radiated wave shown at the upper right. The sound pressure spectrum of this radiated wave, $P(f)$, is the product of the transmission characteristic of the vocal cavities, $T(f)$, and the source spectrum, $S(f)$, which corresponds to the periodic pulse train operated by the laryngeal vibration whose wave form is shown at the upper left. (After Fant, 1960.)

two-resonance type of transfer function curve. As previously stated, such a transfer function is simply a plot for all frequencies of the ratio between the magnitude of the output signal at each frequency and the magnitude of the input signal of the same frequency. The final graph in the figure shows the result of this transfer function acting on the spectrum shown on the left. It is apparent that the spectral distribution of the output sound is very importantly related to the frequency-selective, or resonant, properties shown by the transmission curve.

Several times it has been stated that the pharyngeal-oral tract may be considered as an acoustic transmission line. This descriptive statement is to be contrasted to a different way of thinking of the system, viz., as a system of simple resonators. In the transmission line view the resonant and antiresonant characteristics of the oral tract are related to the dimensions and other characteristics of the complete system. The system of simple resonators concept assigns each of the resonances or antiresonances to a particular division of the vocal tract acting relatively independently of the remainder of the system. At an earlier stage of development of the acoustic theory of speech production, a number of investigators attempted to develop a satisfactory explanation of the properties of the vocal tract in simple resonator terms. We now know that such a conceptualization does not fit the data very well. That is, attempts to account for the variations in the spectral distribution of speech sounds by analyzing the vocal tract as a system of simple resonators have not been successful. On the other hand, work done since about 1950 which has analyzed the vocal tract as an acoustic transmission line has contributed a great deal of information about the

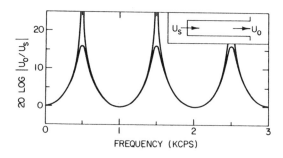

Fig. 4. A plot of the magnitude of the transfer ratio (in dB) as a function of frequency for a transmission line representation of an acoustic tube. The tube represented is of uniform cross-sectional area, is 17 cm in length, and is open at one end. The curve has infinite peaks for the ideal lossless case, and peaks of finite amplitude for the slightly dissipative case, as shown. The bandwidths of all resonance was assumed to be 100 cps. (After Stevens and House, 1961.)

relations between articulatory shaping of the vocal tract during speech and the spectral distribution of speech sounds.[3]

A very simple form of such an acoustic transmission line, together with its transfer function, is shown in Fig. 4. The drawing represents a tube having uniform circular cross-section. It is excited at one end by a volume velocity, represented by U_s in the figure, and has an output volume velocity, signified by U_0. Actually this tube is more nearly analogous to the vocal tract system composed of the pharynx and oral cavities than might at first be apparent. Figure 5 shows a tracing from an x-ray photograph of the vocal

[3] For the interested reader, a more complete discussion of this point may be found in the excellent paper by Stevens and House (1961). Other sources are Fant (1960), particularly Chapters 1.1, 1.3, and 1.4, and Dunn (1950).

tract system. As we know, it is curved rather than straight like the model of Fig. 4, it has numerous small irregularities, and it is by no means circular in cross-section. However, it can be shown that, with respect to the location of most of the resonant frequencies of importance in speech, these differences are of little importance. Up to at least 4000 Hz, all cross-sectional dimensions of the vocal tract, are quite small relative to the wavelengths of sound. Since this is true, the exact cross-sectional shape is a negligible factor in determining the resonant frequencies of significance in vowel sounds, and thus the simplified representation by a circular cross-section, as in the model, introduces no significant error. Moreover, a tube having a certain length will have the same resonant frequencies whether it is curved or straight. Hence, for frequencies lying below 4000 Hz, we can view the vocal tract as adequately represented by a model which is a straight tube rather than a curved one,

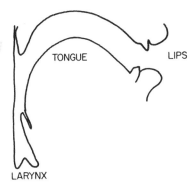

Fig. 5.   Tracing of an x-ray picture showing the midsagittal outline of the vocal tract during the production of a neutral vowel.

and the model will be just as good a representation with a circular as with an irregularly shaped cross-section. Of course, for most vowels the vocal tract will not have a uniform cross-sectional area throughout its length, like the one in the idealized model of Fig. 4, and the variations in cross-sectional area which occur along the length of the tube are important in determining the resonance frequencies. In fact, the length of the tube and the way in which the cross-sectional area varies along its length are the two most important factors which determine the resonant frequencies.

Further consideration of the uniform cross-section tube of Fig. 4 will be useful in illustrating some significant points about such acoustic transmission lines which have application to an understanding of the vocal tract transmission characteristics. It is well known, and taught in every elementary acoustics course, that investigation of the response of such a tube or pipe will show that it has an infinite number of resonances. For a tube that is closed at one end, like that in Fig. 4, the lowest resonant frequency corresponds to a wavelength which is four times the length of the tube; that is, the ratio between tube length and wavelength is one fourth. The successively higher resonant frequencies are those for which the ratios between tube length and wavelength are the successive odd-numbered multiples of this one-fourth relationship, i.e., three fourths, five fourths, etc.

This principle has direct application to the vocal tract. For voiced sounds produced with the velopharyngeal port closed the pharyngeal and oral cavities taken together may be viewed as a continuous tube closed at one end by the vocal folds. Although this tube does not have a uniform cross-sectional area throughout its length, for the schwa vowel it approaches this condition. For adult males this tube has a length, on the average, of about 17 cm, and a uniform cross-section tube of this length will have a transfer function similar to that shown in Fig. 4, with resonant frequencies at 500 Hz, 1500 Hz, 2500 Hz, etc. It is of more than passing interest that these resonant frequencies of the idealized model correspond rather well to values which have been found typical for the schwa vowel of adult males. Although this idealized uniform cross-section does not exactly represent any real case, it can be considered as a prototype from which numerous configurations correspond- ing to the whole range of vowel sounds may be derived. Thus, certain principles which apply to all such cases may be drawn from it. (1) As already mentioned, the complete transfer function will have an infinite number of resonances (although for practical purposes of illustration the figure shows only 3). (2) These resonances will have a certain *average* spacing, approximately 1000 Hz for male voices whose vocal tract lengths approximate the 17-cm length of this tube. The spacings will be farther apart, on the average, and the resonant frequencies will be generally higher for women and children whose vocal cavities are shorter. (3) Lengthening the vocal tract will result in lower frequencies for all resonances and, conversely, shortening the vocal tract will raise all resonant frequencies. It follows that the general levels of the vocal tract resonances and their average spacing depend on the length of the tract. The particular locations of the resonant frequencies for a given vowel will vary considerably depending on the variations in cross-sectional area along the length of the tube which in turn depend on the positioning of the articulators for that vowel. For example, area variations may be introduced by constrictions formed by the lips and jaw, or by narrowing the tube through elevation of the tongue, etc. However, the average spacing due to the length will be maintained.

It is not possible within the limitations of a brief discussion to follow up all of the significant implications of the transmission line model in detail.

However, it may be worth carrying the development a step or two farther. To relate the transfer function of the idealized model to an actual vowel spectrum one needs to apply the characteristics which are imposed by the source spectrum of the vocal fold wave $S(f)$ and to make an appropriate correction for the radiation characteristic $R(f)$. This has been done in Fig. 6, which thus represents the spectrum envelope for the idealized vowel for which the curve in Fig. 4 is the transfer function. The amplitudes of the individual harmonics in the vowel spectrum would, of course, conform to the variation with frequency described by this envelope. The general downward slope of the spectrum envelope is due to the fact that the source spectrum $S(f)$ shows a decrement in harmonic amplitude with increasing frequency. This downward slope is only partially offset by the upward slope of the radiation characteristic curve, $R(f)$.

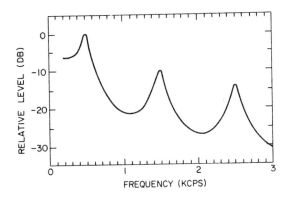

Fig. 6. Hypothetical vowel spectrum envelope constructed by adding together the transfer function for the straight tube shown in Fig. 4, an assumed glottal spectrum envelope and a radiation characteristic rising at 6 dB/octave. (After Stevens and House, 1961.)

Employing these principles of the transmission line model, it is possible to calculate spectrum envelopes for vocal tract configurations having resonances that are appropriate for various vowel sounds. Three such calculated spectrum envelopes for the three vowels, [i], [a], and [u], are shown in Fig. 7. The procedure used in deriving these spectral envelope curves was that of summing pole curves corresponding to the first three resonant modes of the vocal tract for each of the three vowels. (The resonant frequencies employed in these calculations are typical values for these vowels as spoken by adult males.) To the composite curve thus obtained, a correction for the contribution of poles of higher frequency was added, since an acoustic transmission line such as the vocal tract theoretically has an infinite number of resonant modes. The vocal tract transfer function thus obtained was further modified by the addition of curves representing the spectral envelope of the laryngeal source tone $S(f)$ and the radiation characteristic $R(f)$. The reader will doubtless recognize that this process is equivalent to the realization

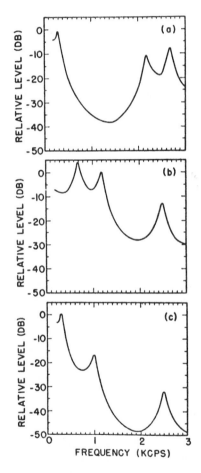

Fig. 7. Computed spectrum envelopes approximating the vowels [i], [a], and [u]. The half-power bandwidth of all resonances were assumed to be 100 cps. (After Stevens and House, 1961.)

of the mathematical equation stated earlier in this chapter (see p. 33). The curves of Fig. 7 are not quite correct with respect to the pole bandwidths, since for the sake of simplicity in calculation, equal bandwidths of 100 Hz were assigned to all poles. The poles corresponding to the low frequency resonances of actual vowels would usually have bandwidths somewhat narrower than this, whereas the bandwidths of the high frequency poles would normally be wider. However, despite this simplification, these calculated spectral envelopes are highly similar to those which experiments have shown to be typical for the respective vowel sounds.

Up to this point the term *formant* has not appeared in this chapter, although this term is very commonly employed in most discussions of the spectral characteristics of speech, especially with respect to vowels. The term has been widely used to refer to the concentrations of energy that are apparent in the spectrographic analyses of vowels, and the frequencies of the amplitude peaks which characterize the spectral distributions of vowels have often been referred to as formant frequencies. However, the term is also used in a somewhat different sense to refer to a resonant mode of the vocal tract. The term was avoided in the foregoing discussion because it has had these two somewhat different and not entirely compatible meanings. From the foregoing discussion it should be clear that the transfer function of the vocal tract is the basic factor which governs the variations in spectral distribution which are important as cues to phonetic distinctions. It may therefore be logically argued that the formant, as a fundamental characteristic of speech sounds, is more properly defined as a property of the vocal tract, i.e., as referring to a resonant mode of the tract, than as a property of the acoustic spectrum. The logic of this position is strengthened by the fact that there is not always an exact correspondence between the pole frequencies of the transfer function which represent the vocal tract resonant modes and the frequencies of amplitude peaks in the acoustic spectrum. Space does not permit a development of the reasons for this lack of correspondence, but a hint or two may be given. It is possible for two resonant modes to so nearly coincide in frequency that the spectrum will not show two distinct peaks corresponding to the two poles. Also, when the system is characterized by antiresonances as well as resonances, it is possible for a pole and zero to occur so close together in frequency that the contribution of the pole will be partially canceled by that of the zero. Even though the cancellation is only partial, the result may be a spectral peak which differs considerably in frequency from that of the pole with which it is associated.

A second reason for preferring to define the term formant as a property of the vocal tract transfer function is that this definition more readily permits the extension of the term to include consonants as well as vowels. Far more laboratory investigations of the spectral composition of speech sounds have been concerned with vowels than with consonants (primarily because of technical problems in the analysis of consonants). Thus, the formant concept was developed in relation to studies of vowels, and has been most often used in this context. However, a beginning has been made in the investigation of the spectral characteristics of both fricatives and stop plosives (Hughes and Halle, 1956; Halle *et al.*, 1957). The concept of formants as it applies to consonant production has also been developed by Fant (1960). His theoretical development shows that the transfer functions of consonants depend both on the articulatory shaping of the vocal tract and on the locus of the input excitation. That is, the transfer function associated with a particular vocal tract configuration for a consonant, such as a postdental fricative, which requires excitation at some midpoint along the tract, will be different from the transfer function when the source of excitation is at one end, as is the case for vowels. Further work on the transfer functions of voiceless fricative consonant sounds has shown that the spectral distribution actually measured for such consonants can be accounted for reasonably well by transfer functions characterized by two poles and one zero having appropriate frequency and bandwidth values (Heinz and Stevens, 1961). It seems apparent, therefore, that the fundamental theory of speech generation, including the concepts of transfer functions and formants, is sufficiently general to account for both consonant and vowel production.

In the foregoing discussion there has been little discussion of the relationship between the fundamental formant parameters (frequency and bandwidth) and the perceptual identification of speech sounds. The relationship between formant frequencies and vowel perception has been extensively investigated. However, data concerning the relationship of bandwidth variations to the perception of phonetic differences are very meager, and only a beginning has been made in the investigation of the relationship of consonant perception to the parameters concerning spectral distribution.[4] Although the purposes of this chapter would not be well served by attempting to review this work in detail, a few summary statements based on presently available knowledge are in point. First, there is a great deal of evidence showing that formant frequencies are very important as perceptual cues to vowel identification and discrimination. Second, the meager information that is available on the subject suggests that bandwidth variations are less significantly related to perceived phonetic differences than are formant frequencies. Although bandwidth variations are perceived by listeners, such variations appear to be more closely related to other perceptual aspects of speech than to

---

[4] Although there has been a considerable amount of experimental work on consonant perception, it has been mainly concerned with other relationships than those considered here. For example, there have been numerous experiments investigating the relationships of consonant perception to such variables as masking of speech by noise, transmission of restricted ranges of frequency, presence or absence of voicing, duration of consonant sounds, and the relationship of consonant perception to interphonemic formant transitions.

phonetic discrimination. For example, experiments in the generation of synthetic speech by means of electrical analogs suggest that the naturalness of the synthesized speech is related to the proper choice of bandwidths for the transfer function and it has been shown that the preference ratings of listeners will vary systematically for vowels which differ only with respect to formant bandwidth (House, 1960). Third, increased bandwidth has been shown to be one of the spectral characteristics which results from the nazalization of vowels, and there is a reasonable presumption that the bandwidth differences contribute to the perception of nasal quality. This relationship will be further considered in the next section.

III. Nasalization of Speech

Nasalization of speech is an important topic for at least two reasons. Nasalization is important in relation to phonetics and phonology, both because some consonants are produced nasally and because in the phonological systems of some languages the nasalization of vowels is phonemically significant. It is also important because excessive nasalization is frequently considered to constitute or contribute significantly to a speech disorder. Our interest in this chapter is, of course, primarily in nasalization as it relates to the speech deviations associated with cleft palate.

In the following discussion we shall be primarily concerned with the nasalization of speech sounds, especially vowels, that are normally produced with little or no coupling between the pharyngeal-oral and nasal portions of the vocal tract system, i.e., with complete (or nearly complete) velopharyngeal closure. Nasalization may be said to occur when this coupling is increased sufficiently to produce a perceptually significant change in the speech signal. Such perceptual differences result from modification of the spectral composition of the speech signals when the transfer function of the vocal cavity system is affected by the coupling between the pharyngeal-oral tract and the nasal cavities. An understanding of the acoustic characteristics of nasalization thus requires consideration of the related transfer function variations.

Fant (1960) devotes a complete chapter in the "Acoustic Theory of Speech Production" to the topic of nasalization, and it is, indeed, a much more complex subject than it might appear to be at first glance. The nasal cavities are very complexly shaped, convoluted cavities whose acoustic characteristics are correspondingly complex. Moreover, the interaction between the pharyngeal-oral tract and the nasal cavities is complexly related to the extent of coupling between them. If the velopharyngeal port is sufficiently open, some of the sound energy will be transmitted via this opening through the nasal cavities and to the outside air. There may, thus, be two transmission channels instead of just one, and the manner in which energy is divided between these two channels is related not only to the extent of the velopharyngeal opening, but also to the articulatory configuration of the oral cavity, e.g., the degree of constriction caused by elevation of the tongue, the amount of lip opening, etc. Consequently, this division of energy will be different for different vowels. In addition the division of energy will be a variable function of frequency. Stated somewhat more exactly, the division of sound energy between the two channels will be related to the opposition to the flow of energy through each. When we are concerned with oscillating signals, such as sound, this opposition to energy transmission is correctly termed impedance (rather than resistance, as it would be if we were dealing with a steady flow), and it is characteristic of the impedance of a transmission channel that it varies with frequency. Since the greater proportion of energy will be transmitted through the channel having the lesser impedance, the division of energy between the two channels will be inversely proportional to the ratio between their respective impedances. This ratio will not only vary for different vowels, but it will be a variable function of frequency.

The complexity and variability of many of the acoustic effects introduced by nasalization have been emphasized in the previous paragraph. Because of such complexity and variability, it is not easy to make a few general statements about the acoustic characteristics associated with nasalization which will be valid for all cases. However, a few relatively general deductions can be made on the basis of acoustic theory. It will, perhaps, be informative to see what these are and to compare these deductions with the experimental data which have been obtained in spectral analysis studies of nasalized speech. In the discussion which follows, the statements concerning experimental data will be drawn from a number of studies, chief among which are those of Curtis (1942), Hattori et al. (1958), Fant (1960), and Dickson (1962). The basic theoretical points have largely been drawn from Fant's development.

One of the important consequences of increasing nasal coupling by opening the velopharyngeal port is that a side branch (the nasal cavities) is added to what would otherwise be a more or less continuous pharyngeal-oral transmission tube. Acoustic theory tells us that one of the consequences to be expected from the addition of such a side branch is the introduction of antiresonances into the transfer function of the system. That is to say, the transfer functions will include the contribution of zeros as well as poles. The frequencies of such zeros will vary somewhat depending on individual differences in structural dimensions, the degree of coupling for a particular case, etc., but Fant's analysis indicates that there are probably two such nasal cavity zeros within the frequency range of significance for vowel sounds. Because their frequencies will vary from one individual to another and in relation to the degree of coupling their exact effect on the vocal cavity transfer function is not easily predicted. Moreover, the effect on the transfer function depends on the relation between the frequencies of these nasal zeros and the poles of the transfer function. If a pole and zero occur at nearly the same frequency some cancellation of the pole by the zero is to be expected. If the zero occurs at a point in frequency remote from any pole, the output spectrum will show a sharp reduction in energy at or near the frequency of the zero. Since the frequencies of the poles of vowel transfer functions, that is to say, the formant patterns, are different for different vowels, the manner in which the formant poles and the nasal zeros interact will not be the same for different vowels. Consequently, we can hardly expect that the spectral analysis of nasalized vowels will reveal a consistent alteration of the spectrum attributable to nasalization, irrespective of the vowel. However, one of the effects that has frequently been noted in experimental studies of the spectral effects of nasalization is an absence of energy, or a gap, at some frequency, or frequencies, of the spectrum.

Another effect that is to be expected as a result of nasal coupling is a substantial increase in the damping of the system. Because of their very complex configuration, the nasal cavities have a large amount of surface in proportion to their volume, and this surface is lined with a rather spongy mucous membrane. Consequently, the absorption of energy by the nasal cavity surfaces is relatively large. So far as nasalized vowel sounds are concerned the spectral effects to be expected from this large damping are (1) an increase in the bandwidths of formants, and a corresponding flattening of formant peaks; and (2) a reduction in the overall energy levels of the vowels. These theoretical predictions are also substantiated by experimental results.

It is also to be expected that there will be additional resonances introduced by nasal coupling, especially if this coupling is great enough for a substantial amount of energy to be diverted into the nasal channel. Because of the large damping of the nasal cavities, it would be expected that the bandwidths of these nasal poles would be relatively large. Fant's theoretical development suggests that for large degrees of coupling, at least, the pharynx and nasal cavities may act as a single continuous tube with a fundamental mode corresponding to the quarter-wavelength resonance of this combined tube. Because such a tube would be quite long, and of constant or nearly constant length, this fundamental resonant mode would be expected to be relatively low and of nearly constant frequency. Corresponding to this prediction experimentally derived spectral data show that a low frequency resonance (250–300 Hz) having relatively large amplitude is characteristic of all nasal consonants. Evidence of this resonance may also be seen in the spectra of many nasalized vowels, although it is neither so clearly apparent or consistent as for nasal consonants, possibly because the proportion of total energy transmitted via the nasal cavities is less for the vowels. On theoretical grounds, one could also expect nasal poles of higher frequency. However, the higher frequency nasal resonances are apparently highly damped due to the substantial energy absorption of the nasal cavities so that spectral peaks corresponding to such high frequency poles are not consistently observed in the analyses of nasalized sounds. The most apparent spectral evidence for them is the appearance of diffuse energy in the spectra of nasalized vowels at frequency locations where energy is of very low amplitude in nonnasal vowels. Hattori et al. (1958) observed such diffuse energy between the spectral peaks associated with vowel formants and attributed it to highly damped, complex nasal resonances.

Among the studies concerned with nasalized speech some of the most interesting and instructive have been those which attempted to simulate the effects of nasalization by means of electrical speech synthesizers. Both Fant (1960) in Sweden and House and Stevens (1956) in this country have performed such experiments. These experiments have the distinct advantage that the variables can be more precisely controlled than is possible with real speakers. Thus, for example, it is possible to observe the effects of changing the nasal coupling in controlled increments. In the interest of reasonable brevity, only the experiments of House and Stevens will be considered in detail.

House and Stevens employed an electrical network which represented in all essential respects the acoustic transmission line model of the vocal tract. The electrical circuits corresponding to the pharyngeal-oral tract consisted of 35 sections, connected in series, each of which was the electrical representation of a segment of the tract having a length of 0.5 cm. Hence, the total electrical network represented a tube having a length of 17.5 cm. Each section representing a 0.5-cm length was designed so that the electrical equivalent of its cross-sectional area could be varied over a range of values that would include the variations in cross-sectional area that will in fact occur in various articulatory configurations of an actual adult male vocal tract. With this model it was possible to simulate to a very good approximation all of the articulatory shape variations (i.e., all of the variations in cross-sectional area along the length dimension) that would be appropriate for the production of various vowels. At a location in this electrical network corresponding to the velopharyngeal port, provision was made for connection to circuits representing the nasal cavities. The electrical coupling between the circuits representing the pharyngeal-oral tract and the circuits representing the nasal cavities could be varied to simulate various areas of opening of the velopharyngeal port.

In the experiments to be discussed the electrical networks representing the pharyngeal-oral tract were adjusted to correspond to the physiological configurations for six vowels. For each vowel configuration the coupling to the nasal cavity analog was varied to correspond to five conditions of velopharyngeal port opening, i.e., no coupling and velopharyngeal port cross-sections of 0.25, 0.71, 1.68, and 3.72 cm². By exciting this system with a complex tone source having characteristics approximating those of the laryngeal excitation vowels with various degrees of nasalization were generated synthetically.

Formal listening tests of these vowels showed that they were judged to be nasal in direct relation to the amount of nasal coupling. Moreover, the nasality judgments were consistent with data on nasalized vowels from natural speech in showing that certain vowels, notably high vowels, such as [i] and [u], were judged to be nasal with very little coupling into the nasal cavities, whereas low vowels, such as [a] and [ɔ], require much greater nasal coupling to be judged as nasal.

Figure 8 presents spectrum envelopes which demonstrate the effects of various degrees of nasal coupling for four of these vowels. It may be noted that the upper two sets of spectral envelopes, which give the data for the high vowels [i] and [u], show a marked effect for even the smallest coupling area. On the other hand, vowels which have more open vocal tract configurations, such as [a] and [ɔ], were much less affected by small degrees of coupling. Note that the changes in the spectral envelopes shown in the lower two graphs of the figure were substantial only for the largest coupling areas. The acoustic data are thus consistent with the listeners' judgments.

Previous discussion of nasalization developed the point that, when the velopharyngeal port is opened, the transmission of energy through the nasal and oral channels will divide in inverse proportion to the impedances of these channels. The experiments with electrical analogs of the oral and nasal tracts provided opportunity for quantitative measurement of these relations. Figure 9 presents the data for two vowels, [i] and [a]. The solid lines numbered 1, 2, 3, and 4 show, as a function of frequency, how the impedance into the nasal tract portion of the electrical model varied with different degrees of coupling. The broken lines represent the impedance into the oral tract measured at the same point, i.e., the point of connection for the nasal tract analog. Note that in the low frequency region of the curve for [i] the oral tract impedance is large compared to the nasal tract impedance, even for the smallest coupling area, whereas for [a] the vocal tract impedance becomes large, relative to the impedance into the nasal tract for larger values of coupling only. Thus, the experiments demonstrate in a manner that would be impossible with human subjects the nature of the relationships which explain why the nasalization effects associated with various amounts of velopharyngeal opening will be different for different vowels.

The spectrum envelopes of Fig. 8 also demonstrate another point that was developed in earlier discussion, i.e., that the damping of the system increases markedly as the nasal coupling becomes greater. This is immediately evident from the flattening of the resonant peaks which is more pronounced

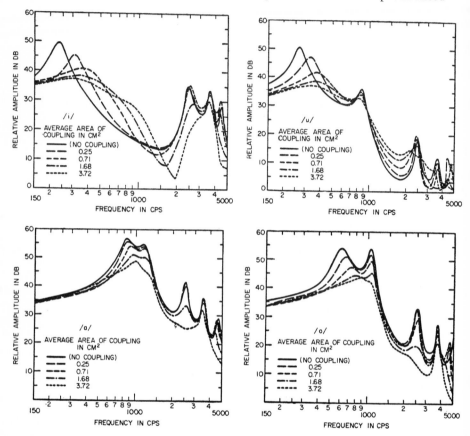

Fig. 8. Spectrum envelopes showing the acoustic effects of varying degrees of nasalization of synthetic vowels generated by an electrical analog of the vocal tract. The curves represent the combined outputs of the pharyngeal-oral tract and the nasal tract for various degrees of coupling. For each set of curves the pharyngeal-oral tract was adjusted to represent one of the four vowels, [i], [u], [a], or [ɔ], as shown on the separate graphs. (Adapted from House and Stevens, 1956.)

with each increase in nasal coupling. In addition to the contribution that this increased damping makes to the perceptual judgment of nasality it may be expected to have a twofold effect. First, the blurring of the resonances may affect the perceptual distinctiveness of the sounds being uttered. Second, the overall intensity of the sound radiated by the speaker will be appreciably reduced. House and Stevens show reductions in the range of 5 to 10 dB for the larger areas of coupling. Reductions in the amplitudes of the first vowel formants are even greater.

Some speculation concerning the implications of these facts for the speaker with a cleft palate, or an inadequate velopharyngeal mechanism,

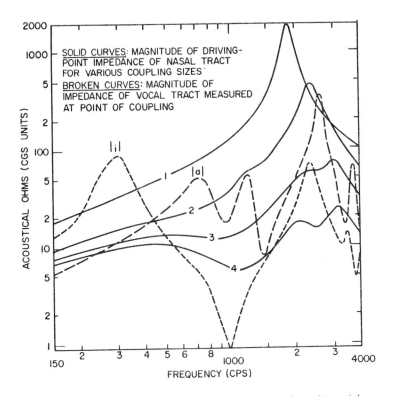

Fig. 9. Magnitude of acoustical impedance of nasal tract and vocal tract (pharyngeal-oral tract) as determined from electrical measurements on the respective analogs at point of coupling. Numbers on solid curves refer to coupling areas as follows: (1) 0.25 cm², (2) 0.71 cm², (3) 1.68 cm², (4) 3.72 cm². (After House and Stevens, 1956.)

may be hazarded. If the relationships that have been demonstrated for large areas of nasal coupling by means of the electrical analog are at all applicable to the situation of the person with a cleft palate, or a velopharyngeal incompetency, it seems obvious that such persons are always confronted with the necessity of speaking with a vocal tract system that absorbs a considerably greater amount of energy than does that of the person with normal oral and pharyngeal structures. To compensate for this he can attain adequate vocal output intensity only by increasing the exciting force from the source, be it the larynx or the noise created by a consonant constriction. Not only will the additional damping of the vocal tract system weaken the vowel sounds and possibly make them less distinct because of the greater formant bandwidths, but it seems likely that the consonant sounds will be weakened also. Although it may be possible for a person with a cleft to make up for some part of this damping of the cavities by driving his vocal system harder, he can do this only by increased expiratory pressure from the lungs and, especially during consonant articulation, by a higher rate of air flow.

It is less clear what compensations may be made for the displacements of the formant peaks shown by the spectral envelopes of Fig. 8 to have been characteristically associated with large amounts of nasal coupling in the synthesized speech experiments of House and Stevens. One suspects, however, that cleft palate speakers may make some kind of such compensations, since spectrographic analyses of the vowels of cleft palate subjects do not show as much dislocation of the formant frequencies as the data from the electrical analog experiments would lead one to expect. It seems probable that cleft subjects may adjust their vocal cavity configurations in some manner which keeps the location of the formant resonances at or near their normal frequency placement. Without more data than we currently have, one can only speculate concerning the specific form that such compensatory adjustments might take. The fact that there is a rather large range of possibilities has, however, been demonstrated by other experiments with the electrical vocal tract analog which have shown that vowel formant frequencies within what appear to be accepted phonemic limits can be generated by a considerable variety of vocal tract configurations (Stevens and House, 1955). Only limited interpretation of these data with relation to the cleft palate problem can be made, because the data were derived from models which simulate the normal vocal tract structure, whereas the cleft palate problem is complicated by an abnormal vocal tract structure with a range of variety and severity of deviations. The research cited certainly indicates that the possibilities for compensatory adjustment are extensive and suggests that investigation of the nature of compensations made by speakers with cleft palate may be worthwhile. A beginning in this direction has been made by using cineradiographic measurements of articulatory configurations together with spectrographic analyses and perceptual judgments of nasalization to study the vowels of a group of cleft palate subjects (Kent, 1966). The cineradiographic data show some evidence for compensatory adjustments of tongue position and lip opening as velopharyngeal coupling is increased. However, considerably more data are needed to provide an adequate description of the nature of such adjustments.

IV. Source Functions

A. THE LARYNX

For all speech sounds which have more or less periodic acoustical wave forms, that is, vowels and voiced consonants, the vocal cavities must be excited by a correspondingly periodic source, viz., the vocal fold vibration. Previous discussion has shown that the spectral characteristics of speech signals which are associated with phonetic variations are primarily related to the vocal tract transfer function which is essentially independent of the laryngeal source. Likewise, the particular spectral effects that act as cues to the perception of nasalization are attributable to modifications in cavity transmission due to nasal coupling. However, the acoustic spectrum generated by the vibrating vocal folds is one of the factors which determines the spectral composition of all voiced speech sounds, and any description of the generation of speech signals must take account of the nature of the laryngeal source. In addition certain aspects of the cleft palate problem can not be fully understood without consideration of the functioning of the larynx as a sound source.

We know that the vocal folds act essentially as a valve. The opening-closing motion of the vocal folds gives rise to a relatively periodic variation in the area of the glottal opening. As a result of interaction between this glottal area variation and the more or less steady subglottic pressures provided by the respiratory mechanism, air is released through the glottis as a relatively periodic train of pulses. This train of pulses constitutes the volume velocity wave which excites the vocal cavities for voiced sounds.

Flanagan (1958, 1965) has shown that, if we know the shape of the curve which describes the periodic variation of glottal area for a particular condition, together with the associated subglottic pressure, it is possible to calculate the shape of the volume velocity pulse, and thus the wave form of the volume velocity pulse train. Figure 10, a graph taken from Flanagan's work, shows these relationships for a single glottal pulse. The symbols F_0 and P_s on the graph denote the fundamental frequency and subglottic pressure, respectively, for the particular phonation, which was a moderately loud tone of relatively low frequency. The glottal area curve, shown by the solid line, was obtained by measuring the glottal areas on successive frames of an ultrahigh speech motion-picture film of the vocal fold vibration taken by indirect laryngoscopy. The dashed line representing the volume velocity pulse was calculated from experimentally derived relations between volume velocity, glottal area, and subglottic pressure.

If the glottal wave form is known it is possible to calculate the corresponding acoustic spectrum. Figure 11 shows the acoustic spectrum calculated from the area curve of Fig. 10. It may be noted that both the shape of the pulse shown in Fig. 10 and the spectrum of Fig. 11 are generally similar to the idealized graphs of the glottal pulse wave form and the acoustic spectrum that were previously presented in Fig. 3. Both show that the excitation due to the vocal fold vibration has its greatest amplitude at low frequencies and that the harmonic amplitudes decrease at higher frequencies. Experimental data have shown that the rate of decrease of harmonic amplitude with increasing frequency varies as the pitch and intensity of phonation is changed, but the general downward slope seen in the spectra of Figs. 3 and 11 is characteristic of laryngeal tones. It may be noted that the idealized spectrum

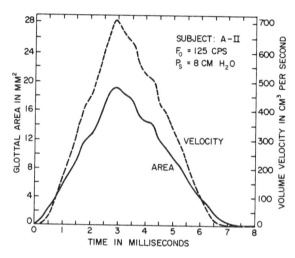

Fig. 10.   Glottal area and computed volume velocity waves for a single vocal period The area wave was derived from high-speed motion pictures of the vocal folds. The volume velocity wave was calculated by taking account of the probable subglottic pressure together with the relation between glottal area and glottal resistance. (After Flanagan, 1958.)

of Fig. 3 shows a relatively smooth decrement in amplitude with increasing frequency, whereas the more precisely determined spectrum calculated by Flanagan for a real case is more irregular, and shows numerous dips or minima. These irregularities in the spectral envelopes for laryngeal tones appear to be characteristic of a wide range of phonatory conditions, although the location and spacing of the minima will change depending on the shape of the glottal pulse. These irregularities in the laryngeal spectrum envelope constitute a complication for experimenters who must attempt to interpret spectral analyses of speech sounds. For example, if the experimenter notes a sharp dip, or gap, in the output spectrum of a particular sound, it may be impossible to interpret this with confidence since it could be due either to an antiresonance in the vocal tract transfer function, or to a minimum in the glottal spectrum. Alternatively, a glottal spectral minimum could by chance coincide closely in frequency with a resonant mode of the transfer function. With respect to the output spectrum which the experimenter is trying to interpret, the result could be a more or less complete cancellation of the transfer function resonance, so that no evidence of this resonance would be seen in the output spectrum. Further discussion of this matter would be out of place in the present context, but it should be apparent to the reader that the interpretation of sound spectra is not a simple matter, since the exact nature of the associated glottal spectrum is generally not known.

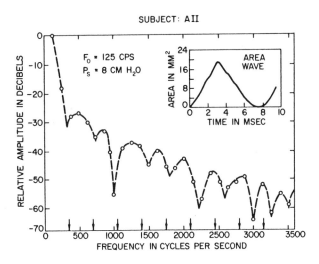

Fig. 11. Amplitude spectrum computed for the area wave shown in Fig. 10. Each point indicates the amplitude of a harmonic of the complex laryngeal tone. (After Flanagan, 1965.)

A matter of more direct interest in the problem of cleft palate speech is the relation of subglottic pressure to the laryngeal vibration. Several investigations, including those of van den Berg (1956), Kunze (1962), and Isshiki (1964), have studied the relationship between variations in subglottic pressure and variations in vocal pitch and vocal intensity. As one might guess, there is a systematic, direct relationship between vocal intensity and subglottic pressure. Higher intensity requires higher subglottic pressure in order for the vocal fold vibration to generate a volume velocity wave of greater amplitude. The results of these investigations also show a direct relationship between vocal pitch (fundamental frequency) and subglottic pressure. The data from these experiments have some possible implications for the problem of cleft palate speech. As was shown in the section on nasalization, one of the significant effects of nasal coupling is to increase the damping, i.e., energy absorption, of the vocal cavity system. It will be recalled that the House and Stevens data show reductions in overall vowel intensity of as much as 5 to 10 dB for the large nasal coupling conditions of their experiments. When one considers that a reduction of 3 dB is equivalent to a loss of half of the sound energy, it is apparent that losses of such magnitude are not trivial. The only way that these losses can be made up is for the input from the source to be increased in proportion. Obviously, for voiced sounds, this means that the vocal fold vibration must generate sound energy at a higher rate and that the subglottic pressure must be correspondingly increased. Isshiki's data show that a 5 dB increase in vocal intensity will probably require more than a 50% increase in subglottic pressure. It seems reasonable to suppose that this increase in subglottic pressure cannot be produced without a very appreciable increase in vocal effort.

One implication is obvious. Consider a hypothetical speaker with a cleft palate who is unable to attain reasonable velopharyngeal closure. Thus, a more or less continuous characteristic of his speech is pronounced nasalization. If our previous reasoning is correct, such a speaker will have to expend more than the usual effort to attain a given level of speech intensity. If, on the other hand, he does not habitually make the necessary additional effort, his average speech intensity level may be too low for good audibility.

An additional implication that may not be entirely obvious is that both the dynamic intensity range and the vocal pitch range of our hypothetical cleft palate speaker are likely to be significantly reduced. Because of the greater energy absorption accompanying nasalization, the greatest subglottic pressure that he can generate, even with maximum effort, will not produce as much output energy from his vocal cavity system as would be the case if he could attain adequate velopharyngeal closure. The logic which suggests a reduction in pitch range is not quite as simple. However, vocal effort and subglottic pressure tend to be closely related to both vocal pitch and intensity. When one increases his effort in order to raise his subglottic pressure and, hence, his intensity level, he involuntarily tends to raise his pitch. Since the speaker with a cleft must generate abnormally high subglottic pressures for all intensity levels, his pitch may be expected to be higher than average for all intensity levels with the result that the lower end of his pitch range may be limited.

No experimental data can be cited to verify these deductions concerning dynamic intensity and pitch range, and, for the present at least, they must be regarded as untested hypotheses, albeit reasonable ones. In the writer's opinion it would be interesting and worthwhile to carry out the experiments required to test these speculations, both to determine their validity and to investigate the extent of such effects should the speculations prove to be well founded.

B. FRICTIONAL AND TRANSIENT SOURCES

The fact that the vocal cavities are excited by noise sources for fricative and stop plosive consonants has been previously discussed. It has also been pointed out that the location of the point at which this excitation occurs is significant in relation to the transfer function of the cavities which determines the spectral distributions of consonants. However, a few additional points may be relevant in the context of this chapter.

The first point to be made is that both the continuous and the transient types of noise sources require relatively high pressures within the oral cavity. At least these pressures must be high by comparison with the oral cavity pressures for vowels. Air cannot be forced through a narrow constriction to produce a voiceless fricative without appreciable oral pressure to create the high velocity air jet which results in the creation of turbulence and thus noise. Likewise, before a transient pulse of air can be released to generate a stop plosive, an appreciable level of pressure must be developed behind the articulatory closure. In both cases the requirement of relatively high oral pressure can be met only if the velopharyngeal mechanism functions to seal off the entrance to the nasal cavities.

The second point concerns the relative resistance to air flow presented by a consonant constriction in the oral tract as compared to the resistance of a small opening of the velopharyngeal port. Hixon (1965) measured the intraoral air pressures and air flow rates for the consonants [s] and [ʃ] for a range of speech effort levels. From these data estimates of the air flow resistance of the consonant constrictions can be calculated. Warren and Deveraux (1966) present data for the resistance of the velopharyngeal port corresponding to a range of orifice areas. Although the absolute values of the two sets of measurements are not exactly comparable, since the conditions of measurement were slightly different for the two studies, relative comparisions of their magnitudes should not be too greatly in error, and will suffice for our purpose. Comparisons between the two sets of data show that the air flow resistance for the [ʃ] constriction is at least two to three times greater than the velopharyngeal port resistance for velopharyngeal orifice areas of 0.2 cm² or larger. For [s] the disparity is even greater. The comparable ratios of [s] constriction resistance to velopharyngeal orific resistance range from 3 to more than 4.5. Thus, even a small velopharyngeal opening having a cross-sectional area of only 0.2 cm² will be critical during the articulation of a fricative. The resistance of even this small an opening into the nasal cavities is so low compared to that of the fricative constriction that a great part of the airstream will be diverted through the nose. The inevitable results are a reduction in intraoral pressure, a weakening of the consonant noise generation due to the reduced air flow through the consonant constriction, and a sharp increase in nasal air flow. The combined outputs of the nasal and oral channels will necessarily be a weakened and distorted version of the fricative consonant.

V. The Respiratory System

In the diagram of Fig. 1 at the beginning of this chapter an analogy was drawn between the breathing mechanism and the power supply which furnishes the electrical energy for an electronic oscillator. Within limits this analogy is reasonable since the function of the respiratory mechanism in speech is to supply the expiratory pressures and the flow of air required for the generation of vowel and consonant sounds. However, the analogy should not be carried too far. Power supplies employed with electronic signal generators are usually designed so that a substantial margin of power is always available in relation to that required at any instant by the generator. The rate of energy flow from such an electronic system is controlled almost entirely by the generator characteristics and is essentially independent of the energy available from the power supply. With respect to the functioning of the respiratory system during speech this is not the case. The respiratory system does not continuously provide a supply of energy much greater than that which may be required at any moment. Rather, the available supply of energy in the form of expiratory pressures and air flow is more or less continually adjusted by actions of the expiratory muscles. Thus, the rate of flow of speech energy is controlled in part by the activity of the respiratory mechanism. The release of energy made available by the breathing mechanism is also controlled in part by the valving actions of the glottis and the articulatory mechanism. For example, variations in vocal pitch and intensity require varying amounts of subglottic pressure, and the respiratory system must adjust accoringly. However, the vocal fold vibration is also controlled by adjustments of the laryngeal muscles. Likewise, fricative and stop plosive articulations require appropriate intraoral air pressures and an adequate flow of air which must be supplied by the breathing mechanism. But the timing of the release of air pressure for stop plosives and the channeling of air flow through a fricative constriction are controlled by the articulatory mechanism. It seems apparent that the control of energy flow in speech calls for a rather precise coordination between the respiratory system and the valving activity of the glottis and articulatory mechanism. At present our knowledge of the details of this coordination is quite meager. Although, as we have seen, we know that variations in vocal pitch and vocal intensity require adjustments in subglottic pressure, we do not know how rapidly subglottic pressure is adjusted during continuous speech. There is some evidence to indicate that the muscular activity associated with expiration may vary from one syllable to another, and that it may be greater for stressed syllables than for unstressed syllables. We do not know whether the respiratory system makes adjustments from one phoneme to another within syllables, or whether the variation in energy flow from one sound to another within a syllable is entirely controlled by the valving actions of the glottis and articulators.

With respect to cleft palate speech previous discussion has shown that, because of the energy losses inherent in the nasalization of speech, the demands placed in the respiratory mechanism may be greater than for nonnasalized speech. Greater subglottic pressures will be needed to increase the energy of the laryngeal vibration. It is also possible that the coordination of the control of energy flow may be affected. Certainly, the valving action of the articulatory constrictions for fricatives and stop plosives is markedly less effective if the velopharyngeal closure is not adequate in that air can escape through the nose. If the articulatory valving actions no longer effectively control the time patterns of expiratory pressure releases and the moment to moment variations in air flow, some substitute means of control must be found. One possibility for a substitute valving action is that glottal or pharyngeal occlusive consonants may replace stop plosives that are normally articulated orally. The air flow regulation associated with fricative constrictions may not have any convenient substitute and the coordination of speech control may suffer accordingly.

With the present state of knowledge, much of the foregoing discussion has necessarily been speculative. It is apparent that much remains to be learned. A good deal of additional experimental work needs to be done before it will be possible to explain adequately the numerous complex effects that may be presumed to result from excessive nasalization of speech. For the person concerned with the speech rehabilitation of individuals having palatal clefts, there is, however, one somewhat comforting fact. All of the consequences of excessive nasalization which the foregoing speculations have indicated as possibilities result from one cause, viz., inadequate velopharyngeal function. The energy losses due to excessive nasalization and the need to compensate for them, the possible disruption of control of expiratory pressures, and the lack of adequate oral pressure for consonant production are all consequences which follow from excessive nasal coupling. The questions and hypotheses suggested by the foregoing speculations should be studied so that we may increase our understanding of the problem of nasalization. However, the basic principle, long known to speech pathologists, that the central problem of controlling nasalization is the problem of achieving velopharyngeal competency, is not likely to be changed by any new discoveries concerning the acoustic processes of speech generation.

REFERENCES

Curtis, J. F. (1942). An Experimental Study of the Wave-Composition of Nasal Voice Quality. Ph. D. Thesis, The Univ. of Iowa, Iowa City, Iowa.

Dickson, D. R. (1962). An acoustic study of nasality. *J. Speech Hearing Res.* **5**, 103–111.

Dunn, H. K. (1950). The calculation of vowel resonances and an electrical vocal tract. *J. Acoust. Soc. Am.* **22**, 740–753.

Fant, G. (1960). "Acoustic Theory of Speech Production." Mouton, The Hague.

Flanagan, J. L. (1958). Some properties of the vocal sound source. *J. Speech Hearing Res.* **1**, 99–116.

Flanagan, J. L. (1965). "Speech Analysis and Synthesis." Academic Press, New York.

Halle, M., Hughes, G. W., and Radley, J. P. (1957). Acoustic properties of stop consonants. *J. Acoust. Soc. Am.* **29**, 107–116.

Hattori, S., Yamanoto, K., and Fujimura, O. (1958). Nasalization of vowels in relation to nasals. *J. Acoust. Soc. Am.* **30**, 267–274.

Hixon, T. J. (1965). Turbulent Noise Sources for Speech: An Aerodynamic Acoustic and Physiologic Study. Ph. D. Thesis, The Univ. of Iowa, Iowa City, Iowa.

Heinz, J. M., and Stevens, K. N. (1961). On the perception of voiceless fricative consonants. *J. Acoust. Soc. Am.* **33**, 589–596.

House, A. S. (1960). Formant bandwidths and vowel preference. *J. Speech Hearing Res.* **3**, 3–8.

House, A. S., and Stevens, K. N. (1956). Analog studies of the nasalization of vowels. *J. Speech Hearing Disorders* **21**, 218–232.

Hughes, G. W., and Halle, M. (1956). Spectral properties of fricative consonants. *J. Acoust. Soc. Am.* **28**, 303–310.

Isshiki, N. (1964). Regulatory mechanism of voice intensity variation. *J. Speech Hearing Res.* **7**, 17–29.

Kent, Louise M. (1966). The Effects of Oral-to-Nasal Coupling on the Perceptual, Physiological, and Acoustical Characteristics of Vowels. Ph. D. Thesis, The Univ. of Iowa, Iowa City, Iowa.

Kunze, L. (1962). An Investigation of the Changes in Subglottal Air Pressure and Rate of Air Flow Accompanying Changes in Fundamental Frequency, Intensity, Vowels and Voice Registers in Adult Male Speakers. Ph. D. Thesis, The Univ. of Iowa, Iowa City, Iowa.

Stevens, K. N., and House, A. S. (1955). Development of a quantitative description of vowel articulation. *J. Acoust. Soc. Am.* **27**, 484–493.

Stevens, K. N., and House, A. S. (1961). An acoustical theory of vowel production and some of its implications. *J. Speech Hearing Res.* **4**, 303–320.

van den Berg, Jw. (1956). Direct and indirect determination of the mean subglottic pressure. *Folia Phoniat.* **8**, 1–24.

Warren, D. W., and Devereaux, J. L. (1966). An analog study of cleft palate speech. *Cleft Palate J.* **3**, 103–114.

CHAPTER

III

Speech Characteristics of Individuals
with Cleft Lip and Palate

Kenneth L. Moll

I. General Incidence of Speech Problems 63
    A. Differences between Subgroups 66
    B. Summary 68
II. Speech Sound Articulation and Intelligibility 68
    A. Measurement Procedures 69
    B. Articulation Skills in Individuals with Clefts 73
III. Nasal Voice Quality 95
    A. Measurement Techniques 96
    B. Nasality in Individuals with Cleft Palates 101
IV. Language Development 108
V. Other Speech Dimensions 110
    A. Vocal Pitch and Intensity 110
    B. Voice Quality 111
    C. Nonauditory Aspects of Speech 112
VI. Summary 112
    References 113

Of the various deviations and deficiencies exhibited by individuals with clefts of the lip and palate, probably the most important are those involving the process of speech communication. Although the existence of speech problems in this population has long been recognized, only during the past 20 to 30 years have they been studied in detail. During this period, however, a great number of research studies have been carried out and a large body of knowledge now is available concerning the speech characteristics of individuals with clefts. The general purpose of this chapter is to summarize these research findings in an attempt to arrive at a more complete and adequate description of the speech problems of these individuals than has previously been available. Information and speculations concerning the

61

possible etiological bases of the speech problems described will be discussed in Chapter IV.

One of the major problems inherent in attempting to summarize information on cleft palate speech involves the decision as to what constitutes a description of speech. As has been pointed out in Chapters I and II, speech can be described acoustically, physiologically, or perceptually. To limit the scope of the present discussion, speech will be considered only as a perceptual phenomenon. Such a viewpoint is adopted on the basis that the primary purpose of speech is *communication* which implies the presence of a listener. The term "communication" should not be confused with "understandability"; ability to understand the words spoken is only one of the perceptual dimensions of speech. Communication also involves the acceptability of the perception. For example, speech may be completely intelligible although extremely nasal. The presence of nasality, however, presumably would be unacceptable to the listener in relation to normal standards and thus could potentially affect general communication between speaker and listener. The perceptual aspects are dependent, of course, on the acoustic signal resulting from physiological activities; however, not all changes in the physiological activities or in the acoustic signal are perceived. Even if they are perceived, the changes are not necessarily unacceptable to the listener and thus may be of little consequence in the communication process. The acceptability of speech can be defined ultimately in terms of the evaluations of listeners in the particular social and cultural milieu in which the speech is used.

In view of the above considerations, this chapter will deal only with information on perceptual aspects of speech. Description in terms of such factors as the "amount of high-frequency energy" or the "competency of the velopharyngeal mechanism" will not be considered. The available information on cleft palate speech will be summarized under the following general headings: (a) general incidence of speech problems, (b) speech sound articulation and intelligibility, (c) nasal voice quality, (d) language development, and (e) other speech dimensions. Techniques of measurement in each of these areas will be described and discussed since evaluation and comparison of research findings necessitates consideration of the specific measurement procedures used. Because of the extreme heterogeneneity of the cleft palate population in relation to such factors as status of physical management or extent of the cleft, differences in speech skills between various subgroups also will be described.

It obviously would be impossible to review all of the available studies in detail. Material to be discussed has been selected to provide for as complete a description of cleft palate speech as possible with recognition of contradictory research results and differences of opinion. Although the description and comparison of available information on cleft palate speech is the primary goal of this chapter, there also is a second goal: to acquaint the reader with deficiencies in present knowledge and with unanswered questions which, from the author's point of view, indicate needs for further research.

I. General Incidence of Speech Problems

In attempting to arrive at an estimate of the incidence of speech problems in the cleft lip and palate population only those investigations which have evaluated the "overall" speech of subjects in relation to normal standards will be considered. Studies dealing with such specific speech dimensions as articulation and voice quality and which, therefore, do not provide information on total speech skills, will be discussed in later sections.

It is impossible to estimate accurately the incidence of deviant speech in the total cleft lip and palate population. There are no reports on the general speech status of individuals with unmanaged palatal clefts or cleft lips only and little data on patients with prosthetic management. Almost all of the available information has been derived from subjects who have had primary surgical repair of the palate or who have undergone some type of secondary surgical procedure. In most instances these data have been reported by individual surgeons attempting to evaluate the success of their operative procedures. Gross classification of subjects into such categories as "normal speech," "good speech," and "bad speech" generally has been used in these studies.

Results of various investigations on individuals with primary surgical repair of the palate are summarized in Table I. Only studies which utilized a category of "normal speech" are included in this table since it was impossible in some instances, such as in the study by Blakeway (1915), to determine the criteria employed for a rating of "good" speech. In addition, only evaluations of speech status were considered.

The most striking feature of the data in Table I is the extreme variability of the results from different studies; reported percentages of individuals with normal speech range from 0 to 90%. Some of this variation undoubtedly represents real differences in speech skills of the groups evaluated. It is likely, however, that much of the variation is related to other factors. There is no assurance that all investigators utilized the same criteria for a judgment of "normal" speech. In addition, such ratings may be particularly subject to observer bias, especially when speech is rated by a surgeon or speech pathologist who may be involved personally in the success of the operative technique and who thus may be unconsciously biased. Another factor which may account for some of the variation in results is that of subject selection. Some

Table I

Percentages of individuals with surgically repaired cleft palates found to exhibit
normal speech in various investigations

Investigator	Year	Number	Normal (%)
Veau	1931	40	00.0
Veau	1931	100	40.0
Veau and Borel-Maisonny	1933	100	62.0
Wardill	1933	38	34.2
Ritchie	1937	100	42.0
Oldfield	1941	73	43.8
Bentley and Watkins	1947	87	52.8
Oldfield	1949	113	61.0
Velander	1952	60	73.3
Battle	1954	37	83.8
Jolleys	1954	128	31.3
Holdsworth	1954	68	69.1
Eckstein and Schuchardt	1955	51	90.2
MacCollum *et al.*	1956		
Selected group		108	70.0
Consecutive series		56	50.0
Reidy	1958	193	77.2
Morley	1962	155	41.0
Calnan	1959	?	75.5
Foster and Green	1960	263	34.2
Glover (prewar)	1961	50	46.0
Glover (postwar)	1961	150	71.0
Lindsay *et al.*	1962	612	39.7

investigators, such as Lindsay *et al.* (1962), presumably utilized all available subjects while others, such as Eckstein and Schuchardt (1955), report only on subjects for whom treatment, including speech habilitation, was completed. The variation in findings which can result from differences in subject selection is demonstrated in the study of MacCollum *et al.* (1956). In a group selected from patients with "good" speech, 70% had speech judged as normal while only 50% of a "consecutive" series of patients were classified as normal.

Differences in such factors as criteria for evaluation of speech and subject selection make it impossible validly to compare or combine results from different studies. Such factors also probably obscure expected trends in the data. For example, although it could be expected, as a result of improvement in surgical procedures and an increase in general medical knowledge, that higher percentages of individuals with normal speech would be reported in the more recent investigations, such a trend is not evident in Table I. In the study of Glover (1961), however, in which subject selection and evaluative criteria were presumably constant, the expected improvement in speech results with time can be seen; only 46% of his prewar patients as compared to 71% of his postwar patients were judged as having normal speech.

Overall speech assessments also have been utilized to evaluate the success of various secondary management procedures. The results of a number of studies, in terms of percentage with normal speech, are shown in Table II. A wide variation in results also can be noted in these data. Such variation again undoubtedly reflects real differences to some degree, although inter-study differences in evaluative criteria and subject selection also may be involved.

Table II

Percentages of individuals found to have normal speech following
different types of secondary management procedures

Investigator	Year	Procedure	Number	Normal (%)
Moran	1951	Pharyngeal flap	35	22.9
Conway	1951	Pharyngeal flap	13	0.0
		Push-back	30	0.0
		Combined	8	100.0
Trauner and Doubek	1956	Push-back	42	29.0
		Obturator	19	21.0
		Trauner operation	89	48.0
Gray and Jones	1958	Pharyngeal flap	20	60.0
Obregon and Smith	1959	Pharyngeal flap	20	35.0
Hamlen	1960	Trauner operation	10	80.0
		Pharyngeal flap	24	58.3
Williams and Woolhouse	1962	Pharyngeal flap	12	25.0
		Hynes operation	12	16.7
Smith et al.	1963	Pharyngeal flap	123	34.2

The extreme variability of results reported in Tables I and II make it impossible to arrive at an estimate of the general incidence of speech problems among individuals with surgically managed cleft palates. It would appear that an average of 40 to 60% of the patients achieve normal speech following primary surgical repair while an additional 30 to 40% exhibit normal speech following some type of secondary management procedure. On the basis of such estimates, and assuming that all patients who do not have normal speech following primary repair receive secondary surgery, it might be concluded that 55 to 80% of individuals with surgically managed cleft palates achieve normal speech. It is obvious, however, that the variability of data among different studies makes this estimate little better than a guess.

Most of the studies summarized in this section had as their primary purpose the evaluation of management results. There appears to be serious doubt concerning the validity of using speech assessments for such evaluation. As pointed out by Smith *et al.* (1963), the existence of nonnormal speech does not mean necessarily that the management procedure has failed; the speech defect may be completely unrelated to the anatomical-physiological deficiency which the procedure is designed to eliminate. When only the overall speech proficiency is evaluated such a possibility usually is not considered.

A. DIFFERENCES BETWEEN SUBGROUPS

Many investigators who have evaluated overall speech skills also have considered differences in results between various subgroups in their samples. The subclassifications most commonly used have been with reference to type of cleft and to age of physical management.

1. *Type of Cleft*

The findings of various studies (Bentley and Watkins, 1947; Lindsay *et al.*, 1962; Morley, 1962; Reidy, 1958; Veau, 1931; Veau and Borel-Maissony, 1933; Velander, 1952) suggest that there are differences in speech status following primary surgical repair which are related to the original extent of the cleft. In general, a greater percentage of individuals with only postalveolar clefts than of those with both lip and palate clefts has been found to have normal speech. The magnitude of the difference reported between the two groups varies from 1.2% (Reidy, 1957) to 29.6% (Bentley and Watkins, 1947). The findings of Glover (1961) and Greene (1960), however, are inconsistent with those of other studies, indicating that normal speech is relatively more frequent in individuals with lip and palate clefts than in those with cleft palates only.

Further breakdown of subject groups according to type of cleft also has been reported (Greene, 1960; Lindsay *et al.*, 1962; Morley, 1962; Veau, 1931; Veau and Borel-Maissony, 1933). In general, within the group with only postalveolar clefts, speech has been judged as normal for a greater percentage of patients with clefts of only the soft palate than of those with clefts which also involved the hard palate. In the cleft lip and palate group speech is normal more often in cases with unilateral than in cases with bilateral clefts. These results suggest that the greater the extent of the cleft the poorer the speech result following primary surgical repair. For individuals who have undergone secondary management procedures, however, no consistent differences in speech results have been found between groups classified according to cleft type (Hamlen, 1960; Moll *et al.*, 1963).

2. *Age of Management*

Most investigators also have evaluated speech status in relation to age of management. The findings are relatively consistent and indicate that a higher percentage of normal speech is associated with earlier ages of operation (Holdsworth, 1954; Jolleys, 1954; Lindsay *et al.*, 1962; Veau, 1931; Veau and Borel-Maissony, 1933). For example, Jolleys (1954) found that 47% of the children managed before 2 years of age and 20% of those managed after this age had normal speech. Lindsay *et al.* (1962) report a percentage of 70.7% for those managed between 1 and 3 years and 60% for those managed later. Although in the latter investigation this difference in percentages was not found to be statistically significant, the consistency of results from different studies suggests that real differences related to age of surgery do exist.

Age of management also has been evaluated in relation to results of secondary procedures; the findings, however, are inconsistent. The results of Moran (1951) and Moll *et al.* (1963) suggest that the relative incidence of normal speech is lower for subjects on whom pharyngeal flaps are performed after the age of 15. Hamlen (1960), however, found no differences which could be related to the age at the time of secondary surgery.

The reader is cautioned against drawing the conclusion that there is necessarily a cause and effect relationship between age of primary palatal surgery and speech proficiency. Although such a relationship may exist, it cannot be demonstrated conclusively from available research data. Investigators who have studied this relationship did not ensure, with respect to other pertinent parameters, that the subject group managed at an early age was similar to the group managed later. For example, if a particular surgeon routinely manages individuals with narrow clefts at an earlier age and if individuals with narrow clefts generally achieve better speech, a relationship between age of management and speech success would be expected on this basis alone, and a causal relationship between age of management and development of adequate speech could not be inferred.

3. *Other Factors*

Overall speech evaluations also have been reported in relation to a number of other factors besides cleft type and age of management. Lindsay *et al.* (1962) relate their findings to the subject's age at time of evaluation and to the presence or absence of previous speech instruction. They found a slight increase in the percentage of subjects with acceptable speech to accompany increased age up to 8 years; at higher ages the percentage was relatively stable. They report that 80% of the patients who had received public school speech correction had acceptable speech in comparison with 52.4% of those who had received other types of speech therapy and 69.9% of those who had received no therapy.

Factors other than those already discussed, such as intelligence, physiological adequacy, and hearing loss, also have been investigated. Results on such factors, however, have potential etiological implications and will be discussed in a later chapter (Chapter IV).

B. Summary

An attempt has been made in this section to summarize research findings on the incidence of speech disorders in the cleft palate population. Although wide variation in research results preclude an accurate estimate of incidence, a number of conclusions may be drawn. First, it appears that there may be real differences in the speech skills of individuals managed in different treatment centers. Second, factors such as cleft type and age of management must be taken into account in any description of the speech characteristics of individuals with clefts.

It should be pointed out that the studies reviewed in this section have been those in which the overall speech of subjects was evaluated. Although some of the investigators (Greene, 1960; Morley, 1962) described the type of speech problem exhibited, such descriptions were very general (for example, articulation defect, nasal voice quality). The usefulness of general ratings of speech in describing communication problems is limited. To arrive at a complete description it is necessary to consider individual speech dimensions in detail. Such dimensions will be discussed in the following sections of this chapter.

II. Speech Sound Articulation and Intelligibility

It is generally agreed (Eckelmann and Baldridge, 1945; Van Riper, 1963; Van Riper and Irwin, 1958) that one of the major speech problems exhibited by individuals with clefts is a deficiency in articulating speech sounds. Although the term "articulation" has a physiological connotation, it is used here only in the perceptual sense. It is defined in relation to whether a speech sound production is or is not judged to be an acceptable sample of the phoneme intended. Although articulation and intelligibility are closely related (Eguchi, 1957; Falck, 1955; Pinson, 1956) and will be considered together here, they do not represent exactly the same speech dimension. For example, a sound production is intelligible if recognized as belonging more to the intended phoneme than to another, but when it is judged by listeners to be an unacceptable sample of the phoneme its articulation is deviant.

A. MEASUREMENT PROCEDURES

No detailed description of articulation and intelligibility measurement techniques will be presented; however, because of the wide variety of procedures used and the frequent disagreement concerning their relative merits, consideration of the general nature of such techniques appears to be necessary.

Procedures which have been used for assessing the speech sound articulation of individuals with cleft palates can be grouped into two general categories: (a) articulation tests, and (b) judgments of overall articulation ability. Even within these categories, however, wide variations in procedures exist. Although all articulation tests involve the evaluation and scoring of individual sound productions, they may differ in numerous ways. Articulation of specific sounds may be assessed in nonlanguage units such as nonsense syllables (Klinger, 1956; McDermott, 1962; Subtelny and Subtelny, 1959), in words (Byrne et al., 1961; Bzoch, 1956; Counihan, 1956; Spriestersbach et al., 1956, 1961; Starr, 1956), or in specially constructed phrases or sentences (McWilliams, 1954; Van Demark, 1964). Some investigators have utilized pictures to elicit the speech productions (Spriestersbach et al., 1956, 1961) while others have used repetition or reading of the speech unit (Van Demark, 1964). Some have scored the responses at the time of testing (Bzoch, 1956; Counihan, 1956; Spriestersbach et al., 1956, 1961); others have scored them from tape recordings (Byrne et al., 1961; Van Demark, 1964). In addition, classifications of types of articulatory errors observed have varied greatly between studies.

Differing techniques also have been utilized for obtaining judgments of overall articulation skills. In some instances, gross categorizations such as "good, moderate, and poor" have been utilized, while in other instances such psychological scaling procedures as equal-appearing intervals (Morris, 1962; Spriestersbach, 1955) or direct magnitude-estimation (Cooker, 1961; Van Demark, 1964) have been employed. Samples which have been utilized include conversational speech (Morris, 1962; Spriestersbach, 1955), reading passages (Cooker, 1961), and repeated sentences (Van Demark, 1964). The number and type of judges used in obtaining such ratings also have differed.

Wide variation in measurement procedures also is evident in the assessment of the speech intelligibility of cleft palate subjects. Overall ratings of intelligibility have been used by some investigators (Bzoch, 1956; Counihan, 1956; Falck, 1955). More frequently, however, listeners have been asked to write down what was heard from tape-recorded speech samples. Such samples have consisted of nonsense syllables (Subtelny et al., 1961), phonetically balanced words or spondee words (Dietze, 1952; Falck, 1955; Fritzell, 1960; Leach, 1957; Wilson and O'Brien, 1953), and specially constructed sentences (McWilliams, 1954). Falck (1955) developed a somewhat different measure of intelligibility which she called "information transfer." This measure involved an examination of listeners on the content of a recorded sample.

The wide range of techniques used to measure articulation and intelligibility presents a number of problems. To the degree that different procedures lead to different findings, this variation makes comparison and combination of research results difficult. It also leads to confusion as to which type of procedure should be selected for use in future investigations. The issues involved in such selection relate primarily to three factors: (a) degree of "subjectivity" or "objectivity" of the measure, (b) measurement validity, and (c) measurement reliability.

1. Subjectivity of Measures

It is obvious that all of the measurement procedures described above involve human listeners, whether it be one examiner scoring articulation test responses or a large group of judges rating connected speech samples. If "subjectivity" is defined as the degree to which human biases and errors of perception might influence measurement, then all of these measures must be considered subjective. This fact, however, has not always been recognized. There often has been a tendency to assume that articulation tests are more objective than judgments of overall articulation ability (Barker, 1960) and that intelligibility measures are more objective than articulation assessments (Fritzell, 1960). Since all procedures involve listeners, however, the validity of such assumptions is questionable.

At the present time, no satisfactory method of assessing articulation and intelligibility without using human listeners is available. It might appear that acoustic analyses of speech could provide more objective measures of these dimensions; however, the wide variation in the acoustic characteristics of correctly articulated speech sounds makes articulation assessment by this method difficult, if not impossible (Fritzell, 1960). In addition, as pointed out previously, not all acoustic variations result in perceptual differences. As a result, it would be necessary to establish a close correspondence between certain acoustic measures and perceptual judgments before acoustic assessment of articulation could be validated. Although gross articulation errors such as omissions of speech sounds might be determined from an acoustic analysis, more subtle types of errors, such as sound distortions, probably could not be detected reliably. Yet, these latter types of errors also can significantly interfere with communication between a speaker and listener.

2. Measurement Validity

The most common criticism (Barker, 1960) of judgments of overall articulation skills has been that they are not "pure" measures of articulation;

that is, listeners' judgments are influenced by other dimensions of speech. There are research data which can be interpreted to support such a contention. Close relationships have been reported (Falck, 1955; McWilliams, 1954; Sherman, 1954; Spriestersbach, 1955) between judgments of such dimensions as articulation, speech defectiveness, intelligibility, and nasal voice quality. Falck (1955) reached the following conclusion from her results:

> It seems quite possible that in reality, although the three experienced judges made separate ratings of intelligibility, defectiveness, and nasality on each of the cleft palate speakers at different times, each clinician based his ratings on the same basic speech characteristics, which might be called deviation from normal.

An alternate interpretation of these data also was recognized by Falck. It is possible that "pure" measures of each of the dimensions are obtained but that the dimensions themselves are inherently related in cleft palate subjects. There appears to be no adequate method for determining which of these interpretations is correct or whether both judgment contamination and real relationships are involved in the high correlations obtained. The recent results reported by Van Demark (1964) suggest, however, that overall judgments of articulatory defectiveness may not be greatly contaminated by other dimensions of speech. Such judgments were found to be highly related (correlation coefficient = .88) to the total number of articulatory errors on specific consonant sounds in the sample judged.

What is not always recognized is that the "purity" of articulation test results and of intelligibility measures other than overall ratings also can be questioned. When scoring an articulation test, how does the presence of voice quality deviations or the overall intelligibility of the speech unit affect the examiner's judgment? Further, intelligibility measures based on such speech material as words, phrases, or sentences are greatly affected by the redundancy of such material. Even phonetically balancing the speech samples does not remove the effect of language redundancy. At this point it has not been demonstrated that articulation test results and intelligibility scores are less contaminated by other dimensions than are overall judgments of articulation or intelligibility.

Another aspect of measurement validity which should be considered is that the validity of a particular articulation or intelligibility measure may depend on the purpose for which it is used. For example, results from word articulation tests have been used (Spriestersbach et al., 1956; Templin, 1957) to arrive at a score which presumably is an index of the individual's general articulation performance in connected speech. There does appear to be a fairly close relationship (correlation coefficients of .70 to .80) between articulation test scores and overall ratings of connected speech, both in subjects with functional articulatory disorders (Jordan, 1960) and in those with cleft palates (Falck, 1955; Morris, 1962; Van Hattum, 1958). These are far from perfect correlations however, since there appears to be only 49 to 64% common variance between the two measures. Weighting articulation test results by frequencies of speech sound occurrence does not improve these correlations greatly (Burgi and Matthews, 1958; Falck, 1955). As Van Hattum (1958) concludes, it appears that "... considerable error would thus be introduced if articulatory ability in connected speech were to be predicted by the results of testing sounds in syllables or single words."

Results of articulation tests also have been used solely to describe an individual's ability to articulate a specific speech sound. Such a use involves an assumption that the test has adequately sampled the subject's productions of that sound. Even if the sound is tested a number of times on the test, the subject's performance on these items may not reflect his ability to articulate the sound in all instances; he may misarticulate all items on the test and yet be able to produce the sound correctly in some contexts (Mc Dermott, 1962). The adequacy of sampling also must be considered in the use of connected speech for articulation and intelligibility measures, since it has been demonstrated (Crosby, 1952) that ratings of the speech of individuals with clefts varies greatly as a function of the type of material used.

The considerations discussed above make it clear that generalization of articulation and intelligibility measures to speech units other than those tested or to all occurrences of the speech unit must be made with caution. They also suggest that the comparison of results obtained by different measurement procedures may not be meaningful, since one might be comparing slightly different dimensions.

3. *Measurement Reliability*

There is sufficient evidence to indicate that all of the articulation and intelligibility measurement techniques discussed provide highly reliable measures. Articulation tests have been found to be reliable in terms of agreement within and between examiners on the correctness of specific sound productions in single words (Byrne *et al.*, 1961; Siegel, 1960; Wright, 1954) and in connected speech (McWilliams, 1954; Van Demark, 1964). Judgments concerning the type of misarticulations are not as reliable as those of correctness of articulation; however, they appear to be of adequate reliability for most research purposes (Van Demark, 1964).

Overall ratings of articulation from connected speech samples also are highly reliable (Morrison, 1955; Prather, 1960). The level of sophistication of the raters has little effect on measurement reliability (Morrison, 1955; Perrin, 1954; Phillips, 1954). Moreover, ratings obtained from tape-recorded samples and from direct observation of the speaker are similar (Leach,

1957; Phillips, 1954). The reliability of various types of intelligibility measures which have been used also is high (Burgi and Matthews, 1958; Bzoch, 1956; Counihan, 1956).

4. *Selection of Measurement*

Essentially all of the wide variety of techniques used to assess speech articulation or intelligibility provide reliable measures, have certain limitations, and are fairly closely interrelated. The preceding discussion was designed solely to acquaint the reader with the fact that there is no one measure which is universally the "best" and that there are a number of unanswered questions concerning measurement methodology which can and should be investigated.

In the final analysis a measurement must be selected for a particular study in relation to the purpose of the study. If data on articulation of specific speech sounds are desired, some type of articulation test must be used. If only an index of general articulation adequacy is needed, an overall rating of connected speech or reading may be sufficient. Although intelligibility measures presumably assess a somewhat different dimension than do articulation measurement techniques, the high relationship between the two types of measures makes this theoretical difference of little practical importance.

One trend in the development of measurement procedures in this area should be noted. Whatever the purpose of the particular study, more recent investigators have tended to attempt evaluation of articulation and intelligibility in speech units more complex than isolated words or nonsense syllables, for example, in spontaneous speech samples or in reading passages. This trend reflects the increased awareness of differences which exist between different types of units and of the fact that the ultimate goal is assessment of these dimensions in speech which is most comparable to that used in the normal communication situation.

B. ARTICULATION SKILLS IN INDIVIDUALS WITH CLEFTS

There have been numerous investigations designed to describe the speech sound articulation of individuals with cleft lips and palates. Although these studies have varied in relation to the specific types of subjects used and the methods of articulation assessment, the results are surprisingly consistent. The research findings can be summarized and discussed under the general headings of (a) general articulation status, and (b) patterns of misarticulations exhibited. Most of the studies which will be discussed have made use of articulation tests (usually word tests) rather than overall ratings of articulation or intelligibility measures. The latter techniques have been used most frequently in studies designed to investigate relationships between articulation or intelligibility and other variables; such relationships are discussed in a later chapter of this book (Chapter IV). Moreover, general ratings of articulation and most intelligibility measures provide no information on the pattern of misarticulations exhibited.

1. *General Articulation Status*

The general articulation status of individuals with cleft lips and palates has been assessed most commonly by a total articulation test score, although the type and length of test used has varied from study to study. The results of all of these investigations (Byrne *et al.*, 1961; Bzoch, 1956; Counihan, 1960; Eguchi, 1957; Klinger, 1956; McWilliams, 1958; Morris, 1962; Spriestersbach *et al.*, 1956, 1961; Starr, 1956; Van Demark, 1964) indicate that individuals with cleft lips and palates, on the average, exhibit a considerable number of errors in the articulation of speech sounds. Reported percentages of correct sound production range from approximately 40 (Starr, 1956) to 80% (McWilliams, 1958). This range of results undoubtedly is related to differences among studies with reference to subjects, the articulation tests used, and other factors. The relationship of articulation performance to these factors will be considered in detail in the next section.

It is obvious that the percentage of items correctly articulated on a test has little meaning unless the measure is compared to normative data or to the performance of a control group on the same test. Such comparison is especially important when subjects with cleft palates who are under 8 years of age are studied, since children without clefts who are below this age also typically exhibit some articulation errors (Templin, 1957). Spriestersbach *et al.* (1956) report that, in relation to the normal, 21 of 25 children with cleft palates were retarded in articulation skills, with 14 of this group exhibiting retardation of 2 years or more. Morris (1962) reports that, on the average, his subjects with clefts also were significantly retarded in articulation skills by comparison of their test results with Templin's data. Counihan (1960) found that only three of his group of 55 adolescent and adult cleft palate subjects exhibited the perfect articulation test performances to be expected for this age group. Nineteen of the group ranked below the norms reported by Templin for 3-year-old children. The validity of this latter comparison might be questioned, however, since the articulation test used by Counihan differed greatly from that used by Templin. Control groups of normal subjects, matched according to factors such as age and sex, have been utilized in only two studies (Bzoch, 1956; Klinger, 1956). Bzoch's cleft palate subjects articulated 50% of the test items correctly in comparison to 79% articulated correctly by the control group. Klinger reports that only 42% of syllables spoken by subjects with cleft palates were correctly transcribed by listeners in comparison to 90% of syllables produced by subjects without clefts. The less than perfect performance of the control groups in these studies underlines the necessity for comparison to normative data before statements are made concerning retardation in articulation skills in the cleft palate population.

From the data summarized above, it can be concluded that, on the average, individuals with cleft palates are retarded in general articulation skills. The importance of the phrase "on the average" in this conclusion should be emphasized. It is obvious, of course, that not all individuals with clefts are retarded in articulation skills; the degree of variation within this population, however, is not always recognized. Spriestersbach et al. (1961) report that articulation test scores for their group ranged from 6 to 100% correct. This range, which represents extreme heterogeneity, is an apt illustration of the wide differences which are to be found in the cleft palate population. Moreover, distributions of articulation scores for groups of individuals with clefts are generally skewed markedly (Spriestersbach et al., 1961); a relatively large number of subjects make scores of 100% while scores for the remaining subjects spread out along the measurement scale. Such observations suggest that measures of central tendency of group distributions are often deceptive if interpreted as describing the articulation of the entire group.

It also is doubtful whether data from the studies reviewed above are truly representative of articulation skills in the total cleft population. In most of these investigations subjects were obtained from among individuals coming to diagnostic or treatment centers. It is likely that, in relation to problems exhibited, such individuals may be quite different from those who do not return to such centers. This inherent selection factor always must be considered, since it may bias the data obtained and thus limit generalization of the findings.

The extreme heterogeneity in articulation skills within the cleft palate population has led to attempts by many investigators to study differences in articulation which may exist between various population subgroups. For this purpose, subjects have been classified into subgroups according to the factors of (a) age at time of testing, (b) type of cleft, (c) sex, (d) type of physical management, and (e) age of palatal management. The results of investigations of articulation differences between subgroups will be summarized here solely to describe more adequately the articulation status of individuals with clefts; hypotheses concerning the etiological significance of such differences will not be discussed.

a. *Age Differences.* The particular level of articulation skill exhibited by an individual with a cleft palate depends, to some degree, on the age at time of testing. Morris (1962) reports that articulation test scores improve with age up to 7 years and that there is little improvement beyond this age. He also reports that older subjects receive more favorable listener ratings of overall articulation than do those who are younger; Morris, however, did not obtain such ratings on children under the age of 5 years. Bzoch (1956) found a similar relationship between articulation and age in younger children with clefts. For the age groups of 3, 4, and 5 years, Bzoch reports correct articulation percentages of 33, 45, and 57%, respectively. It should be noted that, although this increase in articulation ability with age was observed, the differences between the experimental and control groups were essentially the same for all three age levels. Starr (1956), studying subjects in the age range of 6 to 11 years, found no significant differences between adjacent yearly age groups in number of articulation errors; the children aged 6 to 8 years, however, made significantly more errors, as a group, than did the older children. Comparison between the findings of McWilliams (1958) for 17- to 59-year-old subjects and findings for younger groups indicates that adults with clefts of the palate exhibit much better articulation than do children without clefts.

The research findings reviewed suggest that, in general, articulation skills of individuals with clefts of the palate increase systematically with age as do articulation skills of those without clefts; the absolute level of such skills undoubtedly is lower, on the average, however, for individuals with clefts. The only finding not in agreement with this conclusion is that of Counihan (1956), who reports for adolescent and adult subjects with clefts that those over 16 years of age were less proficient in articulation skills (62.4% correct) than those below this age (75% correct). These findings may be the result of the fact that the clefts of the younger subjects were managed more recently than were those of the older subjects and that the younger ones profited from the improvement of physical management skills which occurred with time. This possible explanation of Counihan's findings underlines the difficulties involved in studying articulation differences between cleft palate subgroups; the confounding of other factors with the subgroupings is to a great extent unavoidable. For example, the fact that physical management is more likely to be incomplete for younger subjects may be reflected in relationships observed between age and articulation. On the basis of data on the development of articulation skills in normal children (Templin, 1957), improvement of articulation with age would be expected in the cleft palate population; investigations are needed, however, in which the confounding of biasing variables with age groups is considered and, preferably, eliminated. It is recognized, of course, that complete control of such variables in relation to age groupings would be difficult, if not impossible.

   b. *Type of Cleft Differences.*   A number of investigators (Byrne *et al.*, 1961; Bzoch, 1956; Counihan, 1956; Morris, 1962; Spriestersbach and

Powers, 1959b; Spriestersbach *et al.*, 1961) have studied differences in articulation skills between subgroups classified according to the extent of the original cleft. The findings of some of these studies are summarized in Table III. One observation that can be made from these data is that individuals with clefts only of the lip exhibit essentially no articulation errors (Spriestersbach *et al.*, 1961). The findings of Spriestersbach and Powers (1959b), which are not summarized in Table III, indicate that all of their subjects with clefts only of the lip had normal articulation when evaluated with reference to Templin's (1957) normative data. As a result of this consistent finding, later studies have included only subjects with palatal clefts.

Table III

Mean percentages of articulation test items produced correctly by subject groups classified on the basis of type of cleft

Cleft type	Investigator[a]				
	A	B	C	D	E
General					
Lip only					97.4
Lip and palate	76.7	47.0	68.8	40.1	69.3
Palate only	80.4	33.4	68.1	47.2	61.3
Palate only					
Soft palate			67.4	53.3	65.1
Hard and soft palate			62.3	42.1	57.3
Lip					
Unilateral			70.2	45.1	70.8
Bilateral			62.5	41.5	66.9

[a] Investigators are, from left to right, Byrne *et al.*, 1961 (A); Bzoch, 1956 (B); Counihan, 1956 (C); Starr, 1956 (D); and Spriestersbach *et al.*, 1961 (E).

Research findings on articulation differences between other type-of-cleft groups are inconclusive. In relation to general type of cleft the data of a number of studies (Bzoch, 1956; Morris, 1962; Spriestersbach and Powers, 1959b; Spriestersbach *et al.*, 1961) suggest that children with clefts of both lip and palate may exhibit articulation skills slightly superior to those of individuals with cleft palate only; this difference, however, was significant only in the studies of Bzoch and of Spriestersbach and Powers. Counihan (1956) reports essentially the same articulation scores for the two groups while Byrne *et al.* (1961) and Starr (1956) found slight, nonsignificant differences in the opposite direction (Table III). It should be noted that cleft-type differences in general speech status, which were summarized previously (Section I, A, 1), suggest that the speech of individuals with clefts of both lip and palate is not as good as that of subjects with clefts of the palate only, although findings contradictory to these also have been reported (Glover, 1961; Greene, 1960).

A number of factors may account for the inconsistencies in the results cited above. Again, the possible confounding of other variables with such comparisons between groups should be considered. It is interesting to note that only two investigators found significant differences between cleft-type groups and that these two did attempt to control certain factors. Bzoch (1956) matched complete-cleft and incomplete-cleft groups on the factors of age and sex, and Spriestersbach and Powers (1959b) used a ratio between the obtained articulation score and the score reported for normal children of similar age and sex. The reduction of variability by such procedures probably increased precision of the cleft-type comparisons. Systematic differences between groups in type and age of physical management, which may depend on treatment philosophies in the particular center from which the subject samples were drawn, also may account for contradictory findings from different studies.

From other data summarized in Table III it appears that comparison between subjects with clefts of lip and palate and those with clefts of the palate only may be affected by group composition. These data suggest that, within the palate-only group, those individuals with clefts of the soft palate only exhibit better articulation than subjects with clefts of both hard and soft palate; and that, within the lip-and-palate group, those with unilateral clefts exhibit better articulation than those with bilateral, complete clefts. Although in most instances these differences were not found to be statistically significant, the consistency of the results and their agreement with findings on general speech status summarized previously suggest that real differences may exist between these groups. If this hypothesis is valid, it is obvious that comparison of subjects with complete clefts with those whose clefts are incomplete will be influenced by the manner in which the various cleft subtypes are represented in the two groups. If, for example, a large proportion of an incomplete cleft group had clefts only of the soft palate the group articulation performance probably would be better than it would be if more subjects with clefts of both hard and soft palate were included. This consideration not only may account for contradictary findings from different studies, but it also casts doubt on the meaningfulness of evaluating differences between general-type-of-cleft groups in relation to articulation skills. It would appear that more useful descriptions of articulation proficiency can be obtained with finer subclassifications according to cleft type.

c. *Sex Differences.* Differences in articulation skills between male and female individuals with clefts have been evaluated by only two investigators

(Counihan, 1956; Starr, 1956). In both instances no significant differences between sexes were found. A statement made by Starr should be mentioned, however, since it emphasizes again the possibility of a confounding effect of uncontrolled, irrelevant variables. Although the difference was not significant, he observed fewer articulation errors for females than for males and suggests the explanation that of the 10 subjects who had clefts of the soft palate only and who, probably for this reason, exhibited better articulation, 7 were female.

d. *Type of Physical Management.* Byrne *et al.* (1961) and Spriestersbach and Powers (1959b) report that individuals with unrepaired cleft palates exhibit poorer speech sound articulation than do those who have received palatal management. Although this finding is not surprising, the actual differences reported are not extremely large. Spriestersbach and Powers report mean articulation ratios (observed score/normative score) of .60 for subjects with unrepaired clefts and of approximately .77 for those with repaired clefts. Byrne *et al.* report correct articulation percentages of 54% for subjects with unrepaired clefts and 79% for those with repaired clefts. As Spriestersbach and Powers point out "... the subjects in the unrepaired-palatal-cleft group did have appreciable articulation proficiency."

Byrne *et al.* (1961) also compared subjects with surgical repair of the palate with those who had received prosthetic management and found no significant difference in articulation skills between the two groups. Whether comparisons of such management groups are particularly meaningful seems questionable. The results of such comparisons will provide no information on the efficacy of particular management types unless subjects in each group are assumed to be equal in relevant characteristics before the management is carried out. It would appear that in many instances such an assumption is doubtful. Prosthetic management, for example, may be utilized in a particular treatment center only for the most difficult cases, that is, those with more extensive clefts or those for whom surgery has failed. To the degree that such factors are considered in the selection of cases for particular treatments and to the degree that they are related to postmanagement speech proficiency, differences in speech measures between management-type groups are to be expected on this basis alone and regardless of the particular management types. If such comparisons are made solely to describe the situation in a particular center at a particular time, rather than to make inferences about the relative effectiveness of different management procedures, then the comparisons may be justified. However, such a limitation usually is not imposed in the interpretation of results.

e. *Age of Physical Management.* Articulation skills have been evaluated also in relation to age of physical management which has been, in most instances, surgical repair of the palate. The general trend (discussed in Section I, A) for individuals managed at earlier ages to exhibit better speech also can be noted in studies of articulation proficiency. Counihan (1956), Bzoch (1956), and Eguchi (1957) found slightly better articulation scores or ratings in children whose palate was repaired at a fairly early age. It should be noted, however, that these differences were not found to be statistically significant even when subjects were matched according to age and sex (Bzoch, 1956). The fact that different investigators have classified subjects somewhat differently for such comparisons (for example, before 1 year compared to after 3, before 2 years compared to after 2) makes interpretation of their results difficult. The discussion of factors involved in the inter- pretation of speech differences between age-of-management groups, which was presented in relation to general speech status (Section I, A, 2), also is applicable here.

f. *Summary of General Articulation Skills.* From the review presented above, it is obvious that individuals with clefts are, on the average, retarded in articulation skills. This is not, however, the conclusion that needs to be emphasized. It is hoped that the reader has been impressed mainly with the great heterogeneity of the cleft palate population in relation to general articulation status, the need for further research to define more adequately this variability, and the problems which are inherent in such research because of the possible confounding effects of a great number of variables.

2. *Misarticulation Patterns*

Although a total articulation test score provides information on general articulation proficiency, it does not reveal the pattern of articulation devia- tions: that is, variations among speech sound types or in the types of articula- tory errors. A methodological issue involved in studies of articulatory patterns should be mentioned. As pointed out previously, if a fairly wide range is studied the score distribution in any sample of cleft palate subjects is markedly skewed with a relatively large number of subjects exhibiting perfect articula- tion scores. These perfect scores can interfere with correct evaluation of articulatory variations between categories of speech sounds. The relative differences between categories will not be affected by perfect scores, since their effect is constant for all categories, but, when category differences are evaluated by statistical tests, the perfect scores make a significant result of the test less likely. Elimination of perfect articulation scores from such category comparisons is thus desirable for the simple reason that, in this comparison, the evaluation is relevant only to individuals with cleft palate "who exhibit articulatory errors." Obviously there is no reason to study articulatory patterns among subjects with no articulation problem. Only one investigator (McDermott, 1962), however, has imposed such a limitation on subject selection. It should be emphasized again that this issue becomes relevant only in relation to the use of statistical analyses to evaluate differences among categories.

Most studies of cleft palate articulation have involved consideration of articulatory patterns as well as of general proficiency. The results have consistently indicated that there is an articulation pattern which, in general, is distinctively characteristic of individuals with cleft palate. These findings will be summarized and discussed in relation to the following factors: (a) vowel-consonant differences, (b) manner of consonant production, (c) place of consonant production, (d) voicing, (e) phonetic context, (f) types of misarticulations, and (g) consistency of articulation.

a. *Vowel-Consonant Differences.* Only a few investigators have studied vowel articulation in individuals with cleft palate, possibly because of the difficulty in evaluating articulation of vowel sounds when voice quality is nasal. Since it is generally accepted that vowel nasalization is not phonemically significant in English, attempts usually have been made to evaluate phonemic identity independent of nasalization. Spriestersbach *et al.* (1956) report 96% correct articulation of vowels tested in their study when nasalization was not counted as an error. Bzoch (1956) found some differences between subjects with cleft palate and normal subjects on correctness of vowel sounds, with scores of 89.2 and 96.1% correct, respectively; this difference, however, was much smaller than any observed on consonant sounds. The fact that Bzoch counted as incorrect any vowels observed as having "excessive nasal distortion" may account, of course, for the finding of any difference at all on vowels.

Klinger (1956) investigated a slightly different aspect of vowel productions in cleft palate and normal subjects: the ability of listeners to transcribe correctly vowels produced in syllables. He reports that only 53% of vowel productions by cleft palate subjects were correctly transcribed in comparison to 90% of productions by the control group. Whether this finding reflects the possibility that nasalization can destroy the phonemic identity of the vowel or whether it is due to other articulatory deviations on the vowel is not known. The data of Crosby (1952), however, indicate that vowels produced by individuals with clefts are not deviant in instances where some nasalization of a vowel is the normal situation. She reports that listeners could not differentiate between cleft palate and normal subjects on the basis of recorded speech samples containing only vowel sounds adjacent to nasal consonants. These results and those cited previously suggest that the data of Klinger (1956) may not be representative of individuals with clefts. His subjects, that is, subjects with unrepaired clefts with prostheses removed, may be different from other cleft palate individuals in relation to vowel articulation.

From the previous research it appears that, although vowels often are nasalized, vowel articulation in the cleft palate population is not greatly deviant when judged only on the basis of phonemic characteristics. Since nasal voice quality will be discussed in a later section, subsequent description of articulatory patterns in cleft palate individuals will involve only consonant sound articulation.

b. *Manner of Consonant Production.* Investigators who have considered articulatory variations related to manner of consonant production generally have used the categories of (a) nasals, (b) fricatives, (c) affricatives, (d) glides, and (e) stop plosives. The exact consonant sounds classified in each of these categories have varied to some degree; for example, the /h/ and /hw/ sounds have been classified as fricatives (Spriestersbach *et al.*, 1956), have not been included in such analyses (Spriestersbach *et al.*, 1961), or have been classified into a separate category labeled as aspirates (Bzoch, 1956). In most instances, however, the classification of individual phonemes has been relatively consistent between studies.

The results of various investigations are summarized in Table IV for each manner-of-production category. Although the percentages of correct articulation vary somewhat between studies, the relative ranking of the categories for individuals with clefts is consistent; the highest percentage always is reported for nasal consonants, followed by glides, stop plosives, fricatives, and affricatives in that order. The reversal of fricative and affricative categories in the studies of Pinson (1956) and of Spriestersbach *et al.* (1961) is negligible, since no significant difference between these two sound categories

Table IV

Mean percentages of correct articulation of consonant elements classified by manner of production[a]

Subjects	Nasals	Glides	Plosives	Fricatives	Affricates
Cleft palate (A)	84.8	64.6	44.9	16.4	
Normal (A)	97.5	83.3	88.7	60.5	
Cleft palate (B)	95.0	87.8	72.2	57.3	
Cleft palate (C)	96.0	99.0	86.0	71.0	72.0
Cleft palate (D)	91.0	79.0	71.0	49.0	47.0
Cleft palate (E)	91.1	49.4	41.5	27.9	

[a] Investigators are, from top to bottom in left-hand column, Bzoch, 1956 (A); Counihan, 1956 (B), Pinson, 1956 (C); Spriestersbach *et al.*, 1961 (D); and Starr, 1956 (E).

was found by the latter investigators. The similarity of articulation of sounds in these two classes appears to justify the procedure of combining these categories as used in other studies summarized in Table IV. Only Spriestersbach *et al.* (1961) analyzed intercategory differences statistically. They found that all differences between adjacent categories, except that between fricatives and affricatives, were significant.

Comparison of cleft palate articulation to that of noncleft speakers for each manner-of-production category had been carried out by Bzoch (1956). According to his data (Table IV) the rank order of the differences between the cleft palate and the control groups for the various categories is approximately the same as that of correctness of articulation percentages for the cleft palate subjects. It should be noted, however, that the difference for stop plosive sounds is essentially the same as that for fricatives, although the absolute level of articulation in the cleft group is considerably lower on fricatives than on stop plosives. The data of Counihan (1956) on adolescent and adult individuals with clefts of the palate also can be compared to normative data, with the assumption that normals in this age group exhibit no articulation errors. Such comparisons indicate that greater retardation is exhibited by cleft palate subjects on fricative than on stop plosive sounds. Although this conclusion is not in agreement with the findings of Bzoch, subjects in different age groups were used in the two investigations; Counihan studied cleft palate subjects who were 13 to 24 years while Bzoch studied those from 3 to 6 years. It might be hypothesized from the results of these studies that the difference between normal and cleft palate subjects in articulation of stop plosives decreases with age, while for fricatives the difference stays relatively constant (Table IV). This hypothesis is supported by Bzoch's finding that the gain in correct stop plosive articulation between 3 and 6 years of age was slightly greater for the cleft palate than for the normal group, with gains of 23 and 19%, respectively. Fricative articulation, however, improved with age considerably more for normals, with 39% change, than for cleft palate subjects, with 20% change. Starr (1956) also observed that articulation gains with age for cleft palate subjects varied in magnitude depending on the manner of production category considered. It would appear likely that this trend would continue with age levels not yet investigated and, in fact, become more marked at later ages. There is an obvious need for better definition of how articulation differences between normal and cleft palate subjects for different manner-of-production categories change with age.

Much of the variation in articulation percentages found from study to study probably is due to variations in the age group studied, to the inclusion of subjects with unrepaired clefts in some studies (Bzoch, 1956; Spriestersbach *et al.*, 1956, 1961) and not in others, to differences in articulation testing

methods, and to variations among studies in sound classification. The effect
of this latter factor is illustrated by the finding of Starr (1956) for articulation
of glide sounds. Starr found a much lower percentage of correctly articulated
glides than that reported in other studies despite the fact that he utilized
subjects who were older (6 to 11 years) than those used by some of the
other investigators. However, Starr reported results on only two glide sounds,
the /r/ and the /l/, which are among the most commonly defective sounds
for noncleft speakers (Templin, 1957), while sounds such as the /w/ and /j/,
which usually are not so frequently defective, are included in the glide
category in other studies. This observation emphasizes an important consideration in interpreting articulation data: the results for a particular sound
category may vary greatly depending on the particular sounds included
and the relative number of times each sound is assessed on the articulation
test.

Despite procedural differences between investigations, the results consistently indicate that stop plosives, fricatives, and affricatives are the most
defective sounds in individuals with clefts. Although errors on glides and
nasals also are noted, they are not frequent. A question might be posed
concerning the presence of real differences between cleft and normal individuals in articulation of sounds in these latter two categories. Bzoch
(1956) found such differences for children aged 3 to 6 years, while Pitzner
(1964) reports that data on her cleft palate group did not differ significantly
from normative data on glides and nasal consonants. In the latter study,
however, the vocalic /r/ and /l/ sounds were analyzed separately. For these
sounds Pitzner reports a significant difference between normals and subjects
with cleft palate for a subgroup classified as having inadequate velopharyngeal
function; for the adequate-function group, no significant difference was
observed. Van Demark and Van Demark (1967) investigated articulation
differences between subjects with cleft palate having good velopharyngeal
function and individuals without cleft palate diagnosed as having functional
articulation problems. They found no significant intergroup differences
for any manner of production category except that of glides. Articulation
of glide sounds was significantly better for the cleft than for the noncleft
group. It would appear that further investigation of the articulation of glide,
nasal, and vocalic /r/ and /l/ sounds by individuals with clefts in comparison
with the articulation of speakers without clefts is indicated.

   c. *Place of Consonant Articulation.*   A number of investigators also have
assessed cleft palate articulation in relation to the place in the vocal tract at
which the sound is articulated. Although they made no specific analysis
pertaining to this factor, Spriestersbach *et al.* (1956) report that the eight
most defective consonants are linguadentals and postdentals; these sounds,

however, are also fricatives or affricates. These investigators conclude that the defectiveness of these consonants seems to be related to their manner of production rather than to their place of articulation. They also report that the labial consonants appear to be those most frequently correct in articulation, a finding not in agreement with previous statements in the literature (Berry, 1928).

Counihan (1956) and Starr (1956) assessed articulation differences between consonants classified into the following categories: (a) lip sounds, (b) tongue-tip simple sounds, (c) tongue-tip complex sounds, and (d) back-of-tongue sounds. Counihan concluded that consonants in the latter two categories are more frequently defective than are lip or tongue-tip simple consonants. Starr's findings also indicate that tongue-tip complex sounds are most defective; however, only small differences were observed among the other three categories. These results are confounded almost completely with manner of consonant production, since all of the sounds which were classified as tongue-tip complex are fricatives or affricates. In addition, the other categories each contain a nasal consonant which undoubtedly increases the percentages of correct articulation for these categories.

To avoid the confounding effects of other factors, place of articulation classes must be compared separately for each manner of consonant production. An attempt at such a comparison has been made in Table V. The first data column in this table shows percentages computed by combining the results of various studies (Bzoch, 1956; Byrne et al., 1961; McWilliams, 1958; Spriestersbach et al., 1956; Starr, 1956). The differences in correct articulation percentages between cleft palate and normal groups, reported by Bzoch, also are shown. Combining data from different studies was felt to be justified since there were few differences among studies in the rankings of the various place-of-articulation categories.

The most obvious trend in the data of Table V is that sounds which involve lingual contacts are much more defective in the cleft palate group than are sounds which involve only the lips. This observation is consistent within each manner-of-production category. Among the sounds which involve lingual contacts, however, articulation proficiency does not appear to change consistently with the anteroposterior placement of the contact.

Bzoch's (1956) data on articulation differences between normal and cleft palate individuals (Table V) show essentially the same trend as do data obtained only on cleft palate subjects. The only major reversal occurs in the fricative sounds where the cleft palate group differs more from the normal on the labiodental sounds than they do on the linguadental sounds. Bzoch's data demonstrate, however, that the correctness of articulation of certain sounds (/h/, /w/, /n/, /m/) is essentially the same for the two subject groups. These data also indicate that the linguavelar nasal sound /ŋ/ is rather severely

Table V

Mean percentages of correct articulation, computed by combining
the data of several studies[a,b]

Consonants	M % correct	N and CP difference
Fricatives		
Lingualveolar /s, z/	28.0	53.0
Linguapalatal /ʃ/	43.4	59.9
Linguadental /ө-ʒ/	46.8	24.2
Labiodental /f, v/	56.1	43.3
Glottal /h/	95.2	9.2
Plosives		
Lingualveolar /t, d/	58.8	47.3
Linguavelar /k, g/	60.6	51.7
Bilabial /p, b/	70.8	32.4
Glides		
Lingualveolar or linguapalatal /r, l, j/	75.8	22.3
Bilabial /w/	92.2	1.7
Nasals		
Linguavelar /ŋ/	80.2	47.5
Lingualveolar /n/	92.6	9.7
Bilabial /m/	98.7	4.2

[a] Byrne et al., 1961; Bzoch, 1956; McWilliams, 1958; Spriestersbach et al., 1956; Starr, 1956.

[b] Percentage differences between cleft palate (CP) and normal speakers (N) reported by Bzoch (1956) for children age 3 to 6 years are given in the right-hand column.

defective in the cleft palate group. In light of the relatively high percentage of correct articulation reported for this sound in other studies, this finding may be unique to the age group of 3 to 6 years studied by Bzoch.

Except for suggesting that lip sounds are generally less defective than are lingual sounds, the data concerning place of production contribute little to a description of cleft palate articulation. This may be due to the fact that this variable is relatively unimportant in comparison to the effect of other factors such as manner of production. It also might be hypothesized that even the differences between labial and lingual sounds might be related more to subtle differences in manner of production, which are not taken into account in the usual classifications of this factor, than they are to differences in place of articulation.

d. *Consonant Voicing.* A number of investigators (Bzoch, 1956; Counihan, 1956; Spriestersbach et al., 1956, 1961) have studied cleft palate articulation differences related to consonant voicing. In most instances, voiced-voiceless cognate pairs of fricatives, stop plosives, and affricates were considered. The findings of these studies generally have been consistent in that voiceless consonants appear to be more defective in the cleft palate group than are those which are voiced. In most studies (Pinson, 1956; Spriestersbach *et al.*, 1956, 1961) this difference was found to be statistically significant. Bzoch (1956) also compared cleft palate and normal groups in relation to voiced-voiceless consonant categories. He reports that the articulation difference between groups was much greater on voiceless sounds than on voiced. In addition, the differences between voiced and voiceless sounds were in opposite directions for the two groups; voiced consonants were correctly articulated more often than were voiceless in the cleft palate group with the opposite trend in the normal group. The only research finding in contradiction to these results is that of Cobb and Lierle (1936) who report that, except for the /s/-/z/ consonant pair, voiced sounds are more defective than voiceless.

Spriestersbach *et al.* (1961) have questioned the validity of assessing voiced-voiceless differences in the cleft group by combining fricatives, stop plosives, and affricates. These investigators found that voiced stop plosives and affricates were articulated correctly more often than were voiceless; however, for fricatives, the articulation of voiceless sounds was better than was that of voiced sounds. All of the voiced-voiceless differences were statistically significant. Spriestersbach *et al.* reanalyzed the data of a previous study (Spriestersbach *et al.*, 1956) and again found this reversal of the voiced-voiceless difference on fricatives. They suggest that the differences observed may depend on the age group studied since voiceless fricatives are learned at an earlier age than are their voiced cognates while the opposite is true for stop plosives (Templin, 1957). In an attempt to control the age or maturation factor, Spriestersbach *et al.* (1961) reevaluated the data of Counihan (1956) and of McWilliams (1958) on adolescent and adult cleft subjects "... for whom the period of articulation development was presumably completed." These data indicate that voiceless consonants are more defective than the voiced for fricatives as well as for stop plosives. Spriestersbach *et al.* (1961) conclude that "... voiced fricatives as well as voiced stop plosives are articulated correctly more often than their voiceless cognates when maturation is not a factor."

Although the research results are relatively consistent, further study of the consonant voicing factor is needed to delineate more adequately the effect of age and of other variables on such comparisons. In addition, possible reversals in the voiced-voiceless difference which have been reported for certain cognate pairs (Counihan, 1956) should be investigated.

e. *Phonetic Context.* The effects of a number of aspects of phonetic context on consonant articulation in cleft palate subjects have been studied.

The results of McDermott (1962), Morris *et al.* (1961), and Spriestersbach *et al.* (1956, 1961) indicate that consonants occurring in consonant blends are articulated correctly less frequently than are the same sounds as "singles": that is, the same sounds, but not as part of a consonant blend. Bzoch (1956) reports a greater difference in articulation skills between cleft palate and normal subjects on two-element consonant blends than on consonants as singles. His data also suggest that this difference increases with age. In addition, Morris *et al.* (1961) and McDermott (1962) found consonants to be more defective in three-element than in two-element blends. With reference to a preceding discussion, it might be pointed out that the results of the latter two studies demonstrate the effect of subject selection on statistical analyses. McDermott, studying only the /s/ sound, reports significant differences between singles and blends only after the elimination of subjects who never, and those who always, produced the sound correctly. Morris *et al.* found a difference only for subjects who were classified as having "poor" velopharyngeal function and who, it can be assumed, also had many articulation errors. It is obvious that individuals who make "perfect" scores cannot show context variations.

It has been pointed out by Spriestersbach *et al.* (1956) that the difference in articulation between singles and blends observed in cleft subjects is in the opposite direction of that reported for individuals with functional articulation problems; putting a consonant in a blend may facilitate its correct production by the latter individuals (Spriestersbach and Curtis, 1951). Before such comparison between groups can be made with any certainty it will be necessary to study the performances of these two types of subjects on the same stimulus materials and with age and other factors controlled.

McDermott (1962) is the only investigator who has assessed variations in articulation of speakers with cleft palates as related to the specific consonants in blend with the test sound. He studied the /s/ sound blended with various types of consonant elements. Although no significant differences between contexts were found for the group, McDermott noted that some subjects showed considerable variability with context factors. In evaluating differences among conditions in which a blend sound occurred before as opposed to after the /s/, he reports a significant difference only for blends involving the nasal consonant /n/; he reports more correct productions of the /s/ sound on /-sn/ blends than on /-ns/. Although there were relatively few definitive findings in McDermott's study concerning the effect of specific phonetic contexts, it may be profitable to explore such effects on sounds other than the /s/, which appears to be the most difficult consonant for individuals with clefts.

Another aspect of phonetic context which has been investigated is the position or function of the test sound in the word or syllable. Pinson (1956) and Bzoch (1956) found that, for individuals with clefts, consonants in the medial position in words were more defective than initial or final consonants. For normal subjects, Bzoch reports that final consonants are more difficult. The absolute differences between these categories, however, were very small, 4 to 6%, both for the normal subjects and for those with clefts. Moreover, Counihan (1956) found no significant differences between initial, medial, and final consonant articulation for cleft palate individuals. McDermott (1962), utilizing Stetson's (1951) classification of consonants, evaluated the articulation of /s/ by speakers with cleft palates in relation to whether this sound was "syllable releasing" or "syllable arresting." He reports a significant difference between these categories; articulation was correct more often on syllable releasing sounds. Whether results would be the same for articulation of consonants other than /s/ is not known.

Another aspect of cleft palate articulation which will be discussed here, although it is not necessarily related to phonetic context, is the effect of rate of production on articulation. This factor has been investigated (McDermott, 1962) only for production of the /s/ sound. Correct articulation of this sound was found to decrease significantly as rate of syllable production was increased. There are no data, however, for evaluating the effect of rate on the articulation of other speech sounds by subjects with clefts nor for evaluating the effect of rate on sound articulation by normal subjects or by other types of subjects with articulation deviations.

Summarizing the effects of different aspects of phonetic context on cleft palate articulation is difficult since, with the exception of the difference between singles and blends, most aspects have been investigated in only a few studies. The results, although fragmentary in some instances, do suggest that further exploration of such effects would be profitable.

f. *Types of Misarticulations.* Review of information on the types of articulation errors exhibited by individuals with clefts is complicated by the wide variation among studies in error-type classification. There are, however, a number of general observations which can be made from the research data. These can be discussed best in relation to information on general error types, types of substitutions, and types of distortions.

i. *General error types.* In many investigations (Bzoch, 1956; Counihan, 1956; McWilliams, 1958; Spriestersbach *et al.*, 1956; Starr, 1956) the general error categories of omissions, substitutions, and distortions have been employed. Data from these studies, summarized in Table VI, indicate that the findings from different investigations are not consistent. This may be related to a number of factors. It has been pointed out (Counihan, 1956) that the criteria used for classifying errors into these categories may vary between studies. The distinction between substitutions and distortions, for

Table VI

Percentages of types of articulation errors on consonants as reported
in various studies[a]

| Group | Error | | |
	Omissions	Substitutions	Distortions
Cleft palate (A)	14.1	68.4	17.5
Normal (A)	9.3	72.2	18.5
Cleft palate (B)	0.5	18.3	81.2[b]
Cleft palate (C)	18.5	2.4	79.2
Cleft palate (D)	37.0	35.0	28.0
Cleft palate (E)	4.7	42.8	52.5

[a] Bzoch, 1956 (A) (percentages shown were computed from Bzoch's data on mean number of error types); Counihan, 1956 (B); McWilliams, 1958 (C); Spriestersbach *et al.*, 1956 (D); Starr, 1956 (E).

[b] Includes categories of "indistinct errors" and "emission errors."

example, is difficult in certain instances. Both categories involve substitutions of a sound; the substituted sound, however, is considered a distortion if, in the examiner's judgment, it is not an acceptable example of another phoneme of the language. Some investigators (Bzoch, 1956; Counihan, 1956; Starr, 1956) have classified the production of "pharyngeal fricatives" as substitutions while others may have considered such errors as distortions since there are no pharyngeal fricative phonemes in the English language. Although omissions of speech sounds would appear to be easily identifiable, Van Demark (1964) points out that the distinction between an omission and the substitution of a glottal stop is difficult, especially when observations are made from tape recordings of the speech.

The factor of age appears to be of major importance in studying error types. The data in Table VI reveal a trend for the proportion of distortions of sounds to increase with age. Counihan (1956) and McWilliams (1956), who studied adolescent and adult cleft palate subjects, report higher percentages of distortions than those reported for younger age groups. This trend is not unexpected since there is evidence (Milisen, 1954) of a relative increase in distortion errors and a corresponding decrease in omissions and substitutions with age in children without clefts. It should be noted that, with reference to error types, the only comparison between subjects with clefts and those without was made by Bzoch (1956) for children from 3 to 6 years of age. For these ages the general pattern of error types is similar for both groups. Van Demark and Van Demark (1967) compared a specific subgroup of the cleft palate population, individuals having good velopharyngeal function, with a group of noncleft subjects exhibiting functional articulation errors. All subjects studied were older than 8 years. Statistically significant intergroup differences were found for only one error-type category; the noncleft group exhibited more substitution errors than did the group with cleft palate. It is possible, however, that these findings also may vary with the age group investigated.

A final factor which may account for some of the variability in research findings is that the error types observed may depend on the composition of the articulation test utilized. The misarticulation types observed appear to vary with manner of consonant production and phonetic context. The results of a number of investigations (Bzoch, 1956; Counihan, 1956; Starr, 1956; Spriestersbach et al., 1961) suggest that sound distortions are relatively more frequent on fricative and affricative sounds than they are on other types of consonants. Spriestersbach et al. (1961) also observed that error types varied depending on whether the speech sound was tested as a single or in a consonant blend. For single sounds, distortions were most common on fricatives and afffricates, while substitutions occurred with greater relative frequency on stop plosives. For sounds tested in blends, however, there was an increase in omission errors on both stop plosives and fricatives. This change was accompanied by a decrease in substitution errors on plosives but not on fricatives. From these research findings it appears obvious that the occurrences of different types of errors will depend on the proportions of articulation test items which fall into each manner of production category and on the relative weighting of single and blend items on the test. The fact that Spriestersbach et al. (1956) report a larger percentage of omission errors than do other investigators (Table VI) may be due partially to the nature of their articulation test. The Templin Articulation Test used in this study is weighted heavily with items involving fricatives and plosives in blend with other consonants. To the degree that omission errors occur more frequently and distortions less frequently on blends than on single sounds (Spriestersbach et al., 1961) the finding that omissions are the most common errors in individuals with cleft palates might be predicted for this particular test. This discussion again emphasizes the possible effect on research results of averaging data over categories which may be inherently different with respect to factors discussed above.

ii. Types of substitutions. A number of general conclusions can be drawn from available data on the types of sound substitutions utilized by individuals with cleft palates. The most consistent finding is that the "glottal stop" sound appears frequently in cleft palate speech (Bzoch, 1956; Sherman et al., 1959; Spriestersbach et al., 1961; Starr, 1956). This sound is usually substituted for another stop plosive sound (Sherman et al., 1959; Spriestersbach et al., 1961), although it also may occur as a substitution for a fricative or affricate (Bzoch, 1956; Starr, 1956). Its occurrence on stop plosive test items appears to vary; it is less frequent on stop plosives in consonant blends than on those tested as single sounds (Spriestersbach et al., 1961). Bzoch's data indicate that individuals with clefts exhibit many more glottal stop substitutions than do normal subjects. Sherman et al. (1959) report similar results from a comparison of cleft subjects with individuals with functional articulation problems, although the occurrence of glottal stops in the latter group is greater than might be expected. Van Demark and Van Demark (1967) found no significant difference between subjects with clefts with good velopharyngeal function and subjects with functional articulation problems in relation to number of glottal stop substitutions exhibited. Sherman et al. point out that the glottal stop can occur without being a substitution for another consonant: it occurs, in many instances, as a prevocalic, intrusive sound. Moreover, these investigators found that glottal stops used as intrusive sounds do not appear to be as conspicuous to listeners. The more frequent use of these sounds as substitutions for consonants, rather than as intrusive sounds, may account for the fact that they are perceived more readily in the speech of cleft subjects than in the speech of individuals with functional articulation problems.

Another characteristic of substitution errors in cleft individuals is that the substituted sound tends to have the same manner of production as the test sound (Bzoch, 1956; Counihan, 1956; Spriestersbach et al., 1961). This appears to be true especially for fricative and affricate sounds (Spriestersbach et al., 1961). Bzoch and Starr noted that "pharyngeal" and "velar" fricatives often were substituted for other fricative sounds. Whether the substituted sounds actually are produced, as their labels imply, by lingual approximation to the pharyngeal wall or velum has not been established. As pointed out previously, substitutions of such sounds probably have been classified as distortions in some investigations.

It has been suggested recently that the nature of sound substitution errors in cleft palate speech may be changing. Morley (1962) and Renfrew (1960) note that the frequency of pharyngeal fricative and glottal stop substitutions is decreasing while there appears to be a relative increase in substitutions of sounds which are produced at a more anterior point in the vocal tract. It is possible that this trend is a characteristic only of cleft palate individuals in England, the origin of both of those reports. Studies in this country have not been designed specifically to evaluate changes in the nature of articulation errors with time.

iii. Types of distortions. Two general types of sound distortions have been reported as prevalent in the speech of individuals with cleft palates: those involving nasal emission of air and those on which such emission is not evident. The category labels of "distortions-nasal" and "distortions," used by Van Demark (1964), will be utilized in this discussion also. It should be noted that the perceptual distinction between these two types of distortions may be difficult. The reliability and validity with which such distinctions can be made is not known. In addition, Bzoch (1956) points out that combinations of the two types of errors are possible; that is, nasal emission may be present but may not be the only characteristic distorting a specific sound production.

Although nasal air emission often is considered to be one of the common characteristics of cleft palate speech, distortions-nasal do not appear to be as frequent in individuals with cleft palate as are distortions. Bzoch (1956) reports that 55% of distortion errors are not accompanied by nasal emission. The mean numbers of distortions-nasal and of distortions found by Van Demark (1964) were 9.4 and 11.4, respectively. These findings support earlier statements by Berry (1928, 1949) that distortions without nasal emission occur frequently in cleft palate speech. A possible reason why distortions-nasal are more easily perceived in the speech of individuals with clefts than are distortions is that the former errors do not occur in the speech of normal children. Bzoch (1956) observed no nasal emission errors in his normal control group; the normal subjects, however, exhibited almost as many distortions as the group with clefts. It thus would appear that the presence of distortions-nasal is one of the factors which most consistently discriminate between articulation of the cleft and normal populations.

There also is some evidence that distortions and distortions-nasal occur on different types of sounds. Bzoch (1956) found that most of the distortion-nasal errors observed occurred on fricative and plosive consonants, while the occurrence of distortions was relatively independent of the manner of production of the test sound. Starr (1956), however, reports that both types of errors occur most frequently on fricatives and plosives. The data of Bzoch (1956) also suggest that distortions of the speech sounds of both normal and cleft children decrease with age and that distortions-nasal do not.

As was true for the data on substitution errors, the data of Renfrew (1960) and Greene (1960) suggest that the nature of distortion errors in cleft individuals may be changing. These investigators contend that, in comparison with data obtained in the past, recent results show a decrease in distortions-nasal and a concomitant increase in distortions not involving nasal emission. They note, particularly, a recent increase in "lateral" distortions of sibilant sounds. Evaluation of the reality of this trend will require further investigation.

iv. Summary of misarticulation types. From the available information, it appears that the articulation of individuals with cleft palates is characterized primarily by distortions of speech sounds, often with nasal air emission, and by substitutions and omissions of sounds. The variation of error types with phonetic factors and with age of the subjects should be stressed as well as the need for more consistent definition and identification of the various error types.

g. *Consistency of Articulation.* A final factor which has been investigated is the consistency with which a particular cleft palate individual correctly or incorrectly articulates a specific speech sound. It should be noted that only individuals who correctly articulate a sound 100% or 0% of the time can be said to be consistent. Thus, individuals who misarticulate 50% of the sound productions exhibit maximum inconsistency. As McDermott (1962) points out, consistency of articulation also can be considered in relation to the error types exhibited: that is, in relation to whether the individual consistently uses the same error type on each misarticulation of a particular speech sound. McDermott labeled this latter factor as "error variability."

The information summarized in Section II, B, 2, e on the effects of phonetic context on cleft palate articulation suggests that variability may be found in one subject's performance on a particular speech sound. A number of investigators, however, have studied consistency and error variability specifically. Spriestersbach *et al.* (1956) observed that only 47% of the consonant sounds tested were correctly or incorrectly articulated 100% of the time. Moreover, only 5% of the time did children produce the same type of misarticulation more than twice on a sound. McWilliams (1958) reports similar results and notes that articulation was consistent for more subjects on speech sounds that were more frequently defective. She also points out that the number of times a particular sound is tested is an important factor in interpretation of findings on articulation consistency.

The most comprehensive study of articulation consistency and error variability in the cleft palate population is that of McDermott (1962). He investigated articulation of 180 productions of the /s/ sound, the most defective sound in this population, occurring in various phonetic contexts. McDermott concluded that only 10 of the 54 subjects could be considered to demonstrate a "major degree of inconsistency:" that is, only 10 correctly articulated 40 to 60% of the sound productions. He noted, however, that the group was extremely variable in the types of misarticulations exhibited. Considering the four response categories of correct, omission, distortion, and substitution, he found that 30 subjects exhibited productions of the /s/ sound falling into three or more of these classes.

Another interesting finding in the study of McDermott (1962) concerns the variation in /s/ articulation with changes in the manner in which the sound productions were evoked. The /s/ was produced correctly more often when it was preceded by oral presentation from the examiner than when it was produced spontaneously. This was true whether the sound was elicited as an isolated production, in a nonsense syllable, or in a word. These findings underline the fact that articulation performance in cleft palate individuals is variable and depends on various factors.

It would appear that individuals with cleft palates are relatively inconsistent in articulation of specific speech sounds. Such inconsistency also has been reported in children without clefts (Spriestersbach and Curtis, 1951); however, no comparison of the two groups in terms of relative consistency of articulation has been attempted.

3. *Summary of Cleft Palate Articulation*

The speech sound articulation of individuals with cleft palates often is briefly described by the statement that their speech is characterized particularly by nasal distortions of fricative and stop plosive sounds, the frequent use of glottal stop substitutions, and general inaccuracy of sound articulation. Although such a statement may be valid, the available information which has been reviewed in this section demonstrates that it is greatly oversimplified. The variability in articulation skills between and within cleft palate subjects, the importance of considering phonetic factors and subject groupings, and the lack of information concerning certain aspects of cleft palate articulation make such a statement misleading. Further research is needed before an exact description of articulation skills in individuals with cleft palates can be offered with any certainty.

III. Nasal Voice Quality

In addition to deviations in speech sound articulation, it is generally agreed that individuals with cleft palates also exhibit a voice deviation usually referred to as "nasality" (Eckelman and Baldridge, 1945; Van Riper and Irwin, 1958). Other terms, however, often are used to apply to this phenomenon: for example, "nasal resonance" and "deviation in resonance balance." In light of the conclusion, stated earlier, that speech dimensions must be defined ultimately in terms of listener perception, nasal voice quality is defined best as a perceptual dimension. This fact was recognized by Kantner (1948), who stated, "The final decision as to whether an individual is 'nasal' is still, I believe, to be reached through someone's *subjective* judgment." If the definition of nasality as a perceptual phenomenon is accepted, then it is obvious that only measures which are based on listener perception have face validity as measures of this dimension. Nonperceptual techniques, however, may provide empirically valid measures if it can be demonstrated that they are closely related to listener judgments of nasality.

A. Measurement Techniques

The procedures utilized to assess nasal voice quality in individuals with cleft palates can be divided into two general categories: (a) listener-judgment procedures and (b) "objective" measures of nasality.

1. *Listener-Judgment Procedures*

Consistent with the definition of nasal voice quality as a preceptual dimension, the most commonly used measurement procedures have involved judgments of listeners. One type of judgment procedure which has been used is that of categorization (Bzoch, 1956; Counihan, 1956), a procedure which requires listeners to classify the speech of an individual into such categories as "normal," "mildly nasal," and "moderately nasal." Psychological scaling procedures, discussed earlier in Section II, A, also have been utilized in the assessment of nasality. The scaling procedure of equal-appearing intervals has been used most frequently (Hess, 1955; Spriestersbach, 1955; Spriestersbach and Powers, 1959a; Van Hattum, 1958); other procedures, however, such as direct magnitude-estimation (Van Demark, 1964) and pair-comparisons (Weiss, 1954), also have been used.

Although listener judgments of nasal voice quality have been shown to be adequately reliable (Spriestersbach, 1955; Spriestersbach and Powers, 1959a; Van Demark, 1964), there is some doubt concerning their validity. It would appear that such judgments have obvious face validity for measuring the perceptual dimension of nasal voice quality. It must be assumed, however, that the listeners base their judgments only on perceived nasality; that is, that the judgments are not extraneously influenced by other dimensions. This assumption has been question by Sherman (1954), who concludes:

> Judgments of voice quality in connected speech are probably particularly influenced by the halo effect. Contamination of judgments by irrelevant factors is to be expected. Among possible irrelevant factors are pitch usage, articulation, effectiveness in conveying meaning, cues associated with particular disorders of voice, etc.

Such contamination of judgments is particularly a problem in measuring nasality of cleft palate speakers who often exhibit other speech deviations. As mentioned previously, a number of investigators (Falck, 1955; McWilliams, 1954; Spriestersbach, 1955; Van Hattum, 1958) have demonstrated a fairly high relationship between nasality judgments and articulatory ability of speakers with cleft palates. These findings undoubtedly represent, to some degree, a real relationship between these two dimensions; that is, articulation deficiencies and nasality do tend to occur together in these individuals. It is possible, however, that these findings also reflect some contamination of nasality judgments.

Contamination of voice quality judgments by other dimensions can be minimized by making such judgments from isolated vowel sounds rather than from connected speech. The results of Spriestersbach and Powers (1959a) and Van Hattum (1958), however, indicate that nasality in connected speech cannot be predicted accurately from judgments of isolated vowel sounds. Another method of reducing judgment contamination is to play the speech samples backward, a procedure devised by Sherman (1954). Spriestersbach (1955) has shown that the method of backward play reduces the correlations between nasality judgments and judgments of such dimensions as articulation and effectiveness of pitch usage. The method of backward play has been utilized by a number of investigators (Spriestersbach and Powers, 1959a; Van Demark, 1964) for the study of nasality in cleft palate subjects. It should be noted that this technique involves the assumption that the relevant cues for perception of nasality have not been changed by reversing the time dimension. This is probably a valid assumption, since most investigators (Fant, 1960; House and Stevens, 1956; Smith, 1951) agree that spectral characteristics, rather than variations in the time dimension, give the primary cues for nasality.

2. "Objective" Measures of Nasality

Various types of techniques have been developed to obtain measures of nasality which are presumably more "objective" than listener judgments. These techniques can be grouped into three general categories: (a) techniques for measuring nasal air flow or air pressure, (b) techniques involving measurement of nasal sound pressures, and (c) techniques involving evaluation of the acoustic spectrum.

a. *Measures of Air Flow or Pressure.* A number of investigators have utilized techniques for measuring nasal air flow or nasal air pressure during speech (Bensen, 1951; Hess and McDonald, 1960; Kelleher *et al.*, 1960; Lubker and Moll, 1965; Young, 1953); not all of these investigators, however, assumed that they were measuring nasal voice quality. Such techniques involve the insertion of a nasal olive or tube in the nose or the use of a face mask to cover the nose. The measurement device is either one for measuring air flow (Kelleher *et al.*, 1960; Lubker and Moll, 1965) or one for measuring air pressure (Young, 1953). In some instances (Kelleher *et al.*, 1960; Lubker and Moll, 1965) nasal and oral air flows have been measured simultaneously. The readings from the measurement devices are recorded either directly by the investigator or graphically for later measurements.

If the previous definition of nasal voice quality as a perceptual dimension is accepted, it is clear that measures of air flows or pressures do not in and of themselves have face validity as measures of nasality. It might seem reasonable that the amount of nasal flow or pressure would be closely related to the degree of nasal quality; however, very low correlations have been found between such measures and perceptual judgments of nasality (Benson, 1951). It thus appears that measures of nasal air flow and pressure are not valid as measures of nasal quality. Why, then, have they been used? Their use may be the result of the general confusion of nasal air emission with nasal voice quality. Nasal air emission can be defined physically as the amount of air passing out of the nasal cavities or, in perceptual terms, as the amount of audible nasal emission. These two dimensions may not be the same, and neither appears to be the same as nasal voice quality. Nasal emission in cleft palate speakers has been observed usually during the production of consonant speech sounds. Thus, as McDonald and Koepp–Baker (1951) point out, nasal emission should be considered as part of the articulatory problem and as resulting in distortion of consonant sounds, rather than as a separate entity or as a voice quality.

b. *Measures of Nasal Sound Pressure.* Another technique which has been developed to assess nasality involves measurement of nasal sound pressures by use of a microphone system. Oral and total sound pressures usually have been measured simultaneously. The major problem with such techniques is that they necessitate complete separation of the oral and nasal components of the sound. Weiss (1954) used a probe-tube microphone inserted in one nostril to record nasal sound and a regular microphone to pick up the total sound. Low (1955) and Doubek (1955) utilized mechanical devices, for example, a metal disc, to separate the orally and nasally emitted sound.

Measurements of nasal sound pressure obviously do not have face validity as measures of nasality when this dimension is defined in terms of listener perception. Weiss (1954), however, found a correlation of .95 between the difference in oral and nasal sound pressures and listener judgments of nasality. Low (1955), on the other hand, found a much lower correlation of .50. Doubek (1955) made no attempt to validate his measures against listener judgments, apparently assuming that measures of nasal sound pressure have inherent validity as measures of nasal voice quality. In view of the basic nature of this voice quality dimension such an assumption appears tenuous. Although measures of nasal sound pressure do not have face validity, they may have empirical validity as an index of nasality. This is the case especially for measures determined by Weiss's procedure. As Weiss points out, however, such a measure is only an index; it is not a direct measure of nasal voice quality.

In relation to the reliability of sound pressure measures, Weiss (1954) found fairly good agreement between repeated measures obtained from a graphic record. The repeatibility of such measures on different samples from the same subject, however, has not been determined.

c. *Measures of the Acoustic Spectrum.* In recent years attempts have been made to assess nasality by the use of spectrographic analyses (Hanson, 1964; Millard, 1957). In most instances sonographic records of speech have been inspected for various characteristics which are presumably related to nasality. Again, this technique has no face validity as a measure of a perceptual phenomenon. It also has not been demonstrated to have empirical validity. Some acoustic characteristics have been identified as accompanying nasalization (Fant, 1960; House and Stevens, 1956; Smith, 1951); however, the studies of Dickson (1962) and Hanson (1964) demonstrate that such characteristics do not consistently differentiate nasal from nonnasal speakers as identified by listener judgments and that they do not provide continuous measures of nasality.

The reliability with which decisions concerning nasality can be made from spectrographic records is not known. The records usually have been analyzed by visual inspection only (Millard, 1957) rather than by measurement of acoustic characteristics. It is interesting to note that this presumably more "objective" measure involves human judgments which probably are more difficult than those made in judging nasality from actual speech.

Recently, a somewhat different type of acoustic measure of nasality, a measure based on evaluation of the phase characteristics of the signal, has been proposed (Weatherley-White *et al.*, 1964). The investigators calibrated their instrument, the nasometer, to differentiate between the words "oh" and "nine." Further validation was carried out by utilizing a group of normal children and a group of children with cleft palates. The investigators report that, in general, the instrument differentiated between the two words and the two groups. Several questions have been raised (Moll, 1964) concerning this proposed nasality measure. In the first place, no information is available concerning whether the cleft palate subjects in the validation group were indeed nasal. It cannot be assumed that they were simply because they had cleft palates. In addition, as is obvious from the previous discussion of speech sound articulation, individuals with clefts exhibit speech deviations other than nasality. A feasible hypothesis would be that the instrument differentiated the groups on the basis of articulation rather than of nasal voice quality. Further, differentiation between the words "oh" and "nine" may indicate that the instrument detects the difference between the two vowels /o/ and /aɪ/ rather than between different degrees of nasality. In a later investigation, Weatherley-White *et al.* (1966) demonstrated a relationship between nasometer readings and openings of the velopharyngeal port as measured from cineradiographic films on an adult normal subject. Even if it is assumed that velopharyngeal opening and nasality are related perfectly, the relationship observed by these investigators is only categorical; that is, nasometer readings in a particular direction tend to accompany opening of the velopharyngeal port. It has not been demonstrated, as yet, that such readings can validly and reliably distinguish between degrees of nasality and thus provide a continuous measure of this voice quality.

3. *Summary of Measurement Techniques*

Procedures for assessing nasal voice quality in cleft palate individuals have been discussed in detail because of the almost perpetual controversy concerning the relative merits of subjective and objective measurement techniques and because of the author's conviction that the issues involved in this controversy are not always understood fully.

Despite the possible contamination of nasality judgments by irrelevant dimensions, contamination which can be minimized by the "backward-play" technique, it appears that listener-judgment procedures are the only ones by which direct measures of nasality can be obtained. None of the three types of "objective" measures discussed has face validity for this purpose. Only one of these procedures, the measurement of nasal-oral sound pressures, has been shown to provide measures which are related closely to listener judgments. There is no objection to using measurement of sound pressures or any other procedure to obtain an index of nasality; it cannot be assumed, however, that such measures are somehow inherently superior to listener judgments. To be a valid index of nasality, a measure must be related closely to listener perceptions. If it is contended that "subjective" listener ratings are biased, then it is obvious that any measure which relates closely to such ratings must be biased in the same way.

It should be noted that this discussion relates only to the use of the "objective" measures for assessing nasality. These techniques may be useful and valid for the assessment of other dimensions; for example, the amount of nasal air emission. It also is possible that some index of nasality which is shown to have empirical validity may have practical advantages in comparison with listener-judgment procedures. It appears, however, that nasality judgments obtained by some phsychological scaling procedure provide a more valid and at least as reliable an assessment of this voice quality dimension as is provided by any other technique. By the use of judgment procedures an experimenter recognizes the fact that a listener is always an integral part of the speech communication process. Extreme caution should be exercised in discarding listener judgments for presumably more objective measures which may not be as valid or as reliable. As Kantner (1948) pointed out, in the assessment of nasality the "human ear is the final detector and arbiter."

B. NASALITY IN INDIVIDUALS WITH CLEFT PALATES

Although it is generally agreed that nasal voice quality is quite prevalent among individuals with cleft palates, there are few data on the exact incidence of nasality. Cobb and Lierle (1936) report that all of their 56 subjects exhibited "impaired resonance," while MacCollum et al. (1956) observed nasality in only 29% of their consecutive series of cases. Between these two extreme findings are those of Bzoch (1956), Counihan (1956), and Starr (1956), who report that 62 to 76% of their subjects were judged to exhibit "mild to severe resonance distortion." Such wide variation in results undoubtedly is due to differences in types of subjects utilized, criteria for assessing nasality, and other factors. The only statement that can be made with any certainty is that, on the average, nasal voice quality is more prevalent in the cleft palate population than in the noncleft population; however, it is obvious that not all individuals with clefts are nasal.

Most investigations of nasality in individuals with cleft palates have been designed to evaluate possible relations between variations in nasal quality and other factors. The results of these studies can be discussed profitably in relation to variations in nasality with (a) phonetic factors, (b) vocal pitch usage, (c) vocal intensity, and (d) articulation and intelligibility.

1. Nasality and Phonetic Factors

The most consistent finding concerning nasality variation with phonetic factors is that the degree of nasal voice quality perceived is dependent on the particular vowel sound produced. Hess (1959) and Spriestersbach and Powers (1959a) observed a consistent relationship between nasality in cleft subjects and tongue height on vowels; vowels with high tongue positions, such as /i/ and /u/, were judged as more nasal than low vowels, such as /ɑ/ and /æ/. Van Hattum (1954), however, did not observe a systematic trend in perceived nasality as a function of vowel tongue height. In all three of these investigations, another trend was noted: vowels for which the tongue constriction is in the front of the oral cavity, for example, /i/ and /æ/, were perceived as more nasal than back vowels, for example, /u/ and /ɑ/.

The findings cited above for individuals with cleft palates are not completely consistent with results obtained on subjects without cleft palates. McIntosh (1937) and Lintz and Sherman (1961) found that nasal speakers without clefts exhibited less nasal quality on high vowels than on those produced with a low tongue position. The same relationship was reported (Lintz and Sherman, 1961) for individuals with normal voice quality. In relation to differences between front and back vowels, Lintz and Sherman (1961) report results for normal and so-called functionally nasal speakers which are consistent with findings for individuals with cleft palates: that is, front vowels are perceived as more nasal than back vowels.

The differences in findings for cleft palate and other nasal speakers in relation to nasality variation with vowels should be emphasized. These differences suggest not only that nasal quality may not represent exactly the same phenomenon (Johnson *et al.*, 1963) in both groups but also that they have implications for the description of nasality in speakers with cleft palates. It appears that high vowels are more nasal than low vowels for cleft palate individuals who exhibit hypernasality. For those who are not hypernasal, however, the trend probably is reversed, that is, low vowels are more nasal than high in the same manner as reported for nonnasal speakers (Lintz and Sherman, 1961). Spriestersbach and Powers (1959a) noted that the trend of nasality with vowels varies among cleft palate individuals. A question might be raised concerning the desirability of studying such a trend in the population of all individuals with clefts since it is likely that the trends may be completely reversed for comparisons between certain subgroups.

There is some evidence that nasal voice quality may vary with the consonant context of vowels. For cleft palate subjects, the only study that provides even indirect evidence of context differences in nasality is that of Crosby (1952). Crosby did not obtain measures of nasality; judges were asked only to identify each subject as "cleft" or "noncleft" from tape recordings of speech samples. One finding of this study (reported previously in Section II, B, 2, a) has an implication for the evaluation of nasality: judges could not consistently distinguish cleft palate from noncleft palate subjects on the basis of syllables containing vowels adjacent only to nasal consonants. This result suggests that cleft palate individuals are not deviant, in relation to nasality or any other speech variable, on such syllables. This finding is not surprising in view of the fact that noncleft palate speakers normally exhibit assimilated nasality on vowels adjacent to nasal consonants (McIntosh, 1937).

Systematic study of nasality variation with phonetic context has been carried out by Lintz and Sherman (1961) for noncleft, nasal subjects and for subjects with normal voice quality. These investigators report that consonant-vowel-consonant syllables are judged as less nasal when the consonant is a stop plosive than when it is a fricative; that syllables containing voiceless consonants are perceived as less nasal than are those with voiced consonants; and that voicing appears to have a somewhat greater influence than manner of production. It thus would appear that both the factors of consonant voicing and manner of consonant production affect degree of nasality. These investigators suggest the possibility that changes in degree of nasality dependent upon consonant context may be related to various acoustic characteristics of vowels which change as consonant context changes: that is, that nasality on the vowel may increase as fundamental frequency decreases, as duration increases, and as intensity increases. The effect of these variables on nasality will be discussed in more detail in subsequent sections of this chapter.

It would appear that a study of the influence of consonant environments on nasal quality, similar to that of Lintz and Sherman (1961), should be carried out with cleft palate speakers. A methodological problem, however, essentially prohibits such an investigation. Since articulation deficiencies are prevalent in the cleft palate population, many cleft palate subjects cannot produce some of the consonants; as a result, the findings might be relevant to entirely different consonant contexts than those intended. Since degree of nasality and articulation ability are related in the cleft palate population, the selection of individuals who could produce all of the consonant sounds correctly would bias the data.

2. *Nasality and Vocal Pitch*

Variations of nasal voice quality in individuals with cleft palates have been investigated in relation to vocal pitch level, degree of pitch variability, and effectiveness of pitch usage. Hess (1959) had cleft palate subjects phonate six sustained vowel sounds at habitual pitch and also at a pitch 1.4 times this level. The phonations were then rated for degree of nasality on a 0- to 6-point scale. Hess concludes that less nasality is perceived at the higher pitch level than at the habitual level; the difference in mean ratings for the two levels, however, although statistically significant, was quite small, less than .5 of a scale value. In addition, Hess (1955) did not find a strong relationship between habitual pitch level and the degree of nasality.

Simmons (1955) assessed nasal voice quality on repeated readings of a paragraph by cleft palate subjects under three pitch-inflection conditions: (a) normal inflection, (b) monotone, and (c) exaggerated inflection. No significant differences in mean nasality ratings were found among the conditions, although readings at a monotone were judged to be slightly more nasal than those in the other two conditions, an observation which could be the result of listener reaction to the unnaturalness of monotone.

Spriestersbach (1955) investigated the relationship between nasal quality and what he termed "effectiveness of pitch usage" on connected speech samples from cleft palate speakers. The latter variable was scaled by a group of judges who listened to the speech samples played forward; nasality was judged with both forward and backward play. The correlation between effectiveness of pitch usage and nasality with forward play was a negative .31. This result suggests that less favorable pitch usage ratings are associated to some extent with greater degrees of nasality; the degree of relationship between these two variables, however, obviously is not great. The correlation between pitch usage and nasality with backward play was low, a negative

.15, and not significant, thus providing no evidence of any relationship at all. It is probable, therefore, that the apparent relationship between pitch usage and nasality with forward play is due entirely to contamination of ratings of nasality with forward play by effectiveness of pitch usage.

The data on variations in nasality with changes in vocal pitch in cleft palate individuals are not completely definitive. It does appear that nasality may decrease slightly, on the average, when individuals are instructed to increase pitch level; variations among subjects in degree of nasal quality, however, are not closely related to differences among individuals in habitual pitch level. There also appears to be no consistent relationship between degree of pitch inflection or effectiveness of pitch usage and nasality in cleft individuals. For nasal subjects without clefts there is little empirical information concerning any pitch usage and nasality relationship. It has been suggested, however, that nasality decreases with a decrease in vocal pitch (Holmes, 1932). The only investigation of this relationship was reported by Sherman and Goodwin (1954), who had functionally nasal subjects read a passage at habitual pitch level, at a lower level, and at a higher level. Nasality judgments were made with the samples played both forward and backward. The only statistically significant difference observed was for males on ratings of nasality with forward play; there was less nasality at the lower vocal pitch than at the habitual or higher levels. These authors point out, however, that even this difference was quite small (.65 of a scale value on a 7-point scale). The fact that no relationship was observed between pitch level and nasality rated with backward play suggests again that the relationship between pitch and nasality rated with forward play may reflect only bias or judgment contamination. Sherman and Goodwin conclude that there is "... little evidence to support the hypothesis that there is a relationship between pitch level and perceived nasality." They qualify this conclusion with the statement that lowering the pitch level may be accompanied by a decrease in degree of nasality in some individuals, since this was definitely the case for one of their nasal speakers. It thus appears that if there is a relationship between pitch level and nasality, it is opposite in direction for speakers with cleft palate from that for functionally nasal speakers, that is, nasal quality is decreased with higher pitches in the cleft palate group and with lower pitches in some nasal subjects without clefts.

3. Nasality and Vocal Intensity

Hess (1959) investigated the relationship between nasal voice quality and vocal intensity in cleft palate subjects. Vowels were sustained at sound pressure levels of 75 dB and 85 dB and nasality judgments were made of each phonation on a 7-point scale. The mean difference in degree of perceived nasality between the two levels was statistically significant, with nasal quality rated as less severe at the higher sound pressure level. Again, it should be noted that although the difference was significant, it was small (.25 scale value). The only comparable data on nasal speakers without cleft palates is from the study of Weiss (1954), although 3 of his 17 subjects did have cleft palates. Weiss reports a negative correlation of .57 between judgments of nasality in connected speech and average sound pressure level. This finding is consistent with that of Hess on cleft palate subjects and with the statement of Williamson (1944) that for functionally nasal voices less nasality is perceived at higher intensities.

From the research findings cited above, it appears that nasality decreases with increased vocal intensity for both cleft and noncleft nasal speakers. There are a number of factors, however, which should be considered in interpreting these findings. Hess (1959) points out that, since there are systematic intensity differences between vowels under normal conditions, his requirement that subjects produce all vowels at the same intensities may have biased the data. He observed that many of his subjects had difficulty producing the high vowels, /i/ and /u/, at the 85 dB level, while the low vowels, /ɑ/ and /æ/, were produced easily at this level. Thus it is possible that the phonation of some vowels at a high intensity level was an abnormal situation. Hess suggests that, in future studies, intensity conditions should be determined in relation to the normal intensity of each vowel sound. The results of Weiss (1954) also point up a problem of data interpretation. The relationship observed by Weiss between sound pressure level and nasality may reflect the fact that nasal quality is characterized by a decrease in vocal intensity (Curtis, 1942; House and Stevens, 1956). The interpretation that nasality changes because intensity changes may not be valid. It is obvious that the relationship between intensity and nasality should be studied by having each subject phonate at different vocal intensities, as was done by Hess, rather than to correlate the degrees of nasality with the subject's vocal levels.

4. Nasality, Articulation, and Intelligibility

The relationships between nasal voice quality and articulation or speech intelligibility have been cited in previous discussions of measurement procedures. It appears worthwhile, however, to consider these relationships somewhat more closely. Reported correlations between nasality and articulation or intelligibility are shown in Table VII. It is obvious that the correlation values obtained vary greatly; in most instances, however, there appears to be a moderate relationship between nasality and each of the other two variables. The question as to whether these correlations reflect a real relationship or whether they are due to contamination of nasality judgments by articulation or intelligibility was posed in a previous section of this chapter.

Table VII

Correlations between nasal voice quality judgments and (a)
measures of articulation and (b) measures of intelligibility
as reported by various investigators[a]

Study	Articulation	Intelligibility
A	.49	.78
B	—	.30
C	.66	.87
D	.82	.72
E (1)	.41	.42
E (2)	.56	.54
F (forward play)	.47	—
F (backward play)	.07	—
G	—	.42
H	.42	—
I (sentences)	.64	—
I (vowels)	−.07	—

[a] Counihan, 1956 (A); Eguchi, 1957 (B); Falck, 1955 (C); McWilliams, 1954 (D); Shames *et al.*, undated (E); Spriestersbach, 1955 (F); Subtelny *et al.*, 1961 (G).

The results of Spriestersbach (1955) and Van Hattum (1958) suggest that the relationship between articulation and nasality is due entirely to judgment contamination. For nasality judged during forward playing of the samples, Spriestersbach found a moderate correlation with articulation of .47. When the samples were played backward, a procedure which presumably eliminates judgment contamination, no significant relationship was observed (correlation = .07). Van Hattum concluded that there is no relationship between articulation and nasal quality when the effect of articulation on nasality judgments is minimized by rating only sustained vowels (Table VII).

The data reported by Shames *et al.* (undated) and Van Demark (1964) are not in agreement with the results cited above. In both of these investigations, moderate but significant correlations were found between nasality and articulation judgments (Table VII) even though judgment contamination was minimized by playing the speech samples backward for nasality ratings. It is possible that a significant correlation was not found by Spriestersbach (1955) because of errors of sampling. Van Hattum's (1958) findings may be due to the fact that degree of nasality on isolated vowels is not an adequate index of nasal quality in connected speech (Spriestersbach and Powers, 1959a; Van Hattum, 1958). This point of view is taken since there are a priori reasons for assuming that a real relationship exists between nasality and articulation in cleft palate speakers. Since the primary articulation errors of individuals with clefts are nasal distortions of sounds, it appears logical that individuals who make many such errors would tend to exhibit a greater degree of nasal voice quality than those who have better articulation. For this reason, it is concluded that there is at least a moderate correlation, a correlation not due to judgment contamination, between these two dimensions. The higher correlations obtained by some investigators (Counihan, 1956; Falck, 1955; McWilliams, 1954) undoubtedly reflect a combination of this real relationship and the relationship resulting from judgment contamination.

There are two aspects of the relationship between articulation and nasality which should be noted. Subtelny *et al.* (1961) observed that this relationship seems to be closer at one end of the articulation or intelligibility continuum than at the other. They found that individuals with severe intelligibility losses consistently exhibited hypernasal voice quality; however, not all hypernasal speakers had severe intelligibility losses. The second aspect which should be considered is the finding of Van Demark (1964) that nasal quality is more closely related to certain types of articulation errors than to others. Correlations of .49 to .51 were found between nasality judgments and the number of fricative, stop plosives, and distortion-nasal errors. The correlations of all other types of errors with nasality were less than .30. This finding suggests that the relative frequencies with which different sound types are included in an articulation test will affect the magnitude of the correlation observed. It is obvious, however, that in reality there is only a moderate degree of relationship between nasality and articulation. The observation of Subtelny *et al.* (1961) that there is a difference in the relationship at the two ends of the articulation continuum would preclude a high correlation.

5. *Summary*

From the preceding discussion, it can be concluded that nasal voice quality is exhibited by many individuals with cleft palates. It also was noted that the degree of nasality perceived in the speech of these individuals is less on vowels with low tongue positions and at higher pitch and at higher intensity levels. In addition, although nasal voice quality and articulation ability are related in this population, the relationship is not a strong one. Possibly one of the most important conclusions to be drawn is that nasality does not appear to vary in the same manner for both cleft palate and noncleft palate nasal speakers. Nasality appears to be reduced on vowels with high tongue positions and at lower pitch levels for the latter individuals. As pointed out by Johnson *et al.* (1963), the basic differences between these two groups make generalizations concerning nasality in cleft palate subjects on the basis of data on noncleft palate subjects, or vice versa, of questionable validity.

IV. Language Development

The term "language" is used here to refer to the manner in which verbal units are utilized in spoken communication. In general, language involves the type and the number of such units utilized and the way in which the units are put together in communication. For the purposes of this discussion, a distinction is made between oral language and speech production. The dimensions of speech production, such as articulation ability and voice quality, have to do with the manner in which verbal units are produced. The way in which such units are used, regardless of how accurately they are produced, is considered as language. Many investigators (Morris, 1962; Templin, 1957) have considered articulation skills to represent a language dimension; however, this dimension has been considered separately in a previous discussion. No attempt will be made to defend the validity of the dichotomy between speech production and oral language; it is made here only for purposes of organization.

Techniques for measuring various aspects of language will not be described in detail. McCarthy (1930) and Templin (1957) describe various procedures for measuring such language dimensions as verbal output, language structure, language function, and vocabulary. Summaries of available information on language development in children also are presented by these authors.

Various writers (Johnson *et al.*, 1956; McWilliams, 1956) suggest that certain factors which are present in the cleft palate population may have an adverse effect on development of language; however, until very recently, these speculations had not been tested empirically. Cobb and Lierle (1936) report that 26.8% of their group of 56 cleft subjects exhibited what was called "delayed speech" but these authors do not describe this phenomenon in detail.

Bzoch (1956) attempted to study the language development of cleft palate children, aged 3 to 6 years, by interviewing the parents concerning the child's use of language. On the basis of results of these interviews, Bzoch concluded that the cleft palate children did not differ greatly from normal children in crying or in noncrying vocalizations, in amount of babbling, or in use of "jargon." He found, however, that 43% of the cleft palate subjects were reported to have used their "first true word" after 14 months of age, which was considered to be the upper limit of the normal range. In addition, 50% of the group first used simple sentences after 2 years of age, also considered to represent the upper limit for noncleft palate subjects. From these findings, Bzoch reported that 30 of the 60 subjects were judged to have been delayed in speech development. For only 4 of the children, however, did the parents feel that the amount of talking was less than normal. Bzoch concluded that the findings "... suggest that the delayed speech problem of cleft palate children was not the same as the usual delayed speech problem considered in speech correction texts. It appeared to be more a delay in the timing of early speech development than a delay in the quality and the quantity of expressive language." It would appear that the procedure of obtaining data on language development from parent interviews is subject to certain errors; for example, the parents may not report accurately because of lack of correct recall or because of emotional involvement concerning the questions posed. Despite these possible errors, however, Bzoch's data suggest that some cleft palate individuals may be retarded in language development.

Spriestersbach *et al.* (1958) assessed the language usage of cleft palate subjects by making various measures at the time of examination. They recorded speech samples from 40 children with cleft palates, each sample consisting of 50 responses made by the child to presentation of toys and pictures. The samples were scored to determine mean length of response and structural complexity score. These measures are described in detail by Templin (1957). In addition, the vocabulary of the subjects was assessed by the Ammons Vocabulary Test and by the vocabulary subtest of the Wechsler Intelligence Scale for Children (WISC). The results on all of these measures were compared to available normative data. On the measures of mean length of response the cleft palate subjects were found to differ significantly as a group from the norms for children of similar age and sex. Among the 40 children, 29 had lower mean length of response scores than normals. On the structural complexity score, although the cleft palate subjects were not, on the average, significantly different from normative data, 24 fell below the norm for their age and sex. The cleft palate group made significantly better scores on the Ammons vocabulary test and poorer scores on the WISC vocabulary subtest than did normals. The investigators suggest that these two tests measure somewhat different aspects of vocabulary. Since the subject is required only to point to a picture which matches the presented word, the Ammons test actually measures "recognition" vocabulary. On the WISC the subject is required to define the word so that scores on this test reflect "definition" or "usage" vocabulary. It thus would appear that cleft palate subjects are advanced in recognition vocabulary and retarded in their ability to define words.

Morris (1962) utilized the same type of measurement techniques as Spriestersbach *et al.* (1958) to obtain data on a group of 107 cleft palate subjects. He reports that these subjects, on the average, were significantly retarded on mean length of response, structural complexity, and number of different words used and that they made lower scores on both the Ammons and WISC vocabulary tests. In addition, the cleft palate subjects were more variable than were normals in the length of their responses and they used more one-word responses. From these data, Morris concluded that individuals with cleft palates are significantly retarded, on the average, in communication skills. Morris also assessed differences between cleft-type groups in language development, but found no significant differences between palate-only and lip-and-palate groups on any of the language measures. From an evaluation of relationships among the various measures, he concluded that although interrelationships exist, they are not close enough to justify the use of any one of these measures as an index of overall language skills.

From the studies summarized above, it appears that individuals with cleft lips and palates are retarded to some degree in language development. This retardation seems to exist on almost every dimension measured in the various studies; these children exhibit less verbal output and a more simple language structure than subjects without clefts. It should be noted, however, that few data are available on early language development of cleft palate individuals except for those obtained by Bzoch (1956) from parent interviews. Whether these children are deficient in language skills at very early ages is not well defined. In addition, as with the other speech dimensions discussed, it must be emphasized that the conclusions about retarded language development refer to cleft palate subjects on the average; obviously not all children exhibit retardation in language skills.

V. Other Speech Dimensions

Although deviant articulation, nasal voice quality, and language retardation are the primary speech problems usually considered to be associated with individuals with cleft palates, it has been suggested that deviations exist on other speech dimensions. Such possible deviations can be divided into three categories: deviations in (a) vocal pitch and intensity, (b) voice quality, and (c) nonauditory aspects of speech.

A. Vocal Pitch and Intensity

It has been suggested that individuals with cleft palates are deviant in both vocal pitch and vocal intensity. Berry and Eisenson (1956) state that the speech of a cleft palate child may be described as "... frequently shrill in pitch and sometimes changing with growth to an unnaturally low, gravel voice" and also as "uncontrolled in loudness." Cobb and Lierle (1936) report that a general lack of vocal intensity and pitch variation was noted in the subjects that they studied. Ritchie (1937) mentions that a "flat monotone" intonation pattern is typical of the voices of individuals with clefts.

In general, the suggestions that there are pitch and intensity deviations in individuals with cleft palates are not based on controlled, systematic measurements of these dimensions. The degree and the exact nature of such deviations have not been defined. In fact, it has not been demonstrated that such deviations exist when evaluated by comparison with the pitch and intensity characteristics of normal speakers. There also is no information on the relationships of such deviations to other dimensions of speech. Yet such relationships appear to be important, especially in relation to the dimension of vocal intensity. Since decreased intensity has been found to be characteristic of nasal voice quality (Curtis, 1942; House and Stevens, 1956), intensity deviations might be expected in this population; however, they would not necessarily represent a problem distinct from nasal quality. Procedures are available for systematic measurement of pitch levels, inflectional patterns, and intensity of speech (Steer and Hanley, 1957), and it would appear that definitive studies of pitch and intensity characteristics in the cleft population would provide useful information.

B. Voice Quality

One voice quality dimension, nasality, has been discussed in detail in a previous section; it has been suggested, however, that cleft palate individuals may exhibit other quality deviations. McDonald and Koepp–Baker (1951) state that "faulty phonation," which they say is a problem among these individuals, results in the voice qualities of "breathiness" and "hoarseness." Berry and Eisenson (1956) suggest that cleft palate speech may be "harsh or muffled in quality." Because of such suggestions in the literature, Hess (1959) evaluated the extent to which harshness, hoarseness, and breathiness varies in cleft palate individuals with changes in pitch and intensity. He reports that harshness and hoarseness are reduced at higher pitches and that breathiness is unaffected by pitch. Less breathiness, less hoarseness, and more harshness are perceived by listeners at higher intensity levels. Hess (1955) also observed that vowels with high tongue positions are less breathy than low vowels and that less harshness and less hoarseness are perceived on back vowels than on those produced in the front of the oral cavity.

As with vocal pitch and intensity characteristics, there are no systematic studies which indicate that voice quality disorders other than hypernasality are more prevalent among speakers with cleft palates than among those without clefts. Although the judges used by Hess (1959) rated harshness, breathiness, and hoarseness reliably, these were forced judgments. It is possible that similar ratings might be made for subjects without clefts. Because of the prevalence of nasal voice quality in cleft palate individuals, judgments of the other quality dimensions, even on sustained vowels or with the samples played backward, may be contaminated by the presence of nasality. It would appear that the only possible solution to this problem, at present, is to select only nonnasal cleft palate subjects. It is obvious, however, that such selection would bias the data, since there may be a real relationship between nasality and the presence of the other quality disorders.

C. Nonauditory Aspects of Speech

It has been noted by many authors that unnatural, visible mannerisms often accompany the speech of individuals with clefts. The most common mannerism noted is a constriction of the nasal alae (Berry and Eisenson, 1956; Morley, 1962; Van Riper and Irwin, 1958), although "aversion of the head" also has been reported to exist (Berry and Eisenson, 1956). The incidence of such nonauditory characteristics in individuals with clefts, the effect of such characteristics on listeners, and their relationship to other speech characteristics of cleft speakers have not been investigated.

VI. Summary

From the data reviewed in this chapter, it is obvious that there is a great deal of information concerning the speech characteristics of individuals with cleft lips and palates; there are, of course, obvious gaps in the knowledge of certain of these characteristics. No attempt will be made to summarize the information presented since summaries have been presented at the end of most of the major sections of the chapter. There are a number of general conclusions, however, which should be reemphasized.

It appears that use of the term "cleft palate speech" is essentially meaningless in describing the speech characteristics exhibited by cleft palate individuals. In the first place, it is not really descriptive of the various speech dimensions which are affected. Since any suggested etiologies must explain the variations in speech characteristics which occur between and within cleft palate individuals, a detailed description of the speech problems is very important to the consideration of the etiology of these problems. In addition, the expression "cleft palate speech" seems to mean that cleft palate individuals are all alike in speech characteristics. The available information concerning the manner in which speech problems differ depending on various factors makes it clear that the cleft population is by no means homogeneous in this respect. Although this conclusion appears obvious, it has not always been recognized nor have its implications been considered in describing the speech of individuals with clefts or in hypothesizing about the etiologies of the communication disorders.

A second general conclusion which should be emphasized is the fact that statements which are not based on systematic observations usually are grossly inadequate in describing speech deviations. Until approximately the past 30 years there was little detailed information on speech problems in the cleft palate population; there were only statements to the effect that articulation errors and nasal quality are usually present. The results of many systematic investigations have provided a much better understanding of the nature of the articulation and voice quality disorders. There still has been little systematic research, however, on voice quality deviations other than nasality or on suggested vocal pitch and intensity deviations. It is not enough to suggest that such problems exist; we must try to define the degree to which they exist, the exact nature of the deviations, and how they vary with other factors. The author does not mean to imply that general statements which are not based on systematic observations of fairly large groups of subjects are invalid and useless. Such statements help to define problems for more careful investigation. In almost every area of human behavior there has been a progression from general statements to systematic research on groups, and particularly to the study of variations within groups. This progression has been obvious in endeavors to describe the speech characteristics of cleft palate speakers. The point to be made is that we must not accept general statements as the last answer; we must go farther to test and to define more adequately the speech deviations suggested by such statements.

In preparing this chapter, the author has been somewhat arbitrary in organizing the discussion in relation to his own concepts and biases. For example, nasal emission of air has been considered as an articulatory deviation, although some individuals have considered it as an entity separate from both articulation and nasal voice quality. It is hoped, however, that the preceding discussion has provided a fairly complete summary of available knowledge about the speech and language characteristics of cleft palate individuals, of the problems involved in assessing speech dimensions in cleft palate speakers, and of the issues and questions which, as yet, are unanswered by careful and systematic investigation.

REFERENCES

Barker, J. O. (1960). A numerical measure of articulation. *J. Speech Hearing Disorders* **25**, 79–88.

Battle, R. J. V. (1954). The past, present and future in the surgery of the cleft palate. *Brit. J. Plastic Surg.* **7**, 217–228.

Bensen, J. F. (1951). An Experimental Study of the Relationship Between the Amount of Nasal Emission of Air and Judged Nasality. M. A. Thesis, West Virginia Univ., Morgantown, West Virginia.

Bentley, F. H., and Watkins, I. (1947). Speech after repair of cleft palate. *Lancet* **2**, 862–865.

Berry, Mildred F. (1928). Correction of cleft palate speech by phonetic instruction. *Quart. J. Speech* **14**, 523–529.

Berry, Mildred F. (1949). Lingual anomalies associated with palatal clefts. *J. Speech Hearing Disorders* **14**, 359–362.

Berry, Mildred F., and Eisenson, J. (1956). "Speech Disorders." Appleton, New York.

Blakeway, H. (1915). The operative treatment of cleft palate. *Lancet* **1**, 479.

Burgi, E. J., and Matthews, J. (1958). Predicting intelligibility of cerebral palsied speech. *J. Speech Hearing Res.* **1**, 331–343.

Byrne, Margaret C., Shelton, R. L., Jr., and Diedrich, W. M. (1961). Articulatory skill, physical management, and classification of children with cleft palates. *J. Speech Hearing Disorders* **26**, 326–333.

Bzoch, K. R. (1956). An Investigation of the Speech of Pre-School Cleft Palate Children. Ph. D. Thesis, Northwestern Univ., Evanston, Illinois.

Calnan, J. S. (1959). The surgical treatment of nasal speech disorders. *Ann. Roy. Coll. Surg. Engl.* **25**, 119–141.

Cobb, Lois H., and Lierle, D. M. (1936). An analysis of the speech difficulties of 56 cleft palate and harelip cases. *Arch. Speech* **1**, 217–230.

Conway, H. (1951). Combined use of the push-back and pharyngeal flap procedures in the management of complicated cases of cleft palate. *Plastic Reconstruc. Surg.* **7**, 214–224.

Cooker, H. S. (1961). A Comparison of Articulation Defectiveness Judgments Obtained from Standard Oral Reading Samples and Spontaneous Connected Speech of Speakers with Cleft Palates. M. A. Thesis, Univ. of Iowa, Iowa City, Iowa.

Counihan, D. T. (1956). A Clinical Study of the Speech Efficiency and Structural Adequacy of Operated Adolescent and Adult Cleft Palate Persons. Ph. D. Thesis, Northwestern Univ., Evanston, Illinois.

Counihan, D. T. (1960). Articulation skills of adolescents and adults with cleft palates. *J. Speech Hearing Disorders* **25**, 181–187.

Crosby, C. A. (1952). Audience Differentiation of Recorded Samples of Cleft and Non-Cleft Palate Speech. M. A. Thesis, Univ. of Wisconsin, Madison, Wisconsin.

Curtis, J. F. (1942). An Experimental Study of Wave Composition of Nasal Voice Quality. Ph. D. Thesis, Univ. of Iowa, Iowa City, Iowa.

Dickson, D. R. (1962). An acoustic study of nasality. *J. Speech Hearing Res.* **5**, 103–111.

Dietze, H. (1952). A Study of the Understandability of Defective Speech in Relation to Errors of Articulation. M. S. Thesis, Univ. of Pittsburgh, Pittsburgh, Pennsylvania.

Doubek, F. (1955). Die Prufung der Sprechfunktion bei Gaumenspaltenoperationen. *Fortschr. Kiefer- Gesichts-Chir.* **1**, 104–111.

Eckelmann, Dorothy, and Baldridge, Patricianne (1945). Speech training for the child with a cleft palate. *J. Speech Disorders* **10**, 137–149.

Eckstein, A., and Schuchardt, K. (1955). Ergebnisse bei einseitigen durchgehenden Lippen-Kiefer-Gaumenspalten in kieferorthopadischer und sprachlicher Hinsicht. *Fortschr. Kiefer- Gesichts-Chir.* **1**, 000–000.

Eguchi, B. Y. (1957). An Evaluation of the Speech of a Series of Cleft Palate Subjects Operated by the Wardill Procedure. M. S. Thesis, Pennsylvania State Univ., University Park, Pennsylvania.

Falck, Vilma T. (1955). Selected Factors Related to the Ability of Cleft Palate Speakers to Convey Information. Ph. D. Thesis, Pennsylvania State Univ., University Park, Pennsylvania.

Fant, G. (1960). "Acoustic Theory of Speech Production." Mouton, The Hague.

Foster, T. D., and Greene, Margaret C. L. (1960). Lateral speech defects and dental irregularities in cleft palate. *Brit. J. Plastic Surg.* **12**, 367–377.

Fritzell, B. (1960). Speech improvement following palatoplasty with elongated pharyngeal flap. *Folia Phoniat.* **12**, 118–123.

Glover, D. M. (1961). A long range evaluation of cleft palate repair. *Plastic Reconstruc. Surg.* **27**, 19–30.

Gray, G. H., and Jones, H. W. (1958). Experiences with the posterior pharyngeal flap in repair of the cleft palate. *Am. J. Surg.* **95**, 304–308.

Greene, Margaret C. L. (1960). Speech analysis of 263 cleft palate cases. *J. Speech Hearing Disorders*, **25**, 43–48.

Hamlen, M. (1960). Palato-pharyngeal plasty: speech aspects. *J. Ontario Speech Hearing Assoc.* pp. 17–21.

Hanson, M. L. (1964). A study of velopharyngeal competence in children with repaired cleft palates. *Cleft Palate J.* **1**, 217–231.

Hess, D. A. (1955). The Effect of Pitch and Intensity Level on Perceived Voice Quality of Male Cleft Palate Speakers. Ph. D. Thesis, Pennsylvania State Univ., University Park, Pennsylvania.

Hess, D. A. (1959). Pitch, intensity and cleft palate voice quality. *J. Speech Hearing Res.* **2**, 113–125.

Hess, D. A., and McDonald, E. T. (1960). Consonantal nasal pressure in cleft palate speakers. *J. Speech Hearing Res.* **3**, 201–211.

Holdsworth, W. G. (1954). Early treatment of cleft-lip and cleft-palate. *Brit. Med. J.* **1**, 304–308.

Holmes, F. L. D. (1932). The qualities of the voice. *Quart. J. Speech* **18**, 249–255.

House, A. S., and Stevens, K. N. (1956). Analog studies of the nasalization of vowels. *J. Speech Hearing Diseases* **21**, 218–232.

Johnson, W., Brown, S. J., Curtis, J. F., Edney, C. W., and Keaster, Jacqueline (1956). "Speech Handicapped School Children." Harper, New York.

Johnson, W., Darley, F. L., and Spriestersbach, D. C. (1963). Diagnostic Methods in Speech Pathology." Harper, New York.

Jolleys, A. (1954). A review of the results of operations on cleft palates with reference to maxillary growth and speech function. *Brit. J. Plastic Surg.* **7**, 229–241.

Jordan, E. P. (1960). Articulation test measures and listener ratings of articulation defectiveness. *J. Speech Hearing Res* **3**, 303–319.

Kantner, C. E. (1948). Diagnosis and prognosis in cleft palate speech. *J. Speech Hearing Disorders* **13**, 211–222.

Kelleher, R. E., Webster, R. C., Coffey, R. J., and Quigley, L. F., Jr. (1960). Nasal and oral air flow in normal and cleft palate speech; velocity and volume studies using warm wire meter and two channel recorder. *Cleft Palate Bull.* **10**, 66.

Klinger, H. (1956). A palatographic and acoustic study of cleft palate speech. *Cleft Palate Bull.* **6**, No. 2, 10–12.

Leach, E. A. (1957). Intelligibility of Cleft Palate Speech as Related to Speaker Visibility and Deflection of Nasal Emission. M. A. Thesis, Southern Illinois Univ., Carbondale, Illinois.

Lindsay, W. K., LeMesurier, A. B., and Farmer, A. W. (1962). A study of the speech results of a large series of cleft palate patients. *Plastic Reconstruc. Surg.* **29**, 273.

Lintz, Lois B., and Sherman, Dorothy (1961). Phonetic elements and perception of nasality. *J. Speech Hearing Res.* **4**, 381–396.

Low, G. M. (1955). An Objective Index of Nasality. Ph. D. Thesis, Univ. of Minnesota, Minneapolis, Minnesota.

Lubker, J. F., and Moll, K L. (1965). Simultaneous oral-nasal air flow measurements and cinefluorographic observations during speech production. *Cleft Palate J.* **2**, 257–272.

MacCollum, D. W., Richardson, Sylvia O., and Swanson. L. T. (1956). Habilitation of the cleft-palate patient. *New Engl. J. Med.* **254**, 299–307.

McCarthy, Dorothea (1930). "The Language Development of the Preschool Child." Univ. of Minnesota Press, Minneapolis, Minnesota.

McDermott, R. P. (1962). A Study of / s / Sound Production by Individuals with Cleft Palates. Ph. D. Thesis, Univ. of Iowa, Iowa City, Iowa.

McDonald, E. T., and Koepp–Baker, H. (1951). Cleft palate speech: An integration of research and clinical observation. *J. Speech Hearing Disorders* **16**, 9–20.

McIntosh, C. W. Jr. (1937). An Auditory Study of Nasality. M. A. Thesis, Univ. of Iowa, Iowa City, Iowa.

McWilliams, Betty J. (1954). Some factors in the intelligibility of cleft-palate speech. *J. Speech Hearing Disorders* **19**, 524–527.

McWilliams, Betty J. (1956). Some observations of environmental factors in speech development of children with cleft palate. *Cleft Palate Bull.* **6**, No. 1, 4–5.

McWilliams, Betty J. (1958). Articulation problems of a group of cleft palate adults. *J. Speech Hearing Res.* **1**, 68–74.

Milisen, R. L. (1954). A rationale for articulation disorders. *J. Speech Hearing Disorders* **19**, *Monogr. Suppl. No. 4*, 5–17.

Millard, R. T. (1957). The role of sound spectographic tracing in cleft palate patients. *Cleft Palate Bull.* **7**, No. 2, 7–8.

Moll, K. L. (1964). "Objective" measures of nasality. *Cleft Palate J.* **1**, 371–374.

Moll, K. L., Huffman, W. C., Lierle, D. M., and Smith, J. K. (1963). Factors related to the success of pharyngeal flap procedures. *Plastic Reconstruc. Surg.* **32**, 581–588.

Moran, R. E. (1951). The pharyngeal flap operation as a speech aid. *Plastic Reconstruc. Surg.* **7**, 202–213.

Morley, M. E. (1962). "Cleft Palate and Speech," 5th ed. Williams & Wilkins, Baltimore, Maryland.

Morris, H. L. (1962). Communication skills of children with cleft lips and palates. *J. Speech Hearing Res.* **5**, 79–90.

Morris, H. L., Spriestersbach, D. C., and Darley, F. L. (1961). An articulation test for assessing competency of velopharyngeal closure. *J. Speech Hearing Res.* **4**, 48–55.

Morrison, Sheila (1955). Measuring the severity of articulation defectiveness. *J. Speech Hearing Disorders* **20**, 347–351.

Obregon, G., and Smith, Jeanne K. (1959). The posterior pharyngeal flap palatoplasty. II. An analysis of 29 patients. *Arch. Otolaryngol.* **69**, 174–175.

Oldfield, M. C. (1941). Cleft palate and the mechanism of speech. *Brit. J. Surg.* **29**, 197–227.

Oldfield, M. C. (1949). Modern trends in hare-lip and cleft-palate surgery: with a review of 500 cases. *Brit. J. Surg.* **37**, 178–194.

Perrin, E. H. (1954). The rating of defective speech by trained and untrained observers. *J. Speech Hearing Disorders* **19**, 48–51.

Phillips, Betty R. (1954). An Experimental Investigation of the Relationship Between Ratings of Speech Intelligibility Based on Auditory and Visual Cues and on Auditory Cues Alone in a Group of Cleft Palate Adults. M. S. Thesis, Univ. of Pittsburgh, Pittsburgh, Pennsylvania.

Pinson, A. B. (1956). An Experimental Study of the Palatal Efficiency, and the Articulation, Voice Quality and Intelligibility of Children with Cleft Palate Speech. M. A. Thesis, Bowling Green State Univ., Bowling Green, Ohio.

Pitzner, Joan H. (1964). Articulation Skills for Children with Cleft Palates According to Adequacy of Intraoral Breath Pressure. M. A. Thesis, Univ. of Iowa, Iowa City, Iowa.

Prather, Elizabeth M. (1960). Scaling defectiveness of articulation by direct magnitude-estimation. *J. Speech Hearing Res.* 3, 380–392.

Reidy, J. P. (1958). 370 personal cases of cleft lip and palate. *Ann. Roy. Coll. Surg. Engl.* 23, 341–371.

Renfrew, Catherine E. (1960). Present day problems in cleft palate speech. *Logopeden*, June.

Ritchie, W. (1937). Cleft palate: A correlation of anatomic and functional results following operation. *Arch. Surg.* 35, 548–570.

Shames, G. H., Matthews, J., and Lutz, K. R. (undated). Audible Scales for Measuring Nasal Voice Quality in Adults. Report on Project 289. Univ. of Pittsburgh Speech Department and Office of Vocational Rehabilitation, University of Pittsburgh, Pittsburgh, Pennsylvania.

Sherman, Dorothy (1954). The merits of backward playing of connected speech in the scaling of voice quality disorders. *J. Speech Hearing Disorders* 19, 312–321.

Sherman, Dorothy, and Goodwin, F. (1954). Pitch level and nasality. *J. Speech Hearing Disorders* 19, 423–428.

Sherman, Dorothy, Spriestersbach, D. C., and Noll, J. D. (1959). Glottal stops in the speech of children with cleft palates. *J. Speech Hearing Disorders* 24, 37–42.

Siegel, G. M. (1960). Reliability of measurement in articulation testing procedures: A review of the literature. *Bull. Kansas Speech Hearing Assoc.* 1, 2, 4–11.

Simmons, J. R. (1955). The Influence of Inflection on Ratings of Nasality in Cleft Palate Speech. M. S. Thesis, Pennsylvania State Univ., University Park, Pennsylvania.

Smith, Jeanne K., Huffman, W. C., Lierle, D. M., and Moll, K. L. (1963). Results of pharyngeal flap surgery in patients with velopharyngeal incompetence. *Plastic Reconstruc. Surg.* 32, 493–501.

Smith, S. (1951). Vocalization and added nasal resonance. *Folia phoniat.* 3, 165–170.

Spriestersbach, D. C. (1955). Assessing nasal quality in cleft palate speech of children. *J. Speech Hearing Disorders* 20, 266–270.

Spriestersbach, D. C., and Curtis, J. F. (1951). Misarticulation and discrimination of speech sounds. *Quart. J. Speech* 37, 483–491.

Spriestersbach, D. C., and Powers, G. R. (1959a). Nasality in isolated vowels and connected speech of cleft palate speakers. *J. Speech Hearing Res.* 2, 40–45.

Spriestersbach, D. C., and Powers, G. R. (1959b). Articulation skills, velopharyngeal closure, and oral breath pressure of children with cleft palates. *J. Speech Hearing Res.* 2, 318–325.

Spriestersbach, D. C., Darley, F. L., and Rouse, Verna (1956). Articulation of a group of children with cleft lips and palates. *J. Speech Hearing Disorders* 21, 436–445.

Spriestersbach, D. C., Darley, F. L., and Morris, H. L. (1958). Language skills in children with cleft palates. *J. Speech Hearing Res.* 1, 279–285.

Spriestersbach, D. C., Moll, K. L., and Morris, H. L. (1961). Subject classification and articulation of speakers with cleft palates. *J. Speech Hearing Res.* 4, 362–372.

Starr, C. D. (1956). The Study of Some Characteristics of the Speech and Speech Mechanisms of a Group of Cleft Palate Children. Ph. D. Thesis, Northwestern Univ., Evanston, Illinois.

Steer, M. D., and Hanley, T. D. (1957). Instruments of diagnosis, therapy, and research. "Handbook of Speech Pathology" (L. E. Travis, ed.), pp. 174–245. Appleton, New York.

Stetson, R. H. (1951). "Motor Phonetics—A Study of Speech Movements in Action," 2nd ed. North-Holland Publ., Amsterdam.

Subtelny, Joanne D., and Subtelny, J. D. (1959). Intelligibility and associated physiological factors of cleft palate speakers. *J. Speech Hearing Res.* 2, 353 360.

Subtelny, Joanne D., Koepp–Baker, H., and Subtelny, J. D. (1961). Palatal function and cleft palate speech. *J. Speech Hearing Disorders* **26**, 213–224.

Templin, Mildred C. (1957). "Certain Language Skills in Children." Univ. of Minnesota Press, Minneapolis, Minnesota.

Trauner, R., and Doubek, F. (1956). I. A new procedure in velopharyngeal surgery for secondary operations on too short soft palates. II. The speech results compared with other surgical or prosthetic methods. *Brit. J. Plastic Surg.* **8**, 291–299.

Van Demark, D. R. (1964). Misarticulations and listener judgments of the speech of individuals with cleft palates. *Cleft Palate J.* **1**, 232–245.

Van Demark, D. R., and Van Demark, Ann A. (1967). Misarticulations of cleft palate children achieving velopharyngeal closure and children with functional speech problems. *Cleft Palate J.* **4**, 31–37.

Van Hattum, R. J. (1954). The Interrelationships Among Measures of Articulation and Nasality in Cleft Palate Speakers. Ph. D. Thesis, Pennsylvania State Univ., University Park, Pennsylvania.

Van Hattum, R. J. (1958). Articulation and nasality in cleft palate speakers. *J. Speech Hearing Res.* **1**, 383–387.

Van Riper, C. G. (1963). "Speech Correction: Principles and Methods," 4th ed. Prentice-Hall, Englewood Cliffs, New Jersey.

Van Riper, C. G., and Irwin, J. V. (1958). "Voice and Articulation." Prentice-Hall, Englewood Cliffs, New Jersey.

Veau, V. (1931). "Division Palatine." Masson, Paris.

Veau, V., and Borel-Maisonny, S. (1933). Les resultats fonctionnels de 200 staphylorraphies. *Bull. Soc. Nat. Chir.* **59**, 1372–1382.

Velander, E. (1952). Speech results following cleft palate with or without cheiloschisis. *Brit. J. Plastic Surg.* **5**, 72.

Wardill, W. E. M. (1933). Cleft palate. *Brit. J. Surg.* **21**, 347–369.

Weatherley-White, R. C. A., Dersch, W. C., and Anderson, R. M. (1964). Objective measurement of nasality in cleft palate patients: a preliminary report. *Cleft Palate J.* **1**, 120–124.

Weatherley-White, R. C. A., Stark, R. B., and De Haan, C. R. (1966). Acoustic analysis of speech: validation studies. *Cleft Palate J.* **3**, 291–300.

Weiss, A. I. (1954). Oral and Nasal Sound Pressure Levels as Related to Judged Severity of Nasality. Ph. D. Thesis, Purdue Univ., Lafayette, Indiana.

Williams, H. B., and Woolhouse, F. M. (1962). Comparison of speech improvement in cases of cleft palate after two methods of pharyngoplasty. *Plastic Reconstruc. Surg.* **30**, 36–42.

Williamson, A. B. (1944). Diagnosis and treatment of 84 cases of nasality. *Quart. J. Speech* **30**, 471–479.

Wilson, D. K., and O'Brien, L. W. (1953). An analysis of cleft palate speech without and with dental prosthesis. *Am. Assoc. Cleft Palate Rehabil. Newsletter* **3**, 3–6.

Wright, H. N. (1954). Reliability of evaluations during basic articulation and stimulation testing. *J. Speech Hearing Disorders* **19**, *Monogr. Suppl. No. 4*, 19–27.

Young, N. B. (1953). An Investigation of Intranasal Pressure During the Phonation of Consonant-Vowel Combinations and Sentences. M. A. Thesis, Univ. of Washington, Seattle, Washington.

IV

Etiological Bases for Speech Problems

Hughlett L. Morris

I. Articulation Disorders 121
   A. Anatomical and Physiological Bases 121
   B. Behavioral Bases 140
II. Voice Disorders 149
   A. Pitch 149
   B. Loudness 149
   C. Quality 150
III. Language Development 153
IV. Discussion 156
   A. Articulation 156
   B. Voice 162
   C. Language Development 164
V. Summary 165
   References 165

The task of describing the etiology or etiologies of a speech disorder is not one to be approached casually. First, since speech involves certain anatomical structures, consideration of etiology may involve the description of abnormal structures and their functions. Second, since speech is learned behavior, consideration of etiology may also involve description of the learning process and instances in which the "usual" methods of learning speech do not seem to apply. Finally, combinations of aberrations of the physiological and psychological aspects of speech in many instances may be contributory in "causing" the speech disorder. Thus, there are usually etiologies rather than an etiology when considering any type of speech disorder. These generalizations certainly apply to the communication problems of individuals with cleft palates. Several types of factors need to be taken into account when etiologies of these problems are considered. Some of the etiological factors appear to be related directly to the structural palatal deficiency. Other factors appear related to certain structural defects associated with, but not directly a part of, the cleft of the palate. Still other factors may be related to deviations in the learning process which may in turn be related to the psychosocial milieu within which the individual with a cleft palate functions. Still other factors appear relevant just because the child with a cleft palate is a child and children do not always learn speech in an orderly fashion. Furthermore, some variables may be considered to have stronger etiological significance at certain ages than at others. Lastly, consideration must be given to the possibility that while certain variables, individually, may not be etiologically important, a particular combination of them may be highly contributory in causing the speech disorder.

Various textbooks (Berry and Eisenson, 1956; Johnson *et al.*, 1956; West *et al.*, 1957; Travis, 1957; Van Riper and Irwin, 1958; Morley, 1962; Westlake and Rutherford, 1966) include discussions of factors considered to be causally related to the speech and language problems of speakers with cleft palate. In the majority of these texts the discussions of cleft palate as an etiological factor is relatively brief. In some the subject is treated in more detail and rather careful consideration is given to available research findings. In the several years since many of these texts have been published, however, there has been increasing interest in the area of cleft palate and specifically in the area of the etiology of speech problems of the cleft palate speaker. The result is a considerable increase in the body of information about cleft palate and its effect on speech. The purposes of this chapter, then, are to review in detail the available information on the causes of "cleft palate speech" and to present a point of view based on this information.

In the preparation of this material it has been assumed that the reader is not a beginning student in the study of speech pathology. It is further assumed that in evaluating the material presented here he will rely on a background which has provided him with information about causal factors of speech disorders such as "functional" misarticulations, disturbances in voice quality, and retardation in language development. These deviations will not be discussed here but knowledge of certain relationships developed in the consideration of them will be needed in the interpretation of evidence and in the formulation of inferences presented in this discussion.

Much has been written about the requisites for establishing a causal relationship between two factors. These requisites, in general, include a known relationship between the two factors, a temporal relationship between the two factors, and logical or intuitive support for the relationship in light of other relevant findings. Operationally, however, the statement of a causal relationship between two factors is an inference which often might depend, at least to some extent, upon the person making the inference. Different investigators and their audiences thus, with identical evidence, may not make the same inferences. It is important that this viewpoint be clear throughout the following discussion.

The speech and the language of individuals with clefts have been described earlier in this text. Generally, these individuals, as a group, have (1) defective articulation skills, (2) voice quality which is considered to be nasal, and (3) retarded speech (as children) according to some, or all, of the measures used to evaluate linguistic prowess. For purposes of organization, the etiologies of these facets of speech proficiency will be considered separately although there are, without doubt, several etiological factors which influence all three. The factors to be considered are velopharyngeal competence, oral-facial structures, hearing acuity, psychosocial adjustment, learning, and mental ability.

I. Articulation Disorders

A. ANATOMICAL AND PHYSIOLOGICAL BASES

1. *Velopharyngeal Incompetence*

The case for a causal relationship between velopharyngeal incompetence and the articulation errors which individuals with clefts demonstrate is based on some known relationships among articulation proficiency, intraoral breath pressure, and velopharyngeal competence.

The research findings of Stetson and Hudgins (1930), Hudgins and Stetson (1935), Black (1950), Stetson (1951), Arkebauer (1964), Isshiki and Ringel (1964), and Subtelny *et al.* (1966) indicate that breath pressure is impounded in the oral cavity of the speaker during the production of most of the consonant sounds. Although there is disagreement about the absolute quantities of pressure prerequisite for normal consonant productions, it is clear that fricatives, affricates, and plosives require most pressure; glides and semi-vowels less; and nasal consonants least. The fricatives, affricates, and plosives thus are frequently referred to as the "pressure" consonants. Without intraoral breath pressure, these consonants cannot be articulated. If there is nasal emission of oral pressure, that emission may distort the auditory perception of the "pressure" consonant being articulated.

The process whereby breath pressure is impounded in the oral cavity is not clearly understood. The two avenues through which air pressure from the lungs can be expelled are the mouth and the nostrils. The velopharyngeal mechanism serves to open or close the aperature to the nasal passage. Operationally, three positions of the velum are observed: (1) the velum raises to contact the pharyngeal walls, resulting in an open tract between the oral and pharyngeal cavities; (2) the velum rests against the tongue, resulting in an open tract between the nasal and pharyngeal cavities; and (3) the velum assumes a position between these two, resulting in at least a partial opening of both tracts. Breath pressure is not built up in the oral cavity when the velum rests against the tongue for the obvious reason that in this case air pressure escapes through the nostrils. When the velum is raised to contact the pharyngeal walls, the opening to the nasal passage is occluded, and the air pressure escapes through the oral cavity; with this position of the velum air flow in the oral cavity can be temporarily occluded, then released, as in the production of plosives, or it can be partially blocked as in the production of fricatives. A third position, with the velum between the tongue and the posterior pharyngeal wall and with an opening between the velum and the posterior pharyngeal wall, might reasonably be expected to allow breath pressure to escape through the nostrils. Both clinical and research evidence, however, do show that, under certain conditions, a limited amount of intraoral breath pressure can be impounded under this circumstance. Descriptions of the mechanism, or mechanisms, used to impound air when there is such an opening between the velum and the posterior pharyngeal walls have not been complete and investigation to obtain more information is needed.

Data by which indexes of intraoral pressure are related to velopharyngeal closure are somewhat limited. The results of several studies, cited below, are to be interpreted, however, as indicating the usefulness of information about the relationships between intraoral air pressure and degree of velopharyngeal comptence.

Wildman (1961), using 30 subjects with surgically closed palatal clefts, ages 12 to 20 years, correlated the amount of nasal emission during the production of nonsense syllables, and also the amount during continued blowing, with the size of velopharyngeal aperature shown on x-ray films while the speakers sustained the vowel /u/. Subjects who made sound substitutions, presumably with no nasal leak on those productions, were excluded. Resultant correlation coefficients were .74 for estimating strength of relationship between the size of aperature and emission on syllables and .57 for estimating strength of relationship between the size of opening and emission on continued blowing.

Holt (1959) studied the relationship between velopharyngeal opening, as measured on x-ray films while subjects sustained the vowel /u/, and wet spirometer ratios, that is, vital capacity measurements with nostrils open expressed as a percentage of the same measurements with nostrils occluded. Age and type of management employed for the clefts of the 36 subjects were not reported. The obtained coefficient of .26 was not significantly different from zero.

Buncke (1959), with 38 subjects all of whom had surgically repaired palatal clefts, used a water manometer to study palatal function under the condition of maximum effort and during the production of certain speech sounds. The maximum intraoral pressure, nostrils open, was obtained by having the subjects blow as hard as possible into the manometer. Maximum intraoral pressure, nostrils closed, was assessed by having the subject perform the same task, holding his nose. The maximum intranasal pressure was measured by placing a nasal bulb on the manometer tube and inserting the bulb into one nostril. The subject was then instructed to blow into an occluded section of tubing placed in his mouth with the unplugged nostril manually closed. The intranasal pressure measures were obtained not only for maximum effort but also during the production of /k/, /s/, and /m/ (without the mouthpiece). Lateral, still x-ray films taken during /s/ production were inspected to determine the relationship of the velum to the posterior pharyngeal wall. The subjects were divided into three groups according to judgments of speech proficiency as follows: (1) subjects with normal speech; (2) subjects with speech understandable at conversational levels, but characterized by "discernable stigmata of cleft palate speech"; and (3) subjects with grossly pathological speech. In the group of 14 subjects with normal speech, all showed velopharyngeal closure on x-ray films while only 6 had "normal" manometric readings. In the group of 18 with speech understandable but characterized by cleft palate stigmata, 1 had "normal" manometric readings, 5 had competence on maximum effort or test sounds but not both, and 12 speakers had escape of air during both conditions. In the group of 6 with grossly pathological speech, x-ray films for 3 showed lack of closure (films were not available for the other 3), and no interpretation of manometric performance is reported. Buncke made no generalizations about the relationship per se between the pressure measures and cephalometric observations of velopharyngeal competence. He concluded, however, that cleft palate patients who show manometric evidence of nasal escape of air on maximum effort and with speech, and who show velopharyngeal incompetence on x-ray films, are candidates for further palatal surgery.

Spriestersbach and Powers (1959b) correlated amount of velopharyngeal opening measured from x-ray films taken during the production of /u/ and of /s/ with ratios of wet spirometer and of oral manometer readings. Their groups ranged in size from 23 to 65 and were comprised of children, aged 5 through 15 years, all of whom had had palatal surgery. They computed their pressure ratios by dividing the reading, obtained on the spirometer (or manometer) with nostrils open by the reading obtained with nostrils occluded. The assumption was that, during the condition when the nostrils were occluded, escape of oral air pressure through the nasal passage was prevented, a condition which could be interpreted as a simulation of the occlusion of the posterior orifice to the nasal passage during complete velopharyngeal closure. If the two readings, nostrils open and nostrils occluded, were the same and a ratio of 1.00 was obtained, the subject was judged to have achieved velopharyngeal competence for the task. If, on the other hand, the reading obtained for the nostrils-open condition was lower than for the nostrils-occluded condition and the obtained ratio was less than 1.00 the subject was considered to have demonstrated velopharyngeal incompetence for the task. The obtained coefficients for estimating relationships were as follows: opening on /u/ with wet spirometer ratio, $-.69$; opening on /u/ with manometer ratio, $-.58$; opening on /s/ with wet spirometer ratio, $-.62$; and opening on /s/ with manometer ratio, $-.69$.

That there is a relationship between the ability to impound intraoral breath pressure and the ability to close off the nasopharyngeal orifice is adequately established by these findings; at the same time, however, the far from perfect correlation provides strong evidence that other factors also are important. Generally the techniques used were employed to distinguish between function and physiological event. The assessment of either or both nasal and oral air pressure during blowing, during the production of isolated speech sounds, or during the production of nonsense syllables has been taken to reflect the adequacy of function of the velopharyngeal mechanism. X-ray films, on the other hand, have been employed to evaluate the physiological activity of the mechanism during the same activities. There are disadvantages to both types of measures which will be discussed in some detail later.

Various studies have been designed to investigate the strength of the relationship between size of velopharyngeal opening and articulation skill. Some of these are discussed in the following paragraphs.

Hagerty and Hoffmeister (1954) categorized articulation defectiveness as being none, mild, moderate, or severe. Numerical values were assigned to these categories and correlation coefficients were computed for estimates of relationships between ratings of articulation defectiveness and measure of velopharyngeal distance, that is, the distance from velum to posterior pharyngeal wall, on lateral, still x-ray films. Coefficients between defectiveness and x-ray film measurements were .73 (/u/) and .78 (hissing).

Counihan (1956) used an 83-item articulation test which included consonants, both as singles and in blends, and vowels. Intelligibility of connected speech was rated on a 7-point scale. He measured the distance between the velum and the posterior pharyngeal wall as an index of degree of velopharyngeal competence. Correlation coefficients reported were .33 for articulation test score and velopharyngeal distance and .41 for intelligibility rating and velopharyngeal distance.

Pinson (1956) correlated measures of palatal efficiency with articulation test scores and also with measures of intelligibility. He used measures from

82-item articulation test; measures of intelligibility which were derived from a task in which judges answered questions the subjects had tape-recorded; and measures of palatal efficiency obtained from wet spirometer readings with the nostrils open and occluded. The latter measure was the mean of three differences for three trials for each of the two conditions, each difference being that between the two pressure measures with nostrils open and nostrils occluded. The correlation between the measure of palatal efficiency and each of the two speech measures was .08 for articulation and .03 for intelligibility.

Subtelny and Subtelny (1959) studied the relationships between articulation test scores for various classifications of speech sounds and degree of velopharyngeal constriction as measured on lateral, still x-ray films taken during the production of /u/. The articulation test scores were based upon the subject's ability to produce identifiable consonants appearing in simplified and controlled phonetic environments, that is, nonsense syllables. Judges made phonetic transcriptions of tape-recorded lists. Scores were percentages of consonants correctly transcribed by the judges. The authors have reported as follows:

> On the basis of total number of articulatory errors, subjects with the highest degree of articulatory proficiency were those whose associated velopharyngeal relationships closely approximated the normal. Ten subjects were found to have relatively good articulation. In eight of those 10 subjects velopharyngeal opening did not exceed 1.5 mm. This finding tends to support the premise that articulatory proficiency is associated with near normal velopharyngeal function.

Spriestersbach and Powers (1959b) correlated articulation test scores and also the ratios of these scores to reported norms with breath pressure ratios and with measures of velopharyngeal opening on x-ray films. To adjust for the effects of maturation on articulation proficiency, scores on the test were expressed as ratios of appropriate norms reported for the test. The numbers of 36 plosive items correct and of 36 fricatives items correct from the larger test were used as additional measures of articulatory proficiency. Ratios on an oral manometer and a wet spirometer were formulated by expressing the pressure reading obtained with the nostrils open as a ratio of the reading obtained with the nostrils occluded. Measurements of the velopharyngeal distance on lateral, still x-ray films for /s/ and /u/ were also obtained. Significant coefficients were reported for all pairs of variables with highest coefficients obtained for the relationships between the spirometer ratios and the sores for the two shorter articulation tests involving the plosives and the fricatives.

Subtelny et al. (1961) also studied the relationships between word-syllable intelligibility and the degree of velopharyngeal constriction. Judges transcribed lists of nonsense syllables and words which had been tape-recorded by adults with cleft palate. Scores were in terms of percentage loss of intelligibility. Lateral, still head x-ray films for production of /u/ were used. The following correlation coefficients were reported between measures of velopharyngeal constriction and various intelligibility scores: overall word-syllable intelligibility, .57; plosive intelligibility, .51; glide intelligibility, .35; and fricative intelligibility, .21. All coefficients were significant except the one for fricatives. The authors reported that 92% of speakers with "good" intelligibility either had velopharyngeal closure or missed contact by only 1 or 2 mm. The intelligibility of speakers who missed velopharyngeal closure by distances ranging from 4 to 7 mm was severely defective.

Morris et al. (1961) studied the articulation skills of two groups of children with surgically repaired cleft palate, one group with velopharyngeal competence and one group with velopharyngeal incompetence, as defined by oral pressure ratios and velopharyngeal dimensions from lateral, still x-ray films. The two groups were matched subject-by-subject for age, sex, type of cleft, socioeconomic status, and intelligence. No subject had a hearing loss considered to be educationally handicapping. Comparisons of measurements of facial morphology and ratings of dental models indicated that there were no significant differences between the two groups in facial morphology, continuity of cutting edge of anterior teeth, palatal contour, or anteroposterior relationship of upper and lower incisors. The assumption thus was that any existing variation in articulatory proficiency could best be accounted for by variations in ability to impound air in the oral cavity and thus in ability to achieve velopharyngeal closure. A 176-item articulation test was administered to the subjects. Of those items, 43 were found to be most discriminating between the two velopharyngeal competence groups. Those 43 items consisted of plosives, fricatives, and affricates which require intraoral pressure for normal production. Further analysis of the 176-item test results, not included in the published report, provided evidence the scores for those with good velopharyngeal competence are higher than the scores for those with poor velopharyngeal competence.

Spriestersbach et al. (1961) have reported with reference to proficiency of a large group of children with cleft palate. A 176-item articulation test was employed; the criterion was proportion of items correct. Pressure ratios were computed in the conventional way using a wet spirometer and three subgroups were formed: children with ratios higher than .90, children with ratios of .51 to .89, and children with ratios lower than .50. The differences between the .90-and-above-ratio group and each of the two lower-ratio groups were significant. These investigators conclude that, of the variables they studied, the ability to impound intraoral breath pressure, and thus, inferentially, to achieve velopharyngeal competence, is the variable most closely related to the articulation skills of children with cleft palate.

McDermott (1962), with a sample of 52 children with cleft palate, studied the articulatory proficiency for the phoneme /s/ in relation to several variables. To obtain breath pressure ratios he used an oral manometer with a constant leak or bleed in the pressure system. He used the same classification system for categorizing pressure ratios that Spriestersbach, Moll, and Morris had employed and obtained similar significant intergroup differences and a similar significant difference between the subject group with the highest pressure ratios and the two groups with lower ratios for the articulation of /s/.

Shelton *et al.* (1964) correlated measures of velopharyngeal closure and articulation skill for 31 individuals who had either surgically repaired cleft palates or "palatal inadequacies" without clefts. The obtained correlation coefficient was .52. They used a mean of measurements of velopharyngeal opening from cinefluorographic film and an articulation measure from a test which included a variety of speech sounds.

In a later study, Shelton *et al.* (1965) correlated articulation proficiency measures and several measures which were considered to be indicative of velopharyngeal function. Oral breath pressure ratios were obtained by use of an oral manometer. Readings of nasal breath pressure on a U-tube water manometer were taken during vowels and syllables. A mean measurement of velopharyngeal distance was obtained from measurements of each frame for all phonation in selected isolated sounds, nonsense syllables, and sentences. The highest correlation coefficient (.78) reported for any pair of the four variables was that for articulation proficiency and mean velopharyngeal opening. Other coefficients were considerably lower, ranging from .08 to .29.

Brandt and Morris (1965) correlated velopharyngeal opening and articulation test score for 62 children with surgically repaired cleft palates. The measures of velopharyngeal opening were made from lateral, still x-ray films taken during the phonation of /u/ and of /s/. The articulation test consisted of 109 elements which included fricatives, affricates, plosives, nasals, and glides. Correlations were .60 for /u/ and articulation test score, and .54 for /s/ and articulation test score.

Barnes and Morris (1967) correlated several kinds of manometer ratios with several kinds of articulation test scores for 85 subjects with cleft palate. In general, correlations ranged from .50 to .69, with the highest one between the positive manometer ratio with bleed and a 34-item test of plosive sounds.

Some of the most convincing evidence of a causal relationship between velopharyngeal opening and articulation proficiency comes from information dealing with the dependence of varying relationships between these two factors upon the requirements of certain consonants for intraoral pressure.

Subtelny and Subtelny (1959) investigated the relationships between velopharyngeal measurements and the number of articulation errors on plosives, glides, and fricatives. They obtained correlations between velopharyngeal measurements and number of errors on plosives ranging from .36 to .69. They reported that number of errors on plosives increased appreciably when the velopharyngeal opening exceeded 5 mm. Few errors on plosives were observed when closure of the velopharyngeal space was not complete but nearly so. They interpreted these findings to indicate that complete velopharyngeal closure is not essential for production of plosives but that these consonant sounds could be expected to be defective when the velopharyngeal distance exceeded certain limits. No relationships were demonstrated between palatopharyngeal distance and the number of errors on glides or fricatives. It was also noted that many articulatory errors appeared to be nonrelated to amount of velopharyngeal opening. Further, errors on fricatives occurred almost twice as often as errors on plosives with subjects who showed velopharyngeal openings of 2 mm or less.

Spriestersbach *et al.* (1961) reported mean percentages of consonant elements, classified according to manner of production, which were produced correctly by subjects categorized according to wet spirometer ratios (nostrils open/nostrils occluded). Three pressure ratio groups were used: subjects with ratios of .90 or more, those with ratios of .51 to .89, and those with ratios of .50 or less. For all manner-of-production categories (nasals, glides, stop plosives, fricatives, and afffricates), average scores of the highest pressure ratio group were higher than those of the lower two pressure groups. The differences in articulation performance between the group with highest ratios and the other two groups were, however, much greater for the stop plosives, fricatives, and affricates than for the nasals and the glides. The largest differences among pressure groups occurred on the fricatives. The authors concluded that more stringent oral pressure requirements exist for production of fricatives and afffricates than for stop plosives.

Subtelny *et al.* (1961) investigated loss of intelligibility (not articulation correctness) as a function of velopharyngeal competence. They found that average loss of intelligibility for fricatives increased, almost tripled, from 6.15% for subjects with complete velopharyngeal closure to 17.31% for subjects with small, that is .5 to 3.0 mm, velopharyngeal openings. With the same subjects, they did not find a similar loss of intelligibility for plosives. In addition, the difference in intelligibility of fricatives between speakers with velopharyngeal openings ranging in size from 3.5 to 7 mm and those with openings ranging from 7.5 to 11 mm was large, although the difference in intelligibility of plosives was again negligible.

Pitzner and Morris (1966) compared scores for vowel-diphthong, plosive, fricative-affricate, nasal-glide, and vocalic /r/ and /l/ tests for two groups of subjects classified according to adequacy of spirometer ratios. Forty-six subjects had ratios higher than .90 and 38 subjects had ratios lower than .89. On each of the five subtests, the group of subjects with high pressure ratios obtained higher test scores than those subjects with low pressure ratios. The differences between the two groups were much smaller for the vowel-diphthong and nasal-glide sounds, which are not associated with great amounts of intraoral pressure, than for the plosive and fricative-affricate sounds. The relatively great difference between the two groups on the vocalic /r/ and /l/ subtest is apparently related to faulty learning since those phonemes clearly are not associated with great amounts of intraoral pressure. Pitzner and Morris also compared the articulation skills of the group of subjects with high pressure ratios with articulation skills of normal children and found that except for fricatives and affricates, the two groups, cleft palate and normal, were highly similar. They speculated that the difference on fricatives and affricates might be due to the high incidence of dental problems in the cleft palate group. Such problems, in their opinion, could not be expected to affect the articulation of vowels, diphthongs, plosives, nasals, glides, and vocalic /r/ and /l/ as much as they might affect fricatives and affricates. In the comparison of the data for subjects with low pressure ratios and the nomative data, the subjects with clefts obtained scores on the vowel-diphthong and nasal-glide subtests which were essentially like those scores reported for the normal group of children.

Brandt and Morris (1965) correlated size of velopharyngeal opening measured from lateral, still x-ray films taken during /s/ and /u/ with fricative, plosive, and nasal-glide articulation tests. Correlations between size of opening and test score were comparable in strength for fricatives, .59 and .61, for plosives, .50 and .59, and also, although much lower, for nasals and glides, .06 and .01.

Barnes and Morris (1967) correlated four kinds of manometer ratios with scores on a plosive and a fricative articulation test. For each type of ratio, the correlation was higher with plosives than with fricatives. Representative of the correlations are those for the positive ratio with bleed: .69 for plosives, and .53 for fricatives.

Warren and associates have reported data which are relevant to these findings (1964, 1966). He employed a model in the study of the effects of oral port size on pressure-flow relationships in the upper pharynx. His findings indicate that the differences in measurements of air pressure and air flow between simulated plosives and fricatives are greater for small velopharyngeal orifices than for larger velopharyngeal orifices. He considers an area of velopharyngeal opening of .20 cm^2 as being the cut-off value between the two groupings of large and small openings. This finding is roughly similar to that of Subtelny and Subtelny (1959) and supports the contention that there are differences between plosives and fricatives in associated oral breath pressure.

The above reported findings indicate that those consonants which have relatively high oral pressure requirements for normal production are importantly impaired by velopharyngeal incompetence. Conversely, those consonants which require very little oral pressure are not misarticulated in relation to increase in size of velopharyngeal opening.

Although this discussion refers frequently to amount of intraoral pressure requisite to the production of certain speech sounds, there is evidence to indicate that equal importance must be given to the temporal factor, that is, the length of time during which the pressure is maintained in the oral cavity. Subtelny *et al.* (1966) have reported the use of a measure of duration of pressure; and Arkebauer (1964) has reported the use of a criterion on integrated pressure obtained by tracing, with a planimeter, the area subscribed by the pressure write-out system, thereby taking into account the period of time during which pressure was maintained. Both investigations have demonstrated that more pressure is associated with plosives than with fricatives. For any final conclusions to be reached, additional research is needed.

In summary, the available data indicate that velopharyngeal incompetence results in defective articulation because of the loss of intraoral breath pressure required in the correct production of the majority of consonants in the English language. That a relationship between velopharyngeal opening and articulation proficiency does exist has been established; the strength of this relationship, however, is not, in general, high and is to be estimated by a correlation coefficient of approximately .50. Considering the fact that so many different techniques have been used in the study of the relationship between speech proficiency and velopharyngeal adequacy of cleft palate speakers, it is astonishing that the results are in such good agreement.

One difference among studies is in the criterion employed as a measure of speech proficiency. Several investigators have used measures based upon the number of correct productions of speech sounds in a series of single-word responses; others have evaluated only the intelligibility of the sounds tested; and still others have used psychological rating scales of general defectiveness of articulation during connected speech. Another difference among studies with respect to the criterion of speech proficiency comes from variation in the composition of the speech sample used. In spite of these differences among criteria of speech proficiency, however, results in general indicate that correlation between velopharyngeal incompetence and number of errors on the so-called pressure consonants is higher than correlation between velopharyngeal incompetence and number of errors on glides and semivowels. The consistency of these results, in spite of the varying methodologies, is somewhat surprising and thus may be accepted as strong evidence indicating a real difference.

There are differences also among the measures used to assess velopharyngeal adequacy. Some investigators have used independent measures of oral and nasal pressures and air flow; others have used ratios between the two readings. In addition, the various types of instrumentation which have been used for obtaining pressure measures may have a differential influence upon these measures. Morris and Smith (1962), for example, have pointed out that measures of intraoral pressure will not be the same for an open as for a closed pressure system. Pressure measures also may differ from one study to another with respect to reliability; and, although such differences would not lead to contradictory results, they would probably lead to variations in statistical significance of results. Reliability of measures is often difficult to assess because sufficient information is not available to the reader.

Results of studies employing the general x-ray technique, which has been useful in studying velopharyngeal dimensions, have also differed. To account for some of the differences among results may be variations in procedures for such as the following: positioning subjects for the films; preparation of the films for measurement; choice of landmarks; and measurement techniques.

2. Oral Facial Structures

Many writers have considered and evaluated etiological factors accounting for the speech problems of individuals with cleft palate with particular reference to the importance of oral facial structures such as the lips, the teeth, the hard palate, the oral and nasal cavities, and the two dental arches in relationship to each other.

a. *Cleft Lip.*   West *et al.* (1957) state that the condition of the repaired cleft lip usually disturbs only the sounds involving the upper lip, with the /p/ and /b/ the ones most seriously affected. No research evidence is cited, however. Koepp-Baker (1957) feels that the function of the repaired cleft lip in cleft palate speakers is probably not normal, but qualifies this statement by adding that since lip movement in the articulation of bilabial sound is, in the normal person, relatively gross, the effect of lip deformity is probably less critical than is supposed.

Spriestersbach *et al.* (1961) have reported evidence which indicates that the repaired cleft lip has no effect on speech production. In their study of various subject classifications they concluded that the articulation of children who had had only a cleft lip should not be included in analyses of the articulation skills of children with cleft lip and palate or cleft palate only. Although such specific statements have not been made by other authors, agreement with them appears to be prevalent in recent cleft palate research for, with few exceptions, investigations of speech skills of children with clefts do not include children with cleft lip only.

Further indirect support of the thesis that the cleft lip has little or no effect on speech may be found in the evidence that, as a group, speakers with cleft of the lip and palate show better articulation than speakers with cleft palate only. A possible inference is that cleft lip has a facilitating effect on speech. This, however, seems highly improbable, and careful consideration of the basis for the articulation differences between these groups leads to the more reasonable assumption that these differences may be accounted for by differences in the amount of palatal tissue and that the presence of a cleft lip may be irrelevant. If the surgically repaired cleft lip is of sufficient size and mobility to allow closing and opening the mouth, it probably is not etiologically significant in articulation problems.

b. *Tongue Motility and Carriage.*   Several authors have speculated that the structural deviation of the cleft lip or palate extends to the tongue or that the tongues of individuals with cleft palates do at least show deviant patterns of mobility and coordination important in the etiology of "cleft palate speech." Brown and Oliver (1940) examined the peripheral speech structures of 33 subjects with cleft palate for possible adverse effect of these structures upon speech production. In their opinion, 14 subjects showed tongue activity which they believed would have a possible or almost certain adverse effect on speech. It is important to point out that Brown and Oliver made no attempt to explain why the tongue activities of their subjects were deviant; that is, they did not discuss the question of whether the cause was "organic" or "functional." In addition they did not demonstrate that the tongue activities were indeed deviant: they merely judged that the tongue activities affected speech adversely.

Berry (1949) maintained that many of the articulation errors made by cleft palate speakers are unrelated to the palatal or lip cleft but are caused by poor motility and coordination of the tongue. Data were not reported to support her contentions.

Matthews and Byrne (1953) obtained measurements of tongue flexibility for 19 children with cleft palate and/or lip and for 19 normal children who were matched with the cleft group for age, sex, grade, and level of intelligence. Five nonspeech tasks were devised to assess gross tongue movements and three tasks were employed to assess movements during speech production. No significant differences were obtained between the cleft and noncleft groups for any of the five nonspeech tasks and for one of the speech tasks. The authors conclude that children with clefts do not demonstrate inferior overall tongue flexibility.

Morley (1962), in discussing the matter of abnormal tongue action, has stated that it seems probable that the existence of the cleft palate in some way influences the movements of the tongue tip. The deviant movements, in her opinion, may date even from prenatal life or from compensatory activity developed to assist in sucking during infancy. She also believes in the possibility that the existence of an open cleft of the palate may delay the development of activity in the tongue tip. No data are reported to support these contentions.

In summary, the data reported by Matthews and Byrne provide the only evidence available regarding the matter of deviant tongue structure and deviant tongue motility of cleft palate speakers. Their data demonstrate that cleft palate speakers are able to perform certain nonspeech tasks with the tongue as fast as can normal individuals. The differences between the two groups of speakers for speech tasks can probably be accounted for without reference to any possibility of deviant tongue activity. All of the children with clefts were having speech therapy and indeed had had therapy for an average of 3 years. It seems reasonable to assume that, as a group, they were having difficulty making the speech sounds involved in the assigned speech task (although the authors made no mention of it) and that they may have slowed up the rate of production to produce the best speech sounds of which they were capable. The obvious conclusion, according to currently available information, is that tongue coordination and flexibility are not etiological factors in the speech problems of individuals with cleft palate. That such deviations are characteristic of these individuals seems highly improbable.

Tongue carriage has received most attention as a probable influence upon voice quality. It at least should be considered, however, as of possible importance in relation to articulation proficiency, although at present there is little, if any, evidence of any such relation. As Koepp-Baker (1957) pointed out, there are instances of narrow palatal vaults or shallow vaults which effectively reduce the size of the intraoral cavity and which may result in deviant tongue carriage both in the vertical and the anteroposterior dimensions. Occlusal problems may also affect tongue carriage and thus result in a reduction in the size of the intraoral space, particularly if the maxillary arch fits inside the mandibular arch. Not even for cases where the intraoral cavity is restricted in size and where the tongue is habitually positioned unusually high or unusually posteriorly, however, is evidence available to demonstrate that such malpositioning interferes with normal articulation. Any definite conclusions thus must await investigation planned specifically to answer the indicated questions.

Mention should be made of the recent concern over what is referred to as the tongue-thrust syndrome and its relationship to articulation. The literature contains reports about this phenomenon and its incidence in the "normal" individual. No research data have been reported which suggest that the syndrome is any more characteristic of individuals with clefts than of others.

c. *Dentition.* Dental deviations are viewed by many authors to be an important etiological factor in the speech problems of individuals with cleft palates because of the facts that many children with clefts have malocclusions and that the teeth are considered to have an important role in the production of labiodental, linguadental, and postdental fricatives (Westlake and Rutherford, 1966).

Brown and Oliver (1940) reported that 30 of their 33 subjects had missing teeth or gaps between the anterior teeth, and that 28 had occlusal deviations; they considered both factors might possibly have an adverse effect on speech.

Counihan (1956) studied the relationship between speech performance and a series of judgments regarding size, motility, and probable hazard of various oral-facial parameters to speech. He reported that speakers with dental occlusions which were judged to be of no probable hazard to speech did better in the articulation of tongue-tip sound than did those with occlusions judged to be of a moderate to severe hazard to speech. Similarly, the subject with a maxillary arch judged to be as wide as or wider than the mandibular arch did better on the average than the one with a maxillary arch narrower than the mandibular arch; and the one with a palatal vault which was excessively high or of average height did better on the average than the one with a very low palatal vault. Bzoch (1956), who made studies of subjects with cleft palate generally comparable to the study by Counihan except for the fact that his subjects were younger, did not find the differences Counihan found.

Subtelny and Subtelny (1959) studied the anteroposterior relationship of the anterior teeth and articulation proficiency. Lateral, still x-ray films were taken during occlusion; and the distance between the maxillary and mandibular incisors was measured. The number of articulation errors was not found to be consistently nor significantly related to incisor relationship.

Greene (1960), who studied the articulation of 263 subjects with surgically managed cleft palate, reported that 50 speakers had "lateral articulation" which, in her opinion, was not related to the competence of the velopharyngeal sphincter but to the presence of "oral irregularities." Sibilants, palatal fricatives, and affricates were most commonly involved. She reports further (p. 45) that "... prognosis is improved by orthodontic treatment and by prostheses that fill spaces between the teeth or provide a better contour of the maxillary arch. In some cases orthodontic treatment alone corrects the speech defect."

Foster and Greene (1960) extended the evaluation by Greene (1960) by studying the effect of oral anomalies on the speech proficiency of 102 of Greene's subjects, aged 7 years or more, who were "using the oral cavities in articulation" and who were also receiving treatment in the dental department of their institution. They hypothesized that collapse of the maxillary arch with consequent reduction in tongue space or gaps between upper and lower teeth and that spaces between adjacent teeth in the region of the alveolar cleft might be causally related to articulation errors. Dental casts for patients with lateral and normal articulation were examined. Neither in gaps in occlusion nor in extent of existing alveolar cleft was any difference observed between these two articulation groups; however, a significant difference between the two articulation groups was found in the amount of maxillary collapse.

In an effort to explore and describe factors which might differentiate among speakers who have similar velopharyngeal adequacy but who demonstrate dissimilar articulation skills, seven of whom had adequate velopharyngeal closure and seven of whom had inadequate closure as determined by still x-ray films, Powers (1960, 1962) made observations of 14 individuals with surgically managed cleft palate. Among his observations of the oral structures were ratings made from dental casts with reference to the following factors: anteroposterior relationships, continuity of the cutting edges of the teeth, and palatal contours. Considerable variability was observed among subjects. One subject with good velopharyngeal closure had a relatively low articulation score but misarticulated only the /s/ and /z/. Dental ratings for this subject were below the average ratings for the group and, in Powers' opinion, dentition may have had a detrimental effect on articulation. He compared two subjects with good velopharyngeal closure, one with good and one with poor articulation. Although ratings of continuity of cutting edge were similar for the two subjects, the subject with good speech had essentially normal anteroposterior arch relationships while the one with poor speech was rated as having all upper incisors in lingual version. The subject with good speech was judged to have a deep and narrow palatal contour in contrast to a flat palatal contour for the poor speaker. When two subjects without velopharyngeal closure were compared, however, the subject with poor speech received more favorable ratings of the oral structures than did the one with good speech. The subject with good speech was rated as completely lacking in continuity of cutting edge and as having poor anteroposterior dental relationships.

McDermott (1962), in his study of the production of /s/ by individuals with cleft palate, rated anteroposterior relationships of the dental arches, vertical relationships of the anterior dental structures, continuity of cutting edge of the anterior teeth, and general configuration of the hard palate. Three subgroups of subjects were formed for each of the rated items: subjects with severe deviations, those with moderate deviations, and those with slight deviations. The only significant difference among the three subgroups selected was with respect to the ratings of anteroposterior dental arch relationships.

It seems pertinent to point out in this discussion that, as reported by Bloomer (1957) and by Spriestersbach (1965), although there is a relatively large body of data obtained for the purpose of evaluating the relationship between dentition and speech for noncleft subjects, the evidence in general does not support a conclusion that, on the average, any important relationship exists. Representative of the studies is that reported by Snow (1961). A large percentage of her group of children who had "defective" teeth were able to make correctly the six fricatives which she tested; and a considerable number of children with normal teeth were not able to produce the fricatives correctly. In view of this kind of information, it would seem unreasonable to expect to find evidence of a relationship between dentition and speech for the cleft palate population in general. This is not to say, of course, that defective dentition might not, in individual instances, be of etiological importance as a cause of defective articulation.

Although deviations in anteroposterior and vertical dental relationships and continuity of cutting edges typically are unrelated to misarticulations of persons with cleft palate, specific individuals may lack desired articulation skill because of an overbite or because of missing or malpositioned teeth.

d. *Combinations of Factors.* One point emerges clearly from the above discussion of the effects of deviations of the orofacial structures on speech: that is, consideration must be given to the possibility that, individually, any one factor which has been considered might be unimportant in the production of speech by a person with a cleft but the combined effect of several factors might be very important etiologically. Of relevance are findings reported by Bzoch (1956). Considered singly, no significant differences in articulation proficiency were found in relation to the three variables of velar activity: pharyngeal wall movement, amount of restriction by faucial pillars on velum, and degree of concavity of the posterior pharyngeal wall. Bzoch noted, however, that all subjects in the group who demonstrated good articulation were judged to have fair or good activity of the velum and pharyngeal walls, no binding of the velum by the pillars, and no concavity of posterior wall. He selected 11 children from that group and compared them to a similar group of children who were judged deficient in one or more areas. There was a significant difference in articulation proficiency between the two groups.

Also relevant are data reported by McDermott (1962) and discussed in the preceding section. When the five variables of anteroposterior relationships of the dental arches, vertical relationships of the anterior dental structures, continuity of the cutting edges of the anterior teeth, configuration of the hard palate, and tongue motility were considered individually, a significant difference in proficiency for the /s/ was found only for the comparison between the anterioposterior relationships of the dental arches. When three new subgroups were formed in accordance with results of adding for each subject the scores for all variables, significant differences in articulation proficiency between the severe and the slight and between the severe and the moderate groups provided evidence that the combined effect of several deviations in oral facial structure is, in general, important.

The conclusion from the above discussion, then, is that, while such deviations do not necessarily result in articulation problems for cleft palate speakers as a group, any one of them or any combination of them may be etiologically important in the clinical evaluation of the speech of a person with cleft palate.

e. *Nasal Cavities.* Although relatively little research on the adequacy of the nasal cavities and the effects of nasal cavity deviations on articulation skills has been reported, it seems reasonable to assume that, in some instances, occluded nasal passageways actually assist in correct speech sound articulation. Speakers who would not be able to prevent nasal leak during the production of pressure consonants by means of palatopharyngeal action might achieve partial occlusion because of nasal obstruction or because of development of movement of the alae to occlude the nasal chambers anteriorly. Clinical observation does indeed indicate that such alar movements develop only as a result of velopharyngeal inadequacy. Sometimes the movement is easily observed, with movement not just of the alae but also accompanying movement of the forehead, the brows, and the lips. At other times the action is not visible and can be detected only by feeling alar contractions with the finger tips. Occasionally a speaker is observed who appears to flare the nostrils but who, on further investigation, actually constricts areas of the alar wings posterior to the nares. Nares constriction, then, is simply an attempt to prevent nasal escape of air which normally would be blocked by the action of the velopharyngeal mechanism.

Partial nasal obstruction in the individual may result from a deviated nasal septum, a deviation observed so frequently that it becomes part of the unilateral cleft syndrome. Little is known about the effect of varying degrees of nasal obstruction. Individuals, however, sometimes demonstrate nasal obstruction and/or nares constriction and at the same time produce relatively "normal" direction of air pressure even though not able to achieve velopharyngeal competence according to evidence from x-ray films.

Bzoch (1956) rated, for 55 subjects, degree of nasal obstruction with reference to frontal, still, x-ray films. Of his subject group, 2% had complete obstruction, 8.33% had minor obstruction, and 16.67% had a normally free airway. For evaluation of speech data, Bzoch considered subjects who were rated to have complete, almost complete, or partial obstruction as having "considerable obstruction." Subjects who had minor obstruction and those with a normally free airway were described as having "essentially no obstruction." Subjects with considerable nasal obstruction had significantly better articulation, as measured by an articulation test, and were judged to be significantly more intelligible during connected speech than were subjects with essentially no nasal obstruction. The effect of velopharyngeal competence upon this relationship was not considered in this investigation; but it should be pointed out that approximately half of the subjects exhibited, by measurements from lateral, still x-ray films, openings of 5 mm or greater for the vowel /u/. It thus may be assumed that a considerable proportion of the subjects who showed nasal obstruction by frontal x-ray films also showed velopharyngeal incompetence during the production of /u/.

Powers (1960, 1962) made direct observations of degree of nasal obstruction and alar constriction during speech in his cinefluorographic study of 14 speakers with cleft palate, 7 with good and 7 with poor velopharyngeal closure. While only one subject in the good closure group showed alar constriction, 6 of the 7 subjects in the poor closure group exhibited such behavior. Four subjects were selected for further study: one with good closure and good speech; one with good closure and poor speech; one with poor closure and good speech; and one with poor closure and poor speech. While both subjects with poor velopharyngeal closure demonstrated alar movement, the one with good speech showed more alar movement than the one with poor speech.

The above findings suggest that, in the presence of velopharyngeal incompetence, nasal obstruction and nares constriction apparently may be utilized to assist in impounding intraoral breath pressure for the production of speech sounds and thus should be considered when the articulatory skills of individuals with cleft palates are evaluated.

3. *Hearing Acuity*

The incidence of and the bases for hearing loss in cleft palate speakers have been described elsewhere (Chapter V). In general, a greater proportion of individuals with cleft palate than of those without appear to have hearing losses; typically the losses are fluctuating, conductive, bilateral, and related to middle ear pathology; the incidence of hearing loss for the cleft palate population decreases with age.

Various authors have pointed out that a child with hearing impaired may not use appropriate speech sounds because he has not heard the sounds, or because he has heard them in a distorted fashion during the early language learning years. The degree of hearing loss required to affect the acquisition of speech sounds, however, has not been clearly established. Davis and Silverman (1960) suggest that hearing levels for speech which are 30 dB or more above normal will interfere with the hearing (and learning) of speech sounds. Spriestersbach *et al.* (1962) have defined as educationally significant those losses in the better ear which are 30 dB or greater for the speech frequencies. Certainly there are considerable individual differences among children, whether they have clefts or not, in the ways in which they respond to hearing losses; but a hearing loss of 30 dB or more for the speech frequencies which persists for two or three years before the child is 5 or 6 years of age clearly could result in the retardation of articulation skills.

Spriestersbach *et al.* found educationally significant hearing loss, as defined above, for 8 (5.5%) of a group of 163 children with cleft lip and palate or cleft palate only. Retardation of articulation skills for these 8 children, then, might be attributable to hearing impairment. Five of the children were younger than 6 years; 3 were between the ages of 7 and 12 years.

Graham (1962) obtained audiometric results for 190 children with cleft lip, cleft palate, or cleft lip and palate, who ranged in age at the time of examination from 8 to 22 years. From hospital charts, he obtained for 175 of the children (omitting the 15 children with cleft lip only, all of whom had demonstrated essentially no hearing loss at the time of examination) audiograms which had been recorded when the children were between the ages of 4 and 6 years. Four of the 175 children (2.3%) demonstrated mean losses for 500, 1000, and 2000 cps of 30 dB or greater in the better ear. If it can be assumed that pure tone tests are reliable for children between the ages of 4 and 6 years, it would seem reasonable to believe that approximately 2% of children with cleft palate in this age group are handicapped, because of hearing impairment, in learning speech sounds. With the same criterion for defining hearing loss, 3 (1.7%) of the 175 children had losses when they were 8 years of age or older.

Because audiometric techniques are difficult to use with very young children we have very little data about hearing levels of children with clefts at ages during which language is beginning (18 months to 4 years). Relevant to this discussion, however, are data reported by Graham to the effect that 48% of his 190 subjects had a history of ear disease as reported by the parents. Of the same total group 39.5% had bilateral abnormalities of tympanic membranes as determined during the experimental examination. These data indicate that the children probably had conductive hearing losses during the early years of life even though such losses were not documented at the time.

Sensorineural hearing loss (as opposed to conduction loss) may, of course, be expected to occur in the cleft palate population at least as often as in the noncleft population. Such loss may interfere seriously with the learning of many of the high frequency consonant sounds, depending on the age at which the loss is incurred and upon the severity of the loss. There is no evidence, however, to indicate that sensorineural hearing loss occurs more frequently in individuals with clefts than in those without.

It appears, then, that hearing loss severe enough to impair the development of articulation proficiency occurs for a relatively small percentage of children with cleft palate. However, if a loss does develop it is likely to occur at a young enough age to hinder the acquisition of articulation skills. Since the evidence indicates that the losses for these children are usually transient, probably they typically have no lasting effect on the learning of speech skills. Undoubtedly, however, there are exceptions; and enough children with clefts have educationally significant hearing losses over an extended period of time that this possibility should be carefully considered in a diagnostic evaluation of the child's problems.

B. Behavioral Bases

Some of the misarticulations in the speech of individuals with cleft palate are apparently functional, that is, unrelated to anatomical and physiological anomalies. Spriestersbach et al. (1961) reported differences in articulation proficiency within a group of subjects who had pressure ratios of .90 or more, a ratio presumably representing adequate or nearly adequate for velopharyngeal closure. While many in the group had essentially no articulation errors, others did have errors and one subject produced only 36% of the articulation test items correctly. Possible anatomical and physiological bases other than velopharyngeal incompetence which might account for the misarticulations of these subjects were not specifically evaluated, but the findings indicate that there may have been behavioral as well as structural bases for the articulation errors. The behavioral bases to be considered here are psychosocial and learning factors, which, although they are to be discussed separately in the following sections, are quite probably strongly related to each other.

1. Psychosocial Bases

Before discussing the influence of such variables as personality, attitudes, and emotional adjustment upon the acquisition of speech sounds by persons with cleft palate, it seems appropriate to point out that the effect of such factors upon the development of articulation proficiency of "normal" speakers is controversial. Research has usually been for the purpose of evaluating either the adjustment of the child himself or the patterns of parental personality and the general emotional environment within which the child with functional misarticulations lives. There is little directly pertinent research evidence to support the contention that functional articulation disorders may be caused by personality maladjustment. There is, however, some disagreement about this point. McCarthy (1954a, p. 623), in her extensive treatment of language development in children, presents a summary "... of a number of significant contributions in this area which the writer believes point to an emotional and functional explanation of most of the language disorder syndromes and indicate that these emotional disturbances are for the most part environmentally determined."

Although many authors have speculated on the possibility that the impaired speech of children with cleft lip and palate probably results in some degree of maladjustment, there is little evidence to support the contention. Sidney and Matthews (1956) reported that children with clefts do not differ from normal children on standardized personality tests, a teacher's rating scale of social adjustment, or a sociometric questionnaire. Palmer and Adams (1962) found no differences between cleft palate and normal children on projective test drawings of faces. Watson (1964) also found no differences in personality adjustment among boys with cleft lip and palate, boys who were chronically physically disabled, and normal boys. Watson (1964) is the only investigator who obtained ratings of articulation defectiveness for cleft palate subjects for the purpose of evaluating the possibility of relationship between adjustment and speech proficiency. He reports obtaining nonsignificant correlation coefficients for estimating the relationships between the speech ratings and the five adjustment scales of the Rogers Personal Adjustment Inventory.

It may be concluded, then, that if children with clefts are maladjusted because of impaired speech, facial disfigurement, or some other abnormality associated with cleft palate, the personality testing instruments which have been used do not reflect that maladjustment. Further, if proficiency in articulation skills in the cleft palate population is influenced by personality maladjustment, it has not yet been demonstrated. This does not preclude the possibility, of course, that in specific individuals such relationships may exist and should be considered.

A somewhat stronger case can be made to support the idea that parental adjustment may have some influence upon the acquisition of speech sounds. Wood (1946) has reported a study on environmental factors and emotional adjustments of children with functional misarticulations and of their parents. Scores on personality tests, when compared to test norms, indicated emotional maladjustment on the part of one or both parents. Mothers were more maladjusted than fathers. Case histories revealed frequent disruptions in the home resulting from the absence of both parents from the home or their separation or divorce. The parents were also found to have few interests outside the home; they tended not to employ "good" child-rearing practices; and they used overly severe techniques of child discipline. No control group was employed. The study was extended to include speech therapy for the children, the mothers of half of the group receiving extensive parent counseling and those of the other half not. The children whose mothers received counseling improved in speech more rapidly than did those whose mothers received no counseling. Results reported by Egbert (1955) in general support Wood's findings. Moll and Darley (1960) found, according to results obtained with standardized attitude scales, that mothers of children with functional misarticulations had higher standards and were more critical of their children's activities than mothers of a control group of children.

Goodstein (1960) and Spriestersbach and Powers (in press) report data concerning the attitudes and expectations of parents of children with clefts. Goodstein found no evidence that parents of children with cleft palates are on the average different from parents of normal children in their responses to the Minnesota Multiphasic Personality Inventory (MMPI). Spriestersbach and Powers, however, found that parents of children with cleft palates, when interviewed, express higher standards for their children and tend to be more defensive about their children than do parents of normal children. The discrepancy between the two studies is probably the result of difference in techniques. It seems likely that there are real differences in adjustment between parents of normal children and parents of children with clefts but that these differences are highly specific and that an inventory scale such as the MMPI is not useful for revealing them. The interview technique, however, does apparently reveal some differences. Neither Goodstein nor Spriestersbach and Powers correlated parental adjustment scores with the children's articulation proficiency scores, and it is possible that such a procedure might provide additional evidence one way or the other.

The hypothesis that psychosocial factors may be etiologically significant in accounting for the functional articulation errors of cleft palate speakers cannot at this time be refuted. If there is any validity to the notion that parental attitudes can affect the learning of speech skills of normal children, the same is probably true for children with cleft palates also. In few other clinical diagnoses is there as much likelihood of finding parental feelings of guilt, rejection, and overcompensation, any one of which would influence the interpersonal relationships between parent and child and in turn affect communication skills of the child.

2. *Learning Factors*

Pitzner and Morris (1966) compared proficiency on several articulation tests for cleft palate children with high manometer ratios and cleft palate children with low manometer ratios with normative data for those articulation tests, taken from Templin (1957). Among their findings was the indication that cleft palate children who do not demonstrate velopharyngeal competence (the low manometer-ratio group) show significantly poorer scores on an articulation test composed of vocalic /r/ and /l/ than do normal children. The scores of cleft palate children who demonstrate velopharyngeal competence (the high manometer-ratio group) did not differ from the normative data. It is difficult to account for this difference in terms of velopharyngeal competence, since there are indications that the vocalic /r/ and /l/ have little requirements for intraoral breath pressure and hence velopharyngeal competence. The best explanation seems to be a difference in learning.

Since there are few research data regarding the importance of learning factors and the conditions which facilitate the learning of speech for the normal child, or, for that matter, for the child with structural deviations such as cleft palate, the bulk of the writing on learning factors has been theoretical in nature and has been based, for the most part, on a priori reasoning. McCarthy (1954a) has presented an extensive review of the relevant literature and has described the importance of such factors as imitation, auditory reinforcement, and the role of models.

Other variables operative in the learning process also may affect the way in which children with cleft palate learn speech sounds. For example, there appears to be relatively good agreement that, in general, however it comes about, young children who are learning to talk are greatly influenced with reference to the frequency of effort that they make and also with reference to the selectivity of their responses by the speech they hear. Over a period of many months they appear to show better and better approximation of the model set for them; the better the approximation, presumably the greater the reinforcement of the response. Consider the dilemma of the child with an unrepaired cleft palate, or a repaired cleft which does not function adequately, who, because of structural inadequacies, is not able to produce the majority of the consonant sounds which he hears. It may be that he "learns" to equate his "best" attempt in producing a specific speech unit with the productions which he hears and goes on, as it were, from there. Or it may be that in his failure to improve his approximations of the models he hears, he tends to withdraw from the activity and makes fewer attempts to perfect his skills on those units which he can approximate quite well, that is, phonemes which do not require such a great amount of intraoral pressure.

There is support for this contention in some of the data reported by Brandt and Morris (1965). Subjects in their group which had large velopharyngeal openings, generally larger than 8.00 mm, showed larger openings on /s/ than /u/ while the reverse was true for subjects with small velopharyngeal openings. One interpretation of this finding is that the children with large velopharyngeal openings were so discouraged in their productions of /s/ that they made little effort to achieve closure of the velopharyngeal port and so showed little movement of the mechanism. Their expectations for an acceptable production of /u/ however were higher and so they showed more movement of the mechanism than they had for /s/. This observation has been referred to by several authors as the "psychological" or "discouraged" /s/.

Related to this discussion is the consideration that parents may be told by various authorities that their child is not capable of normal speech production before the palatal cleft is physically managed. Again, the authority in question is undoubtedly talking about the fact that the child is not able to impound sufficient intraoral breath pressure for those pressure consonants which require it, and that the parents should not expect him to be able to produce these sounds. The authority may fail to mention that not all speech sounds have the same requisites for intraoral pressure and that the child will be able to learn speech sounds such as vowels, nasals, and glides despite the structural inadequacies that he may have. The parent, not knowing this, may adopt the attitude that his child simply "can't talk well" and thereupon employs lower speech standards and accepts less critically the attempts which the child makes at talking. In turn, the child may not be stimulated, either verbally or through more subtle cues, to pursue the process of approximating the speech exhibited in his environment and may be content to achieve at a lower level of skill than normally would be expected.

Morley (1962) contends that some children with cleft palate apparently hear no differences between their speech and the speech of individuals without clefts or at least do not express such feelings verbally. Their inability to distinguish between their own speech and the speech of others, according to her, results in the perseveration of faulty articulation patterns which frequently are not related to the palatal cleft per se. She writes (p. 135):

> So a form of speech will develop, through stages similar to the normal certainly, but with marked deviation from the normal in the result obtained; and, as previously described, it is the continued reproduction of faulty speech movements which steadily and surely builds up those incorrect speech habits which, in later years, are so difficult to eradicate. Also, not only is the ear of the child becoming accustomed to the sound he hears himself producing, but these auditory images are being inevitably correlated in his mind with the normal sounds he hears around him and which he is attempting to imitate.
>
> It is due to these facts that the child with a cleft palate is usually completely unconscious of any difference between the sounds he makes and the sounds he hears from others. He only becomes conscious of his defect when he is old enough to realize that he differs from other children in his ability to make himself understood or

when his companions ridicule his attempt at speech.... In this way such patients differ entirely from a stammerer, who is, except in rare instances, acutely aware of his speech disability. As the perseveration of these faulty speech associations increases the difficulties of patient and speech therapist alike, the age at which treatment is commenced is of the greatest importance.

On occasion, however, clinicians observe a relatively young child with a cleft palate who shows minimal speech skills, who reportedly uses gestures as a major method of communication, and who in general has withdrawn from activities which involve speech. The child may even comment during the examination that "I can't say that." Although this type of child does not comprise a majority in the cleft palate population, and although the withdrawal may be made for reasons other than failure at articulation tasks, the inference can be made that some of these children recognize their limited skills in speech activities and deliberately and effectively withdraw from such situations. This withdrawal with fewer attempts at approximating appropriate speech patterns results in more retardation in speech skills because of the attitudes of the child towards speech than because of any structural deficiency.

There are additional variables of learning which are considered to be etiologically important and which are specifically related to the cleft palate. One such variable is age of surgery (or in the larger sense, age of physical management) of the palatal cleft. This may be considered to be related to learning articulation skills under the assumption that the earlier the structural deviation is treated, that is, under the condition that the treatment is successful, the more likely is the child to learn appropriate articulatory movements. On the other hand, children with unmanaged palatal clefts learn inappropriate patterns of articulation, which may be modified after management, that is, after the child is able to impound adequate intraoral breath pressure. Morley (1962, p. 138) advocates this position when she writes:

In cases operated upon between one and two years of age, when, although speech is not yet established, it may be assumed that the child has already learned some incorrect habits for the production of many consonants sounds, it is found that, given a successful surgical result, normal speech may be attained without the aid of special training.

Morley believes that the longer surgery is delayed after the age of 2 years, other factors being equal and with successful surgical results, the longer will it be before normal speech is attained. As supporting evidence for her position, Morley cites a report by Jolleys (1954) and operative results obtained by Braithwaite in Newcastle-upon-Tyne. Wardill (1937) also took a position comparable to Morley's, but did not report supporting data.

Jolleys studied 254 subjects who had palatal surgery at various ages and with two general types of surgical techniques. A total of 132 subjects had a lip-and-palate cleft; 122 had a cleft palate only. Speech proficiency was rated on a 4-point scale. In general, the Von Langenbeck technique was used on the majority of the subject group and at various ages, mostly after the age of 2½ years. The remainder of the subjects had management of the type typically used by Veau and by Wardill with the anterior cleft closed at about 5 months of age (along with the cleft lip repair) and the posterior cleft repaired at about 18 months of age. The speech of 90% of the group with surgery before the age of 2 was rated as "good" or "perfect" (as opposed to "bad" or "fair") while that of only 37% of the group with surgery after the third birthday was rated as "good" or "perfect." Jolleys attributes the superiority in speech function of the earlier surgery group to greater palatal length, better muscular development, and increased mobility, all of which, in his opinion, may be related to the early establishment of natural function. He also reported that better speech results were obtained for postalveolar cases than for children with complete (lip-and-palate) clefts.

Pitzner and Morris (1966) report data with reference to articulation proficiency and age of management. They divided their high manometer-ratio group (ratios of .90 or higher), as mentioned previously, into two subgroups according to age of physical management. A total of 17 subjects had been managed before the age of 30 months, while 29 subjects had been managed after the age of 30 months. The difference between the two groups on mean age of management was significant. The two groups were roughly comparable in intelligence, sex distribution, socioeconomic status, type of cleft, and type of management. Since the two groups were not comparable in age when they were tested, the criterion score for articulation proficiency was defined as the difference between the obtained score and the appropriate test norm for that age. The mean difference between the obtained scores and the test norms was not significant for the subjects who had management before the age of 30 months but was significant for the subjects who had management after the age of 30 months. These findings were interpreted to indicate a trend toward greater speech proficiency with younger age of management.

There is little evidence to refute the hypothesis that, other things being equal, early physical management of the palatal cleft results in the learning of more appropriate patterns of articulation and hence greater speech proficiency. The point is, of course, that frequently other things are not equal! There are no reports of investigations in which results are reported for large groups of children whose clefts were managed by the same surgical or prosthetic technique and who were randomly assigned, regardless of variables such as type and extent of cleft and quantity of soft tissue, to one of two groups: one group to have early management; and the other group, late management. Jolleys' results are less convincing than they would be if it could be ascertained that there was no tendency to assign children with generally less severe clefts to the early surgery group and to defer surgery until later for the children with more severe clefts. If such was not the case, his results could be interpreted to indicate that severity of cleft rather than age of surgery may be predictive of speech success. In any event, while the notion that providing adequate physiological function at an early age facilitates the acquisition of articulation skills is entirely plausible, recognition must be given to the fact that age of surgery may be influenced by other variables which may bias the results.

Another variable related to the considerations of learning speech sounds by individuals with inadequate oral structures is that of compensatory articulatory movements. Clinical observations reveal that frequently children who are unable because of inadequate physical structures to produce normal speech sounds often do attempt to compensate for the inadequate structures by adjusting the movements and positions of the articulatory mechanisms. It has been observed, for example, that children with open clefts frequently occlude the cleft with the tongue, at least partially, during speech. The use of nares constrictions, discussed earlier, is a compensatory mechanism for speakers with inadequate velopharyngeal closure. In a sense, for the same group of speakers, the use of the pharyngeal fricative or of the glottal stop is compensatory, since these sounds are produced because normal fricatives and plosives are not possible. In fact, recent studies of the speech physiology of these speakers (Spriestersbach and Moll, 1964) reveal that compensatory mechanisms are far more common and significant in maintaining acceptable speech than had previously been suggested. The important point about such behavior is that it is learned as a compensation for structural inadequacies and may continue after the structures are no longer inadequate. In these instances the articulation may be considered deviant, not because of the cleft palate, per se, but because inappropriate patterns of movement had been learned at an earlier age. The question of determining whether misarticulations are related to structural deviations or are functional in nature, and presumably easily modifiable, is of prime importance to the speech diagnostician and is discussed in detail in Chapter VIII.

3. *Mental Retardation and Brain Injury*

The intellectual development, the social maturity and adjustment, and the educational attainment of children with cleft palate have been considered elsewhere. In general, indications are that children with cleft lip and palate are significantly impaired, on the average, in their intellectual development and that the impairment is most substantial in the area of verbal intellectual skills (Goodstein, 1961). The effect of this impairment on speech proficiency for the cleft palate population is not clear. One might expect, however, that the intellectual impairment would result in speech being learned, on the average, at a slower-than-normal rate. The intellectual impairment thus would be an etiological factor in learning speech. On the other hand, as Goodstein points out, problems in oral communication could result in retarded development of verbal intellectual skills; if this is the case, the speech problem would be a factor influencing the level of learning of verbal skills. Further consideration of this point is beyond the scope of this discussion and, for the present purpose, only the effect of intelligence upon the learning of speech will be considered.

Consider, for example, the finding that 60% of Goodstein's cleft-palate group had full-scale IQ's of 90 or higher on the Wichsler Intelligence Scale for Children (WISC). Certainly one would not expect that intellectual functioning would be of etiological significance in accounting for the poor articulation skills for such a group. An additional 25.7% had IQ's between 80 and 89; the remaining 14.3% had IQ's lower than 79. There is no research evidence regarding minimal level of intelligence for "normal" acquisition of speech sounds. It is difficult to contend, however, that children with IQ's between 80 and 89 would be retarded in articulation skills because of mental retardation. If that is true, then, only 14.3% of the cleft palate population might demonstrate retarded articulation proficiency for reasons of intelligence. The tenth percentile rank is assigned to an IQ of 81 by Wechsler (1949) for the WISC and, according to Terman and Merrill (1960), 8.23% of the 1937 standardization group for the Stanford-Binet scale had IQ's under 80. Thus only 4 to 6% more children with clefts have intelligence levels which may be considered, conservatively, as etiological factors in learning speech skills than would be the case for the total population of children.

There are a limited number of reports regarding the strength of the relationship between intelligence and articulation proficiency for cleft palate children (Morris, 1962), for normal children (Winitz, 1964), and for children who are mentally retarded (Riello, 1958). In general, there appears to be some correlation between the two variables for all three subgroups. Comparisons among groups, however, could be misleading because of the differences in the way they were selected. If differences exist, they probably demonstrate the similarity in this regard between the cleft palate and normal groups, rather than between the cleft palate and educable mentally retarded groups. It is concluded then, that, as a group, mental retardation is not an important etiological factor in affecting the way in which the cleft palate population acquires articulation skills.

Brief mention must be made of the factor of brain injury, although there have been no research reports about investigations of this factor and few authors of textbooks have included considerations of it. Suffice it to say that incidence of brain injury or neuropathology is probably not smaller in the cleft palate population than in the normal population and so must be considered in the evaluation of individual speakers.

II. Voice Disorders

A. PITCH

Suggestions have been made in the literature to the effect that individuals with cleft palate may show restricted pitch variation and that they may frequently demonstrate pitches which are shrill and which sometimes change with growth to an unnaturally low pitch.

If anatomical and physiological bases for the above-mentioned pitch deviations exist, those bases have not been described in the literature. Certainly there is no evidence that laryngeal size is atypical for this group. Hypotheses about laryngeal function of individuals with cleft palate will be presented later, but they are theories at best, with no documentation to support the notion that such deviations in laryngeal function result in abnormal pitch levels or pitch variability for this population.

Consideration must be given in discussions such as this to behavior which may be compensatory in nature. It is suggested that in those instances when a child uses a monotonous pitch level or when he uses an atypical pitch level he may simply reflect, by an effort to be less conspicuous, his awareness of his difficulties in communication. Again, however, such compensations are probably not typical of the cleft palate population in general.

B. LOUDNESS

There is no evidence of direct anatomical or physiological bases for inappropriate loudness levels in the speech of individuals with cleft palate. Curtis (1942) made spectrographic analyses of speech samples of subjects with velar insufficiency, velar paralysis, and open cleft palate. His findings indicate that the intensities of high frequencies are attenuated in those speech samples. The findings of Curtis may be relevant to the extent that attenuation in high frequencies results in the perception of decreased loudness levels. The relationship between the two parameters is far from clear, however.

Decreased loudness levels, if or when used by individuals with clefts, may be related to a motivation on the speaker's part to make his communication problem less apparent or less conspicuous, as already hypothesized with reference to pitch usage. He may simply speak more softly in the attempt to call less attention to his speech problem or, extending the theory further, to himself as a person. Hypotheses such as this are difficult to test but must be considered.

C. QUALITY

The cleft palate population has been reported to demonstrate deviations in voice quality, particularly nasality, by many authors. There is not a great deal of research reported about the etiologies of those deviations, however.

1. *Nasality*

The quality deviation most frequently identified with the cleft palate population is excessive nasality. It is important to note in this discussion that apparently excessive nasality and one type of misarticulation for this group are often confused or are often described so carelessly that confusion results. Nasal emission consists of a leak of oral air pressure during the articulation of consonants; excessive nasality consists of an undesirable degree of nasal resonance which is present during phonation of vowels. In considering the etiology of the two disorders, a further distinction must be made between variables related to the shaping and coupling of resonance cavities and those related to the articulation of the air stream.

It is not the purpose of this discussion to describe the etiology of "functional" nasality nor to present a detailed discussion of resonance theory. The discussion will concern only possible etiologies of nasality for individuals with cleft palate.

Certainly the anatomical-physiological basis most frequently associated with nasality in this population is that of velopharyngeal incompetence. In general the same techniques are used and the same limitations apply in studying competence related to nasality as those techniques which are used and those limitations which apply in studying articulation.

Kodman (1951) obtained for eight subjects ratings of nasality and measurements taken from still x-ray films of distance between the posterior pharyngeal wall and the posterior margin of the obturator. Nasality was judged on a 3-point scale, and the difference between the two groups who were judged *most* and *least* nasal was not significant with reference to the mean obturator-pharyngeal wall distances.

Hagerty and Hoffmeister (1954) studied 44 subjects with surgically repaired cleft palate. Distances between the velum and pharyngeal wall were measured from still x-ray films taken during the production of /ɑ/, and also during the production of a "hissing" noise. Nasality was rated as none, mild, moderate, or severe. Values of *none*, 1, 4, and 9 were assigned those ratings, respectively, and were used in a correlation procedure to relate nasality to velopharyngeal distance. Correlations of .60 for /ɑ/ and .78 for "hissing" were obtained.

Although the use of categorical data in a product-moment correlation technique can be questioned, this study was one of the first of its kind and made an important contribution at the time.

Holt (1959) used approximately the same technique as Hagerty and Hoffmeister except that nasality was apparently judged on a 4-point rating scale. X-ray films for /u/ were used for the measurement of physiological closure and wet spirometer ratios were used to assess velopharyngeal function. Correlation coefficients of .04 for velopharyngeal dimension and judged nasality and .13 for velopharyngeal function and judged nasality were reported. Again, the appropriateness of the use of such a restricted scale (4 points) is questionable in a product-moment correlation technique.

Spriestersbach and Powers (1959a) correlated wet spirometer ratios with nasality ratings obtained by use of a 7-point scale and backward play to avoid contamination of the judgments by articulation errors of the recorded speech samples. Fifty subjects were used and nasality ratings were obtained for samples of connected speech as well as samples of seven isolated vowels. The coefficients were $-.33$ for connected speech and ranged from $-.06$ to $-.45$ for the seven vowels.

Counihan (1956) used nasality ratings of connected speech (backward play) and measurements of the velopharyngeal distance from still lateral x-ray films for /u/. The correlation coefficient between the two variables was .51.

Subtelny *et al.* (1961) correlated velopharyngeal distances for x-ray films taken during /u/ and nasality rated on a 4-point scale. The obtained correlation coefficient was .53. Again the problem of the restricted range of the scale must be considered.

Clearly, the variable of velopharyngeal incompetence is related to judged nasality in speech. The best evidence indicates that the strength of that relationship is probably to be estimated by an *r* in the order of .30 to .60.

Counihan (1956) investigated the role of several other anatomical and physiological bases of possible etiological significance in causing nasality. Connected speech samples for 55 subjects were judged for nasality on a 7-point scale. The variables of velar mobility, velar length, adenoid convexity, nasal obstruction and two dimensions of facial growth were rated either by direct examination or from still, lateral x-ray films. Descriptive categories were used for the ratings, such as *none, mild, moderate,* and *severe*. In most instances the number of categories for a variable did not exceed three. Mean nasality ratings for the descriptive categories were compared. No differences were significant except two between the categories concerning velar length. Subjects with velar lengths judged to be adequate and those with velar lengths judged to be short were rated less nasal than were those with velar lengths judged to be very short.

McDonald and Koepp-Baker (1951) suggested that elevation of the mandible and the dorsum of the tongue are causally related to nasality. They offered no documentation for their position but formulated several hypotheses, based on clinical and limited research findings, which emphasized the importance of oral structures other than the velum and pharyngeal wall in causing nasality. It should be noted that Buck (1951) reported that his cleft palate group showed lower tongue positions than did the normal group. Unfortunately he did not evaluate the relationship between nasality ratings and tongue elevations. However, the description of the ratings assigned his subjects with clefts indicates that the group as a whole showed speech that was moderately to markedly nasal (19 of his 20 subjects received average ratings of 4 or above on a 7-point scale). These data suggest that depressed, not elevated, tongue positions may be associated with hypernasality. The difference between the two findings probably is to be explained with reference to the types of subjects studied and differences between subject groups in velopharyngeal competence. Buck's subjects had physically managed cleft palate and, if the ratings of nasality can be used as an index of velopharyngeal function, probably had problems of gross incompetence, as a group. McDonald and Koepp-Baker, on the other hand, were referring in large part to data reported by Hixon who used nasal subjects who had no clefts, and who probably had borderline or minimal problems of velopharyngeal incompetence.

It should be noted that there are physiological relationships between the lingual and palatal structures, that nasal speakers without clefts may use relatively great physical efforts to achieve velopharyngeal closure, and that these efforts may be associated with elevated tongue positions. In contrast, individuals who have had structural defects and who continue to demonstrate gross velopharyngeal incompetence are not able to achieve closure even with their greatest efforts, and probably do not demonstrate the kind of palatal movement, and hence the kind of tongue elevation, that the nasal speakers without clefts exhibit. Typically, tongue position during vowel production is lower for the group with clefts than for the nasal speakers without clefts perhaps for the reason that the maintenance of a relatively open oral passageway may tend to minimize the nasalization which would occur without such a compensation.

Considering the amount of literature about tongue carriage, mouth opening, and hypernasality, it is surprising that so little research on these factors has been conducted. Clearly, additional research is needed in this area and it should take into account the variable of velopharyngeal competence. Size of mouth opening might also be considered. Cinefluorography may be particularly useful in such investigations.

There are apparently no research reports which suggests psychosocial or learning bases for nasality in individuals with clefts. In certain instances chronic hearing losses or low intelligence or motivation levels may be relevant in the acquisition and retention of such a quality but there is no evidence to support the hypothesis that these factors are etiologically significant.

2. *Other Quality Disorders*

There have been suggestions in the literature that individuals with cleft palate have voice quality deviations other than nasality. McDonald and Koepp-Baker (1951) advanced the hypothesis, without direct documentation, that an important part of the defective quality of cleft palate speech is the result of faulty phonation. This quality, in their opinion, results from an ineffective use of air which adds a feature similar to breathiness to the overall quality, and which prevents the speaker from producing sounds with a wide acoustic spectrum. They cite as evidence the findings of Curtis (1942) which include the observation that high frequencies are markedly attenuated in the nasalizations produced by speakers who showed pathologies of velar insufficiency, velar paralysis, and open cleft palate. McDonald and Koepp-Baker speculate that the attenuation of high frequencies observed by Curtis may have been the result of faulty phonation rather than of a damping effect of certain resonators. From clinical observation they report a tendency for cleft palate speakers to have voices which may be described as being hoarse, suggesting that the hoarseness may be due to a tissue pathology alone, perhaps generalized from severely disturbed nasal and pharyngeal mucosa, or to a tissue pathology in combination with the aberrant use of the larynx as an articulator of speech sounds, referring apparently to the use of glottal stops by many speakers who show velopharyngeal incompetence. The have been no recent investigations of their hypothesis.

III. Language Development

There is no evidence to indicate that there are additional anatomical-physiological bases for the retarded language development of cleft palate children other than those bases discussed in accounting for lack of articulation proficiency in this population. Morris (1960, 1962) reports significant correlations between articulation skills and measures of language development based on analysis of language samples including such measures as mean length of response and vocabulary comprehension. These correlations indicate that speakers with more defective articulation may simply not talk as much or know as many words as speakers with less defective articulation. Since velopharyngeal competence has been demonstrated to be etiologically significant in the articulation errors of the child with a cleft palate, it follows that velopharyngeal competence is also related to verbal output and vocabulary size. Such a notion has not been directly investigated but seems reasonable. Furthermore, by the same reasoning, hearing acuity, malocclusion, or other structural deviations may influence the growth of language skills in the cleft palate population.

There is evidence, however, that for children with cleft palate there are other bases for retardation in linguistic skills in addition to those discussed earlier for retardation in articulation proficiency. The additional bases are discussed here rather than earlier since they are considered to have major impact on the total development of oral communication skills, grossly defined, rather than on articulation proficiency, per se. These bases, suggested by Morris (1960), may be considered to be psychosocial in nature since they are related to attitudes of parents toward the child with a cleft and his needs; to experiences which take place at a relatively early age of the child with a cleft; and to the effects of these attitudes and experiences on the development of the child's language.

McCarthy (1954a, b) presents extensive reviews of data which, in her opinion, emphasize the importance of the psychosocial environment of the infant and young child during the language learning years. Differences can be clearly drawn between the psychosocial environment for "normal" development as described by her and that environment in which young children with clefts may spend their early childhood. McCarthy describes the kind of nurture which she relates to "normal" linguistic development. This nurture includes not only the physical surroundings and procedures for infant care but, more importantly, the attitudes which the mother reflects in that care. She writes (1954b):

> The very way she approaches motherhood,... whether she feels adequate to care for him, or whether she is tense, worried, and uncertain in everything she does for him, whether she is happy and talks to him as she goes about her tasks or pushes the baby carriage, whether she is silent and preoccupied while giving physical care or is impersonal and merely allows the child to vegetate most of the time are the kinds of things which are important in determining whether his language development will thrive, or be stunted, or distorted in some unfortunate way.

Consider the data reported by Spriestersbach and Powers (in press) who conducted extensive interviews with a large group of mothers of children with cleft palates and a comparable group of mothers of normal children. Of 112 mothers, only 18 were able to use regular nursing nipples, either as purchased or with enlarged holes, as the major feeding technique. None was able to use breast feeding as the major technique. A total of 94 used, as major feeding techniques, special devices which ranged from a special nipple with a suction plate and rubber flange for covering the cleft to an eye or medicine dropper. More mothers with children who had clefts reported feeding problems such as "gas in stomach, choking because the milk flowed too fast," and "vomiting or spitting up" than did the mothers of normal children. Feedings, on the average, were reported to take longer with the children with clefts. Comparing their children to others the same age, more mothers of the cleft group rated their babies as crying more during the first three months of life than did the control mothers. Both the experimental and control mothers listed colic as a probable cause of crying but more mothers of children with clefts listed hunger as a probable cause of crying than did the mothers of normal children. It seems evident from these data that often a mother of a young child with a cleft, in contrast to a mother of a normal infant, undoubtedly faces feeding problems which make child care exceedingly more difficult to manage and which may indeed result in anxiety on her part.

Also, with reference to general attitudes, consider the fact that of 169 mothers of children with clefts interviewed by Spriestersbach and Powers, 85 had never been acquainted with persons who had clefts and presumably had only general information about the anomaly or may have had none at all. Further, of the 84 who had been acquainted with persons who had clefts, 48 considered that person to be "handicapped" because of his cleft. For that group, then, the stage is set for the expectation of "difficulty" with the child, and, probably, for the expectation that their child will be "handicapped" throughout life. If the parents do not view their child as "defective," they may view him as being "special" and may react to him in unrealistic ways even at a very early age.

Another consideration involves the effect upon the child of hospitalization for management of the cleft or for other reasons. In the majority of treatment centers children with cleft lips have lip surgery during the first three months of life. The period of confinement may range from 2 to 4 weeks, depending on recovery and on the number of surgical techniques used. If there are nutritional problems, the infant may be hospitalized for a longer period of time. McCarthy (1954a) reviews the findings reported by Aldrich and his associates and by Irwin and his associates which indicate that even at that early age, several weeks of hospitalization may influence the development of linguistic skills. Aldrich and his associates found that babies under 30 days of age who were in hospital nurseries had 11.9 periods of crying per day (over 3 minutes) while babies of the same age in home situations showed such crying behavior only 4 periods per day. In general, there was a decrease of 51.4% in the amount of crying when comparisons were made between the hospital and home situations. Irwin and his associates noted evidence of retarded development in frequency and variety of phonemes in orphange children as compared to children in their own homes as early as the first two months of life. The discrepancies between the two groups became more marked by the sixth month of life. Other investigators have reported comparable findings. From this rather indirect evidence, it is reasonable to expect these psychosocial factors to influence the acquisition of language by the child who has a cleft palate.

It was suggested previously in this chapter that hearing loss incurred during the early years could impede the development of articulation skills. Such a loss could undoubtedly affect language learning also, particularly in combination with other factors. There have been no research reports about relationships, however.

IV. Discussion

In this section, the objectives are, first, to present a general overview of the etiological factors important in the consideration of the speech problems of individuals who have or have had a cleft palate and, second, to present a point of view with reference to the inferences which can be made on the bases of the research reports reviewed in previous sections of this chapter. The reader should keep in mind that these inferences are made by the writer according to his interpretation of the data and should be evaluated as such rather than as first-order facts.

A. ARTICULATION

The findings indicate that for the cleft palate population the most important etiological factor in causing articulation problems is velopharyngeal incompetence. The requirement of intraoral pressure for normal speech sound articulation is established and the requisite of the capability of velopharyngeal competence for achieving intraoral pressure is accepted by most investigators.

Clearly, however, there is not a one-to-one relationship between degrees of articulation proficiency and velopharyngeal competence. That is, increases in velopharyngeal opening do not result necessarily in proportional increases in the number of articulation errors. Lack of a finding of such a one-to-one relationship is undoubtedly to be accounted for to some extent by the fact that factors other than velopharyngeal competence affect the articulation of speech sounds. Another possibility has been suggested elsewhere (Spriestersbach and Powers, 1959b; Spriestersbach *et al.*, 1961; Spriestersbach 1964): that is, that the relationship between the two factors is curvilinear rather than linear. The data of Subtelny and Subtelny (1959) also suggest the possibility of curvilinearity, at least for the fricatives. Also, according to their data, there may be a size of velopharyngeal opening past which intraoral breath pressure adequate for fricatives is not impounded and, indeed, past which a further increase in size of opening does not contribute additionally to their misarticulation.

There is evidence that, clinically, the effect, beyond a certain point, of varying degrees of velopharyngeal incompetence on articulation proficiency may be considered to be essentially the same, regardless of the size of opening. For example, Spriestersbach et al. (1961) compared the articulation skills of three groups of speakers who varied according to wet-spirometer ratios. One group had ratios of .90 and higher, that is, complete or nearly complete closure for the task; one group had ratios of .50 or lower, that is, as measured, gross inadequacy for the task; and the third group had ratios of .51 to .89, that is, more competence than the poorest group but less than the best group. The scores, expressed as mean percentages, for general articulation proficiency were as follows for the three groups: ratios of .90 or higher, 81.40; ratios of .51 to .89, 61.00; and ratios of .50 or lower, 57.91. Clearly, the two lower groups were very much alike in articulation skills and both groups showed lower levels of achievement in those skills than did the highest group. If the variable of velopharyngeal competence is linear in its relationship to articulation proficiency, one would expect the middle group (.51 to .89) to demonstrate more defective articulation than the highest group but better articulation than the lowest group.

Two recent investigations have included techniques for describing the nature of the relationship between articulation proficiency and velopharyngeal opening. Shelton et al. (1964) correlated measures of velopharyngeal closure and articulation skill for 31 subjects who had either surgically repaired cleft palate or palatal inadequacies without clefts and obtained a coefficient of .52. They tested for linearity of regression and the hypothesis of linearity was rejected at the 1% level of significance. From the same data, a correlation ratio (or eta) of .78 was obtained, which was significant at the .1% level. They conclude, then, that the relationship between the two variables is nonlinear.

Brandt and Morris (1965) correlated two measures of velopharyngeal opening and four measures of articulation proficiency. They also computed a correlation ratio (eta) for each of the relationships. Only the correlations for the relationship between plosive articulation and velopharyngeal opening for /u/ were significant; correlations for the relationships between opening on /u/ and /s/ and total articulation, fricative articulation, nasal/glide articulation, and between plosive articulation and /s/ were not significant. They concluded that, except for /u/ and plosives, the relationship between velopharyngeal opening and articulation proficiency is linear. Their conclusion, then, is in disagreement with that of Shelton, Brooks, and Youngstrom.

In the report by Brandt and Morris, two explanations of the above-mentioned difference in findings are offered as being plausible. The first is that the measures of velopharyngeal opening used in the two studies are not similar. Brandt and Morris measured the opening from a single observation from a still, lateral x-ray film taken during the phonation of /s/ or /u/. In the research report by Shelton and his associates, a mean was obtained of measurements of opening for every film frame taken while the subject repeated three sentences, seven phonemes in isolation, four nonsense syllables, and while he counted from 1 to 6. This measure, then, took into account velopharyngeal openings on a variety of vowels and consonants in several contexts.

A second explanation, one which seems to have more face validity than the first, is that the subject groups in the two investigations differed in amount of velopharyngeal opening and that that difference influences the linearity of the relationship observed. That is, the sections of the curve representing the relationship was not the same in the two studies. The subject group studied by Shelton and associates typically showed, by their measure, small velopharyngeal openings. A total of 24 of their 31 subjects had openings which were smaller than 2.00 mm. Openings for the group ranged from .08 mm to 9.40 mm. In contrast, subjects studied by Brandt and Morris had relatively large velopharyngeal openings. Openings for the entire group ranged from 0 to 17.5 mm, and only 18 of the 62 subjects had openings smaller than 2.00. Furthermore, 21 of the 62 subjects had openings larger than 9.00 mm, the largest opening shown by any subject in Shelton's group. The Shelton study, then, may be relevant only for subjects with relatively small openings. Information from the Brandt study may be relevant only for subjects with larger velopharyngeal openings.

There is need for further research in this area to describe more completely the relationships between the variables of velopharyngeal competence, intraoral breath pressure, and articulation skills. Particular interest centers about the requirements for intraoral breath pressure for normal articulation of consonants and the degree of velopharyngeal competence for the creation of the intraoral breath pressure. It may be that, as Kaltenborn (1948) and later McDonald and Koepp-Baker (1951) speculated, there is a critical point in the degree of nasopharyngeal closure for nasality, and that the same critical point operates also for articulation. Relative to this point are the observations which have been reported from cinefluorographic data to the effect that normal speakers do not always demonstrate velopharyngeal closure during the production of pressure consonants. There appears to be variation for normal speakers in the degree of velar contact depending on phonetic context.

All things considered, however, the existing evidence supports the contention that velopharyngeal closure must be *achievable* for the production of consonants in connected speech. It may be that velopharyngeal closure is not always demonstrated, however, when sounds are articulated normally. It may be that, during normal speech, amounts of intraoral pressure adequate for consonant articulation are created instantaneously not by closure of the nasopharyngeal port but by variations in air pressures and rates of air flow. The position is taken, however, that the speaker must be able to obtain closure of the nasopharyngeal port during the rapid-fire movements of connected speech and that inability to do so will result in impaired articulation characterized by nasal emission of air.

The position is also taken that the importance of velopharyngeal competence is the same regardless of status of physical management of the palatal cleft or indeed whether there is a cleft of the palate at all. Inability to occlude the velopharyngeal port, the resulting leakage of air through the nasal passages, and the perceived nasal emission accompanying the articulation of the consonant sound will result in impaired speech. This inability to occlude the velopharyngeal port may be caused by a physically unmanaged palatal cleft which clearly cannot be occluded during speech activities or it may be caused by a leak of air pressure at some point around the margins of the obturator bulb in this instance when the cleft has been obturated. The inability to occlude the velopharyngeal port may occur in the case where the palatal cleft has been surgically repaired but in which the repaired palate is too short or too immobile; or it may occur if the nasopharynx is too deep for the length or motility of the palate or it may occur in the case where secondary palatal surgery, such as the pharyngeal flap, has been performed but in which the lateral openings between the flap and the pharyngeal walls are still too large to be occluded by movement of the palatal and pharyngeal structures during speech activities. The inability to occlude the velopharyngeal port may occur also in the case where there has never been a cleft of the palate but where there is an apparent shortness or immobility of the palate. In the above series, it is interesting to note that only two of the above-mentioned types of speakers actually *have* cleft palate. Two other types *have had* cleft palate but currently do not. The fifth type has not ever *had* a cleft. This suggests that the term "cleft palate speech" is inappropriate with reference to speech characterized by inadequate intraoral breath pressure during speech. A more appropriate description might be speakers who show velopharyngeal incompetence for speech.

As we have seen, learning can be another important etiological factor in accounting for the articulation errors of an individual who has, or has had, a cleft palate. It should be made clear that two possibilities exist regarding the acquisition of inappropriate articulation movements on the part of a child with anatomical physiological deficiencies. The first is that, although he has such deficiencies, faulty learning which is completely unrelated to these deficiencies can take place: that is, presumably he could demonstrate the same functional articulation problems as might a child without anatomical deficiencies. The second possibility is that, as Morley and others have pointed out, the child, or adult, may adopt patterns of articulation which compensate for the anatomical-physiological deficits but are not directly related to them. That the behavior is functional can be supported by the observation that eliminating the anatomical-physiological deficits does not always change the behavior.

As an example, consider a child with velopharyngeal incompetence who demonstrates, among other errors, distorted /r/, /ɚ/ and /ɝ/ and a substitution of a glottal stop for the plosive /k/. Both types of articulation errors may have been learned. The use of the glottal stop for the /k/ may have come about because the child was not able to impound an adequate amount of intraoral pressure for an acceptable /k/, and because he rejected the faulty /k/ in favor of glottal stop for the reason that the glottal stop sounded better or more normal to him. The response then became generalized and in subsequent behavior the glottal stop was consistently substituted for the /k/. Clearly, the individual easily could have continued to use the /k/ which was characterized by nasal leak of oral breath pressure. The glottal stop error for /k/, then, is related both to the velopharyngeal incompetence and to inappropriate learning.

The examples of distorted /r/, /ɚ/ and /ɝ/ were chosen for this discussion because the requirements for intraoral breath pressure for these phonemes are apparently not as great for the stop-plosives or fricatives. Presumably these errors are related to tongue placement only and are learned. Such inappropriate articulatory behavior may be observed as often in individuals with velopharyngeal competence as those with velopharyngeal incompetence and are considered not to be related, either directly or indirectly, to the anatomical-physiological deficiency.

Consider again the child described above. Even after the velopharyngeal incompetence has been successfully managed the child still demonstrates the two types of errors, the distorted /r/, /ɚ/ and /ɝ/ and the substitution of a glottal stop for /k/, because meeting the anatomical-physiological deficit did not change the behavioral aspects of the problem. If the child can now obtain velopharyngeal closure, there is an anatomical-physiological basis for helping the child acquire a more appropriate /k/. The fact that he can achieve adequate closure, however, does not facilitate efforts to improve productions of /r/, /ɚ/ and /ɝ/.

Support for the contention that velopharyngeal competence and learning, or maturation, are the two most important etiological factors in accounting for the articulation problems of individuals with clefts is given indirectly by findings reported by Van Demark (1964). He employed a multiple correlation procedure to investigate the possible contributions of 14 articulation measures in predicting severity of articulation defectiveness. His subjects were 154 children with cleft palate. Although he did not employ measures of velopharyngeal competence or maturation, their possible etiological importance is indicated by his identification of two clusters of variables which related best to the ratings of articulation defectiveness. One of these clusters consisted of the variables of plosive misarticulations, fricative misarticulations, distortions-nasal, substitutions-nasal, and ratings of nasality. On the basis of evidence reported by other investigators, Van Demark considered this cluster to represent a velopharyngeal closure factor. A second cluster consisted of the variables of glide misarticulations, nasal semivowel misarticulations and substitutions, and was identified by Van Demark to represent a maturational or learning factor. With the use of the two variables of plosive misarticulations and glide misarticulations, a fairly high multiple R of .883 was obtained. With the inclusion of the remaining nine variables the multiple R was increased only slightly, by .046.

Beta weights for the two variables (stop-plosive misarticulations and glide misarticulations) were .626 and .356. The squares of the beta weights give an estimate of the relative contribution of the variable in accounting for the variance of the dependent variable (here, articulation defectiveness). It appears, then, that velopharyngeal closure might contribute possibly more than three times as much as maturation in the prediction of the degree of articulation defectiveness.

Further validation of the two clusters comes from factor analyses of the above-discussed data (Van Demark, 1966). In these analyses two additional variables were added: manometer ratio and age. The measures obtained with the manometer were reported to be closely related to the velopharyngeal closure factor. The variable of age was highly associated with the maturation factor. Van Demark also reported on the interrelationships among the variables for each of three subgroups: subjects with manometer ratios of .90 and higher, those with ratios between .51 and .89, and those with ratios of .50 and lower. Velopharyngeal closure was not as highly related to severity of misarticulation for the group with the highest manometer ratios as for the two groups with lower pressure ratios.

With reference to the other factors considered in this discussion of articulation problems of an individual who has or has had a cleft palate, factors such as hearing acuity, intelligence, emotional adjustment, and oral-facial deviations, the position is taken that any of these could be etiologically significant in specific instances but that they are not primarily important in causing the articulation problems of this subject group as a whole. Or, said in another way, these factors should be evaluated for the individual with a cleft palate in the same way that they should be considered for the individual without a cleft palate. However, the attachment of special signific-ance to these factors for the cleft palate population in particular does not seem justified at this time.

A word should be added here about the possibility referred to earlier, the possibility that several otherwise insignificant factors may have a cumulative effect which is etiologically important. Research evidence was cited previously in relation to the judged effect of several structural and behavioral deviations. Consider a 7-year old child with velopharyngeal competence and a rather marked occlusal problem. He is able, with considerable care, to compensate for the dentition problem and to make acceptable sibilants. However, he does not always exercise this care and frequently does not make acceptable sibilants during speech. Soon he finds it more difficult to make compensations and, on more and more attempts, uses poorer and poorer approximations of these speech sounds. Is the articulation problem caused by the occlusal problem or by faulty learning? Maybe both, in combined effect. Might he have responded the same way at a younger or older age? Probably not. Was his occlusion the same at a younger age and will it remain the same at older age? Probably not. But, at this very point in time, the occlusal problem and his attitudes about his abilities result in faulty articulation. Undoubtedly such interactions among factors occur more frequently than is generally suspected. They are, of course, difficult to document but should certainly be considered in discussing the etiology of articulation problems for this population.

B. VOICE

There is a consensus among most investigators that hypernasality is the most important deviation in voice production and quality for the cleft palate population. Furthermore, it is apparent that the single most important etiological factor for this nasality is velopharyngeal incompetence. The recognition of the importance of this factor does not mean, however, that other factors, such as mouth opening and tongue height, need not be taken into account in specific instances. Indeed, any anatomical-physiological variable which might influence the shaping or coupling of the resonance cavities could presumably play a significant role. Nevertheless, there is not research evidence that documents the importance of such factors for cleft palate speakers as a group as there is for so-called functionally nasal speakers. It should be remembered that there is considerable evidence that nasality for functionally nasal speakers is dissimilar to nasality for the cleft palate speakers. Spriestersbach and Powers (1959a) obtained scale values of nasality for six vowels in isolation for 50 children who had cleft palate. Some subjects had had physical management and others had not. It is presumed therefore that they ranged from velopharyngeal competence to gross incompetence. The rank ordering of vowels from least to most nasal was as follows: /ɑ/, /ʌ/, /ə/, /ɛ/, /u/ and /i/. Tongue height, then, appeared to be an important variable related to the perception of nasality: low vowels were judged least nasal and high vowels were judged most nasal.

Lintz and Sherman (1961) obtained scale values of nasality for seven isolated vowels for 10 adult male speakers who had been diagnosed as functionally nasal. The rank ordering to the vowels from least to most nasal was as follows: /u/, /ʊ/, /ʌ/, /i/, /ɛ/, /ɑ/ and /ə/. Again, tongue height appeared to be an important variable related to perception of nasality but in opposite direction to that for cleft speakers: high vowels were judged least nasal and low vowels were judged most nasal.

The difference in the findings for the two subject groups is probably related to differences in amount of velopharyngeal opening for the noncleft and cleft groups and to the relationships between the lingual and velopharyngeal structures. Indications are that the cleft palate group studied by Spriestersbach and Powers had problems of gross velopharyngeal incompetence; by and large the size of velopharyngeal opening probably did not vary much during phonation of the six vowels which they studied. Considering the concept of critical point of closure (which has been discussed in detail previously), the opening of the oral cavity was greater in proportion to the opening to the nasal cavity for the low vowels than for the high vowels and so the low vowels were judged less nasal in quality than the high vowels. In contrast, the functionally nasal speakers, without cleft palate, studied by Lintz and Sherman, probably showed considerable variation in velopharyngeal closure during the production of vowels. Obtaining closure may be easier for high vowels for that subject group since the dorsum of the tongue is high and since, as postulated previously, there are physiological relationships between the lingual and velopharyngeal structures. For high vowels, then, the size of the velopharyngeal space is decreased and the vowels are judged nonnasal. For low vowels, the dorsum of the tongue is low, and the velopharyngeal structure must work in opposition to it in order to elevate to close the velopharyngeal port. In that instance, the speaker finds it difficult to occlude the velopharyngeal port and the low vowels tend to be nasal.

Additional research needs to be done to test this hypothesis. Functionally nasal speakers and nasal speakers with cleft palate might be matched with regard to amount and pattern of velopharyngeal competence. If the variable of velopharyngeal competence is of major importance, the two subject groups, matched in that way, should show similar patterns of judged nasality.

Similarly, there is need for investigations regarding other factors which may contribute to nasality in the cleft palate population. It may be that interrelationships exist among several such factors which need to be taken into account. For example, the variable of tongue height has been considered as a possible etiological factor for nasality, and misarticulation, for the cleft palate population. The results of those investigations of the role of tongue carriage have been relatively inclusive. It has been suggested (Powers, 1962; Spriestersbach, 1965) that relationships exist between tongue height and amount of velopharyngeal closure, and that studying tongue height of various velopharyngeal closure subgroups may be productive. Other such relationships may exist.

C. LANGUAGE DEVELOPMENT

The important etiological factors in retarded language development of children with cleft palate are velopharyngeal incompetence and its effect on articulation (which has been discussed previously), and lack of stimulation from adults either because of hospitalization or because of parental attitudes. The possible effect of parental attitudes is seen in the fact that the language retardation is most apparent, according to data reported by Morris (1962), at relatively early stages of development: that is, before the age of 5 or 6 years. The period of time from birth until the child is 5 must surely be the one during which the parents feel the most anxiety, need for overprotectiveness toward the child, and guilt about the child, his cleft, his appearance, and his care. By the time the child is past 6, the parents' fears may be somewhat allayed by management which has taken place, or they may have adapted to the problem to a greater extent than they had earlier. The parents may also be less anxious about the child since, by the time he is 6, his general ability to communicate may have improved considerably. Data reported by Morris (1962) indicate that although children with clefts are retarded in the level of achievement in language skills throughout the age range from 5 to 16 years, there is nevertheless a steady increment of skills during that period.

It is interesting to note that although their general level of language achievement continues to improve with age, children with clefts who are older than 8 years obtain lower scores on measures of verbal output and spontaneity than do younger children with clefts. This reverse in the trend could be interpreted to mean that children with clefts begin in their early teens to become more acutely aware of their differences from normal individuals and tend to withdraw from speaking situations. Data reported by Spriestersbach and Powers (in press) support that interpretation. In their group of 175 families with a child with a cleft and 175 control families, the parents of children with clefts rated their children as being more shy than did the parents of normal children. Furthermore, the difference was more marked for parents of older children than for parents of younger children. A case can be made for the contention that, as the child with a cleft lip and palate gets older, he becomes increasingly aware of the differences between him and his peers. That awareness, particularly if the differences are relatively great, may serve to curb spontaneity even more than that which typifies the usual adolescent and young adult period of life. More research is needed.

V. Summary

In large part, the articulation, voice, and language problems of individuals with cleft palate are causally related to many factors which are important in considering the etiologies of the speech and language disorders of other clinical populations. These factors include level of intelligence, hearing acuity, amount of stimulation, and dentition. Some of these factors are relevant for the child with a cleft palate just because he is a child. Others, such as dentition and amount of language stimulation, may be of more significance for the child with a cleft than for the normal child because the cleft palate in many instances has an effect on the development of dentition and, indirectly, on the amount of language stimulation which the child receives.

Of greatest significance is the difficulty which individuals in this population typically have in achieving velopharyngeal competence and the deficiencies in intraoral breath pressure which result. These deficiences in pressure result in distorted consonant productions, that is, impaired articulation, and in an unusual amount of nasal resonance on vowels, that is, hypernasality. To the extent that communication is impaired by these disorders during the early age of the child with a cleft palate, the development of general language proficiency may also be retarded.

REFERENCES

Arkebauer, H. J. (1964). A Study of Intraoral Air Pressures Associated with Production of Selected Consonants. Ph. D. Thesis, Univ. of Iowa, Iowa City, Iowa.

Barnes, Ida J., and Morris, H. L. (1967). Interrelationships among oral breath pressure ratios and articulation proficiency for individuals with cleft palate. *J. Speech Hearing Res.* **10**, 506–514.

Berry, Mildred F. (1949). Lingual anomalies associated with palatal clefts. *J. Speech Hearing Disorders* **14**, 359–362.

Berry, Mildred F., and Eisenson, J. (1956). "Speech Disorders." Appleton, New York.

Black, J. W. (1950). The pressure component in the production of consonants. *J. Speech Hearing Disorders* **15**, 207–210.

Bloomer, H. H. (1957). *In* "Handbook of Speech Pathology" (L. E. Travis, ed.), pp. 608–652. Appleton, New York.

Brandt, Sara D., and Morris, H. L. (1965). The linearity of the relationships between articulation errors and velopharyngeal incompetence. *Cleft Palate J.* **2**, 176–183.

Brown, S. F., and Oliver, Dorothy. (1940). A qualitative study of the organic speech mechanism abnormalities associated with cleft palate. *J. Speech Hearing Disorders* **5**, 265–270.

Buck, M. W. (1951). An X-ray Study of Cleft Palate, Oral, and Pharyngeal Structures, and Their Functioning During Phonation. Ph. D. Thesis, Univ. of Iowa, Iowa City, Iowa.

Buncke, H. J., Jr. (1959). Manometric evaluation of palatal function in cleft palate patients. *Plastic Reconstruc. Surg.* **23**, 148–158.

Bzoch, K. R. (1956). An Investigation of the Speech of Pre-school Cleft Palate Children. Ph. D. Thesis, Northwestern Univ., Evanston, Illinois.

Counihan, D. T. (1956). A Clinical Study of the Speech Efficiency and Structural Adequacy of Operated Adolescent and Adult Cleft Palate Persons. Ph. D. Thesis, Northwestern Univ., Evanston, Illinois.

Curtis, J. F. (1942). An Experimental Study of Wave Composition of Nasal Voice Quality. Ph. D. Thesis, Univ. of Iowa, Iowa City, Iowa.

Davis, H., and Silverman, S. R. (1960). "Hearing and Deafness," rev. ed. Holt, New York.

Egbert, J. H. (1955). The Effect of Certain Home Influences on the Progress of Children in a Speech Therapy Program. Ph. D. Thesis, Stanford Univ., Stanford, California.

Foster, T. D., and Greene, Margaret C. L. (1960). Lateral speech defects and dental irregularities in cleft palate. *Brit. J. Plastic Surg.* **12**, 367–377.

Goodstein, L. D. (1960). MMPI differences between parents of children with cleft palates and parents of physically normal children. *J. Speech Hearing Res.* **3**, 31–38.

Goodstein, L. D. (1961). Intellectual impairment in children with cleft palates. *J. Speech Hearing Res.* **4**, 287–294.

Graham, M. D. (1962). A Longitudinal Study of Ear Disease and Hearing Loss in Patients with Cleft Lips and Palates. M. S. Thesis, Univ. of Iowa, Iowa City, Iowa.

Greene, Margaret C. L. (1960). Speech analysis of 263 cleft palate cases. *J. Speech Hearing Disorders* **25**, 43–48.

Hagerty, R. F., and Hoffmeister, F. S. (1954). Velo-pharyngeal closure: an index of speech. *Plastic Reconstruc. Surg.* **13**, 290–298.

Holt, D. L. (1959). A Study of the Relationship between Velopharyngeal Closure and Observed Nasality (in Cleft Palate Children.) M. A. Thesis, Univ. of Nebraska, Omaha, Nebraska.

Hudgins, C. V., and Stetson, R. H. (1935). Voicing of consonants by depression of larynx. *Arch. Neerl. Phon. Exptl.* **11**, 1–28.

Isshiki, N., and Ringel, R. (1964). Air flow during the production of selected consonants. *J. Speech Hearing Res.* **7**, 233–244.

Johnson, W., Brown, S. F., Curtis, J. F., Edney, C. W., and Keaster, Jacqueline (1956). "Speech Handicapped School Children," rev. ed. Harper, New York.

Jolleys, A. (1954). A review of the results of operations on cleft palates with reference to maxillary growth and speech function. *Brit. J. Plastic Surg.* **7**, 229–241.

Kaltenborn, A. (1948). An X-ray Study of Velopharyngeal Closure in Nasal and Non-nasal Speakers. M. A. Thesis, Northwestern Univ., Chicago, Illinois.

Kodman, F. (1951). A Radiographic Psychophysical Study of the Nasality of Eight Cleft Palate Subjects Fitted with a Speech Appliance. M. A. Thesis, Univ. of Pittsburgh, Pittsburgh, Pennsylvania.

Koepp-Baker, H. (1957). *In* "Handbook of Speech Pathology" (L. E. Travis, ed.), pp. 597–607. Appleton, New York.

Lintz, Lois, B., and Sherman, Dorothy. (1961). Phonetics elements and perception of nasality. *J. Speech Hearing Res.* **4**, 381–396.

McCarthy, Dorothea. (1954a). *In* "Manual of Child Psychology" (L. Carmichael, ed.), rev. ed., pp. 492–630. Wiley, New York.

McCarthy, Dorothea. (1954b). Language disorders and parent-child relationships. *J. Speech Hearing Disorders* **19**, 514–523.

McDermott, R. P. (1962). A Study of /s/ Sound Production by Individuals with Cleft Palates. Ph. D. Thesis, Univ. of Iowa, Iowa City, Iowa.

McDonald, E. T., and Koepp-Baker, H. (1951). Cleft palate speech: An integration of research and clinical observation. *J. Speech Hearing Disorders* **16**, 9–20.

Matthews, J., and Byrne, Margaret C. (1953). An experimental study of tongue flexibility in children with cleft palates. *J. Speech Hearing Disorders* **18**, 43–47.

Moll, K. L., and Darley, F. L. (1960). Attitudes of mothers of articulatory-impaired and speech-retarded children. *J. Speech Hearing Disorders* **25**, 377–384.

Morley, Muriel E. (1962). "Cleft Palate and Speech," 5th ed. Williams & Wilkins, Baltimore, Maryland.

Morris, H. L. (1960). Communications Skills of Children with Cleft Lips and Palates. Ph. D. Thesis, Univ. of Iowa, Iowa City, Iowa.

Morris, H. L. (1962). Communication skills of children with cleft lips and palates. *J. Speech Hearing Res.* **5**, 79–90.

Morris, H. L., and Smith, Jeanne K. (1962). A multiple approach for evaluating velopharyngeal competency. *J. Speech Hearing Disorders* **27**, 218–226.

Morris, H. L., Spriestersbach, D. C., and Darley, F. L. (1961). An articulation test for assessing competency of velopharyngeal closure. *J. Speech Hearing Res.* **4**, 48–55.

Palmer, J. M., and Adams, M. R. (1962). The oral image of children with cleft lips and palates. *Cleft Palate Bull.* **12**, 72–76.

Pinson, A. B. (1956). An Experimental Study of the Palatal Efficiency, and the Articulation, Voice Quality and Intelligibility of Cleft Palate Speech. M. A. Thesis, Bowling Green Univ., Bowling Green, Ohio.

Pitzner, Joan H., and Morris, H. L. (1966). Articulation skills and adequacy of breath pressure ratios of children with cleft palates. *J. Speech Hearing Disorders* **31**, 26–40.

Powers, G. R. (1960). A Cinefluorographic Study of the Articulatory Movements of Selected Individuals with Cleft Palates. Ph. D. Thesis, Univ. of Iowa, Iowa City, Iowa.

Powers, G. R. (1962). Cinefluorographic investigation of articulatory movements of selected individuals with cleft palates. *J. Speech Hearing Res.* **5**, 59–69.

Riello, A. (1958). Articulatory Proficiency of the Mentally Retarded Child. Ph. D. Thesis, New York Univ., New York, New York.

Shelton, R. L., Jr., Brooks, Alta R., and Youngstrom, K. A. (1964). Articulation and patterns of palatopharyngeal closure. *J. Speech Hearing Disorders* **29**, 390–408.

Shelton, R. L., Jr., Brooks, Alta R., and Youngstrom, K. A. (1965). Clinical assessment of palatopharyngeal closure. *J. Speech Hearing Disorders* **30**, 37–43.

Sidney, R. A., and Matthews, J. (1956). An evaluation of the social adjustment of a group of cleft palate children. *Cleft Palate Bull.* **6**, 10.

Snow, Katherine. (1961). Articulation proficiency in relation to certain dental abnormalities. *J. Speech Hearing Disorders* **26**, 209–212.

Spriestersbach, D. C. (1964). *In* "Reconstructive Plastic Surgery" (J. M. Converse, ed.), Chapter 41. Saunders, New York.

Spriestersbach, D. C. (1965). The effects of orofacial anomalies of the speech process. *In* "Proceedings of the Conference: Communicative Problems in Cleft Palate." *ASHA Rept.* **1**, 111–128.

Spriestersbach, D. C., and Moll, K. L. (1964). "Speakers with Cleft Palates," Research film. Univ. of Iowa, Iowa City, Iowa.

Spriestersbach, D. C., and Powers, G. R. (1959a). Nasality in isolated vowels and connected speech of cleft palate speakers. *J. Speech Hearing Res.* **2**, 40–45.

Spriestersbach, D. C., and Powers, G. R. (1959b). Articulation skills, velopharyngeal closure, and oral breath pressure of children with cleft palates. *J. Speech Hearing Res.* **2**, 318–325.

Spriestersbach, D. C., and Powers, G. R. (in press). "The Cleft Palate Problem." Univ. of Iowa Press, Iowa City, Iowa.

Spriestersbach, D. C., Moll, K. L., and Morris, H. L. (1961). Subject classification and articulation of speakers with cleft palates. *J. Speech Hearing Res.* **4**, 362–372.

Spriestersbach, D. C., Lierle, D. M., Moll, K. L., and Prather, W. F. (1962). Hearing loss in children with cleft palate. *Plastic Reconstruc. Surg.* **30**, 336–347.

Stetson, R. H. (1951). "Motor Phonetics—A Study of Speech Movements in Action," 2nd ed. North-Holland Publ., Amsterdam.

Stetson, R. H., and Hudgins, C. V. (1930). Functions of the breathing movements in the mechanisms of speech. *Arch. Neerl. Phon. Exptl.* **5**, 1–30.

Subtelny, Joanne D., and Subtelny, J. D. (1959). Intelligibility and associated physiological factors of cleft palate speakers. *J. Speech Hearing Res.* **2**, 353–360.

Subtelny, Joanne D., Koepp-Baker, H., and Subtelny, J. D. (1961). Palatal function and cleft palate speech. *J. Speech Hearing Disorders* **26**, 213–224.

Subtelny, Joanne D., Worth, J. H., and Sakuda, M. (1966). Intraoral pressure and rate of flow during speech. *J. Speech Hearing Res.* **9**, 498–518.

Templin, Mildred C. (1957). "Certain Language Skills in Children, Their Development and Interrelationships." Univ. of Minnesota Press, Minneapolis, Minnesota.

Terman, L. M., and Merrill, Maud A. (1960). "Stanford-Binet Intelligence Scale." Houghton, Boston, Massachusetts.

Travis, L. E. (1957). "Handbook of Speech Pathology." Appleton, New York.

Van Demark, D. R. (1964). Misarticulations and listener judgments of the speech of individuals with cleft palates. *Cleft Palate J.* **1**, 232–245.

Van Demark, D. R. (1966). A factor analysis of the speech of children with cleft palate. *Cleft Palate J.* **3**, 159–170.

Van Riper, C. G., and Irwin, J. V. (1958). "Voice and Articulation." Prentice-Hall, Englewood Cliffs, New Jersey.

Wardill, W. E. M. (1937). The technique of operation for cleft palate. *Brit. J. Surg.* **25**, 117–130.

Warren, D. W., and Devereaux, J. L. (1966). An analog study of cleft palate speech. *Cleft Palate J.* **3**, 103–114.

Warren, D. W., and DuBois, A. B. (1964). A pressure-flow technique for assessing velopharyngeal orifice area during continuous speech. *Cleft Palate J.* **1**, 52–71.

Watson, C. G. (1964). Personality adjustment in boys with cleft lips and palates. *Cleft Palate J.* **1**, 130–138.

Wechsler, D. (1949). "Manual for Wechsler Intelligence Scale for Children." Psychological Corporation, New York.

West, R., Ansberry, M., and Carr, Anna (1957). "The Rehabilitation of Speech." Harper, New York.

Westlake, H., and Rutherford, D. (1966). "Cleft Palate." Prentice-Hall, Englewood Cliffs, New Jersey.

Wildman, A. J. (1961). Analysis of tongue, soft palate, and pharyngeal wall movement. *Am. J. Orthodont.* **47**, 439–461.

Winitz, H. (1964). Research in articulation and intelligence. *Child Develop.* **35**, 287–297.

Wood, K. S. (1946). Parental maladjustment and functional articulatory defects in children. *J. Speech Hearing Disorders* **11**, 255–275.

V

Audiological and Otological Considerations

William F. Prather and C. M. Kos

I. Introduction 169
II. Incidence of Hearing Loss and Aural Pathology 170
   A. General School-Age Population 170
   B. Cleft Palate Population 171
III. Incidence of Hearing Loss and of Aural Pathology in Relationship to Other Variables . . . . : 174
   A. Intelligence 174
   B. Type of Cleft 175
   C. Degree of Cleft 176
   D. Sex 177
   E. Type of Physical Management and Age at Surgery 177
   F. Associated Congenital Anomalies 181
   G. Eustachian Tube and Palatal Muscle Function 182
   H. Adenoids and Tonsils 187
   I. Nasal Obstruction, Swollen Turbinates, and Sinuses 189
   J. Allergy 191
   K. Age 191
   L. Reflux of Food and Other Matter 193
   M. Upper Respiratory Infections 193
IV. Discussion and Implications for Management 194
   References 198

I. Introduction

The primary purpose of this chapter is to draw together, to relate, and to summarize available information important to useful audiological and otological descriptions of individuals with cleft palate. Since there is a high relationship between hearing loss[1] and aural pathology and since some

---

[1] Throughout this chapter, unless noted otherwise, all hearing levels are expressed in decibels re the 1951 ASA audiometric zero.

authors use the two terms interchangeably, incidence of hearing loss and of aural pathology are discussed as one unit. It is possible, however, to find individuals with a hearing loss but with no aural pathology demonstrable by otological examination. Conversely, it also is possible to find individuals with aural pathology but with no hearing loss, at least as measured by some of the more commonly accepted standards.

In any attempt to describe or to discuss the hearing status of any individual, many problems soon become apparent. A description of hearing acuity for a given person is obviously not merely a categorical statement that "he hears" or "he does not hear." It is, in part, a description of how much he hears. It is also a description of what kind of loss he has and of the extent to which his loss is progressive, reversible by medicine or surgery, and amenable to "improvement" by amplification, or other "rehabilitation."

Inherent dangers exist, obviously, in generalizing from a description of the hearing of one individual within a group for the purpose of describing hearing for the group on the average or as a whole, even when this group is fairly homogeneous with respect to traits associated with hearing problems. To reverse this process, however, is common practice, since whatever is most characteristic of the group constitutes the best estimate of what will be characteristic of an individual within the group. The average accuracy of such estimates increases, of course, with greater size and greater homogeneity of the group. In publications dealing with the problem of hearing for individuals with cleft palate, unfortunately, predictions for all individuals of a certain group are sometimes made without due regard to the very simple fact that the data for a group are always, to some extent, variable and without appropriate evaluation of the scientific rigor with which the group data were compiled and interpreted.

The following subsections are for organizational purposes and are not intended to be mutually exclusive. Hearing loss and aural pathology in individuals with clefts appear, in fact, to be so confounded with other interrelated parameters that to consider any one of these by itself could be misleading. However, interrelationships among parameters will be pointed out insofar as possible and it will be important to the reader when any one parameter is discussed categorically to keep these interrelationships in mind.

II. Incidence of Hearing Loss and Aural Pathology

A. GENERAL SCHOOL-AGE POPULATION

Since it is not the purpose of this chapter to review all of the pertinent information and data regarding hearing surveys in the general population and to discuss completely the varying definitions of "hearing impairment," the reader is referred to Davis and Silverman (1960, pp. 242-264) for a more complete report. The American Medical Association, however, generally recognizes that hearing "impairment," at least for medical purposes, is a hearing loss of more than 15 dB (see footnote 1) for the average over frequencies 500, 1000, and 2000 Hz. A gross estimate of the incidence of hearing impairment among school-age children by this definition and by results of early surveys is approximately 5%. For a hearing loss of 10 dB or more, with various frequency criteria, the incidence according to results of various public school surveys has been reported as anywhere from 4 to 17% (Hearing Conservation, 1962).

Eagles *et al.* (1963) has reported on the incidence of aural and related pathology from data collected on 4078 children, aged 5 to 14 years and representing a cross-section of the Pittsburgh elementary public school population. Of these 4078 children 15% were classified as "otoscopically abnormal." For 20% of these children so classified otoscopic findings were indicative of acute and chronic ear disease and for the remaining 80% were indicative of past pathology.

B. CLEFT PALATE POPULATION

For information on incidence of hearing loss or aural pathology among those with cleft palate as reported in the literature prior to 1940 the reader is referred to the review by Skolnik (1958).

In a comparison between children with cleft palate and children with functional articulation problems, Gaines (1940) reported that the children with cleft palate had the higher mean percentage of hearing loss for the frequencies 512 to 2048 Hz and that they also demonstrated more individual variation in degree of loss and more inflammation of the middle ear. Wagner (1941) reported a "probable higher incidence" of hearing loss in 50 cleft palate subjects than in "normal" children.

Sataloff and Fraser (1952), who defined "hearing loss" as a loss of 15 dB or more for two or more frequencies at octave points between 250 and 8000 Hz, found a hearing loss, usually bilateral, for over 90% of a series of children with cleft palate. They also reported finding pathological changes in both middle ears for all children in the series.

From a study of 50 cleft palate children Gannon (1950) has reported for the better ear average over the speech frequencies that 66% had no loss (0–10 dB), 18% had a "slight" loss (10–20 dB), 12% had a "moderate" loss (20–30 dB), and 4% had a "marked" loss (30 dB or more).

Means and Irwin (1954) have reported that 59.4% of 225 cleft palate children failed to pass a sweep-check test at 15 dB, that is, failed to hear four out of six octave frequencies between 250 and 8000 Hz at this level.

Holmes and Reed (1955), who studied 26 cleft palate subjects, stated that over the speech frequency range 62% had a loss greater than 10 dB in one or both ears and 46% had a loss of 20 dB or more. They also stated that 62% of their subjects showed scarring or retraction of the eardrum. Referring to the fact that chronic middle ear changes (eardrum perforations, fibrosis, and adhesions in the middle ear) had occurred, they said that it became especially important to study and understand these hearing losses since, as seen in these patients, the losses were of a permanent, untreatable nature.

Counihan (1956) reported that in a group of 55 adolescent and adult cleft palate subjects only one had a loss in the better ear of more than 20 dB at any frequency between 125 and 8000 Hz.

Berry and Eisenson (1956) stated that of the 383 children they had observed between 1946 and 1955 less than 60% suffered from a "recognizable" handicap in hearing.

Lis et al. (1956) stated that at their Cleft Palate Center 40% of all children with "palatal disturbance" had a hearing loss in one or both ears of at least 15 dB in the speech frequency range.

Miller (1956) reported that 54% of 35 cleft palate subjects, aged 3 to 23 years, had a loss of 30 dB or more at at least one of the octave frequencies between 125 and 12000 Hz. He further noted that the most common conductive loss was in the high frequencies (8000 to 12000 Hz).

Halfond and Ballenger (1956a, b) found a significantly greater incidence of active middle ear pathology and tympanic membrane scarring for 37 subjects with clefts of the lip and palate and with a demonstrable hearing loss, that is, a loss of 20 dB or more in both ears at any two or more of the octave frequencies from 125 to 8000 Hz, than they found for 32 subjects with clefts of the lip and palate and with no hearing loss by their definition. Between these two groups they found no differences in the incidence of eardrum perforations, of middle ear fluid, or of narrow external auditory meati; they also found no differences in the frequencies of a history of earaches, of running ears, or of mastoiditis. Although the incidence of hearing loss was not studied as such, they were of the opinion that over 50% of their total number of cases had medically significant losses, an incidence that was "much higher than previously reported." Recognizing that even in their so-called "no-hearing loss" group there were many individuals who had hearing losses by criteria less stringent than theirs, they estimated that the incidence of hearing loss in their cases could be as high as 75% or more.

Skalbeck in 1956 (cited in Casteel, 1960) reviewed 127 medical records of children with cleft lip and palate and found that for 64% aural pathology had been reported.

After examining 295 patients with clefts Whaley (1957) reported that 25% of them had impaired hearing.

For 63 subjects with clefts Drettner (1960) found that 56% had tympanic membrane changes.

Skolnik (1958), who over an 8-year period had seen 401 patients with clefts of the lip and palate or palate only, reported that 45.8% had ear pathology, with the pathology unilateral in 16.8% of the cases and bilateral in 83.2%. Although he does not state what test frequencies are included in his analysis, he reported that of the 288 pathological ears (not patients) that could be accurately tested, 11.1% had no hearing loss, 56.2% had a mild hearing loss (loss than 30 dB), 28.4% had a moderate hearing loss (between 30 and 60 dB), and 4.3% had a severe hearing loss (over 60 dB). Perceptive hearing loss was noted in only 5 cases; all other losses were of the conductive type, with the predominant loss in the low frequencies and usually bilateral with a similar pattern in both ears. A close relationship was noted between the degree of middle ear disease and the degree of loss.

Tangen (1960) has reported on complete otological histories and examinations of 65 children with cleft palate who were referred for reasons other than ear complaints. He found that ear pain (at some time during the life of the child) was the most common complaint in the histories, occurring for 75.4% of the cases. Ear discharge was reported for 30.8%. By results of examination all children had an abnormal appearance of the tympanic membranes, which were usually lusterless, thickened, and opaque. Sluggish motion of the tympanic membrane was noted in 33.1%, retraction in 23.8%, scarring in 19.2%, calcium plaques in 8.5%, increased vascularity in 7.7%, and perforations in 4.6%. Of the total number of ears 44.6% were considered pathological. Tangen also noted a "definite preponderance" of secretory otitis media. Skolnik (1958), however, found no evidence of difference in frequency of occurrence between purulent and catarrhal otitis media in his cases.

Graham (1963), reporting on 190 subjects with clefts of the lip and/or palate, found 48.4% with a history of ear disease. Of 29 subjects with clefts of the palate only and 146 subjects with clefts of the lip and palate 57.1% and 51.0%, respectively, had a history of ear disease.

For 163 cleft palate children, aged 2 years, 9 months, to 15 years, 11 months, Spriestersbach et al. (1962) reported incidence figures which ranged from 74.1% for a loss at any one of six frequencies, 250 to 8000 Hz, of 10 dB or more in the worse ear to 3.2% for an average loss over all frequencies, 250 to 8000 Hz, of 30 dB or more in the better ear. Both the incidence of loss and the magnitude of threshold deviations were significantly greater in the youngest age group (33 to 71 months) than in any of the older age groups (see Section III, K).

It is clear that hearing loss and aural pathology incidence data obtained from samples of the population of children with all types of cleft palate are not the most useful for the purposes of comparison with the population without clefts. These are not to be expected to be the same for various subclassifications of children with clefts. For the entire population of children with clefts, however, in comparison to the population of children without clefts, at least three general patterns emerge: (1) the incidence of hearing loss, regardless of definition, is greater among children with clefts than among those without; (2) the incidence of aural pathology is greater among children with clefts than among those without; and (3) the hearing losses of children with clefts are primarily bilateral and conductive in nature.

III. Incidence of Hearing Loss and of Aural Pathology in Relationship to Other Variables

From the above discussion arise several questions important to audiological and otological considerations with reference to cleft palate: (1) How does the incidence of hearing loss and/or aural pathology vary with cleft palate subclassifications? (2) What factor or factors account for the higher incidence of hearing loss and aural pathology in the cleft palate population and to what extent and how are these factors related to each other as well as to the overall problem? (3) Since hearing losses of children with cleft palate are primarily conductive in nature, to what extent, in general, is the hearing loss and/or aural pathology preventable or amenable to treatment? It is to these other variables and their relationship to the incidence of hearing loss and aural pathology, then, that we now must turn.

A. Intelligence

Means and Irwin (1954) divided 225 cleft palate children, aged from 3 years and 9 months to 16 years, into two groups, one with hearing losses and one with no hearing losses. The former group consisted of those children who had a loss of 25 dB or more at the frequency 250, 500, 1000, or 2000 Hz or 30 dB or more at 4000 or 8000 Hz. They reported a significant difference between these two groups with respect to IQ, with 52% of the group with no losses and 37% of the group with losses having IQ's of 100 or more. This finding, however, does not provide evidence for a specific conclusion with reference to intelligence. It is possible that the group with losses included a higher proportion of subjects with clefts of the palate only. As Goodstein has reported in Chapter VI, this subgroup scores significantly lower on intelligence tests than either of the other two subgroups, cleft of the lip only and cleft of the palate and lip. Further research is needed to determine whether intelligence level is functionally related to hearing level.

B. Type of Cleft

Skolnik (1958) reported a maximum frequency, that is, 73%, of ear pathology for submucous cleft palates and a minimum, 31% for clefts of the hard and soft palates. He stated, however, that it is not feasible to use his frequency data for comparisons among different types of clefts without considering the age factor. For preschool children he noted the smallest incidence of ear pathology in those who had clefts of both hard and soft palates but for school-age children he noted no substantial difference in incidence among cleft types. Among the 133 cases of unilateral cleft lip and palate, 62 had ear pathology. For 21 of these the pathology was unilateral or definitely more pronounced in the ear opposite the side of the cleft; 7 had pathology in the ear on the same side as the cleft; and the remaining 34 had bilateral ear pathology.

Drettner (1960) noted a significant difference in incidence of hearing impairment or aural pathology between two cleft-type groups, 63 subjects in all. Of those with clefts of the lip and palate and of those with clefts of the palate only, 74 and 43%, respectively, were considered to have tympanic membrane changes or hearing impairment or both. There was no relation, however, between the side of the cleft and the side of changes in the ear.

Phillips in 1956 (cited in Casteel, 1960) stated that he found that hearing loss varied with the type of cleft. For 75 cases with cleft lip or cleft palate only incidence of hearing loss was about 5%, but for clefts of the lip and palate the incidence of hearing loss was 83% of those patients tested at ages up to 5 and 75% of those tested at later ages up to 20. Masters et al. (1960) noted, however, a higher incidence in those with clefts of the hard and soft palate than in those with clefts of the lip and palate. Spriestersbach et al. (1962) did not find a significant difference between cleft palate-only and cleft lip-and-palate groups with respect to incidence of hearing loss, but the observed difference was in the direction of the cleft palate-only group having a greater incidence of loss.

Graham (1963) found no hearing loss (15 dB or more in the speech frequencies) for subjects with cleft of the lip only but did find losses for 37.9% of the subjects with cleft palate only and for 38.3% of the subjects with cleft lip and palate. On the basis of these findings he concluded that "the presence of the palatal cleft appears to be the primary factor related to a higher incidence of ear infection and hearing loss in the population with the cleft anomaly."

Goetzinger et al. (1960) found no significant variation in hearing levels among the cleft palate classifications studied in adult subjects.

In summary, then, the incidence of hearing loss and aural pathology appear to vary with the type of cleft, but the nature of the relationship is not clear. Skolnik (1958) found the highest incidence of ear pathology in those with submucous clefts but maintained that his incidence figures were confounded with the variable of age. In preschool-age children, however, he noted the smallest incidence of ear pathology in those children who had clefts of both the hard and soft palate, but in school-age children the incidence was similar for all cleft groups. Some investigators have noted a higher incidence of hearing loss and aural pathology in those with clefts of both the lip and palate (Phillips in Casteel, 1960; Drettner, 1960) while others have noted at least a trend for a greater incidence in the palate-only group (Spriestersbach et al., 1962; Masters et al., 1960). Various factors, such as age and management differences, undoubtedly tend to influence results and may, at least in part, account for apparent inconsistencies among incidence data. Of some relevance here may be an observation by Drettner (1960) who found a higher incidence not only of hearing loss but also of nasal obstruction in those with clefts of the lip and palate than in those with clefts of the palate only (see Section III, I). Spriestersbach et al. (1962) observed that in those patients who have clefts of the palate only and also associated anomalies incidence of hearing loss was significantly greater than for those patients in the same cleft group but without other anomalies. This difference in incidence of hearing loss between those with other anomalies and those without was not observed in the group of patients with clefts of both the lip and palate (see Section III, F).

C. DEGREE OF CLEFT

Gannon (1950) found no correlation between the degree of the palatal cleft and the amount of hearing loss and concluded that the important factor was the "mere presence" of rather than the degree of the cleft. Likewise, Holmes and Reed (1955) found no relationship between the severity of the primary deformity and the degree of loss. Masters et al. (1960), however, found the highest incidence of hearing loss in subjects with "wide" clefts of the hard and soft palates.

Halfond and Ballenger (1956b) found no difference between their hearing-loss and no-hearing-loss groups of children with cleft palate either in the "openness" of the palate or in the distance of the palate from the posterior wall of the pharynx. They suggested that "openness" of the palate was not a factor which influences the incidence of loss in individuals with clefts. Skolnik (1958) reported that for 47 "definitely wide" clefts, not amenable to surgical closure, 44% of the subjects had ear pathology and 56% had normal ears. Immediately prior to surgical closure for 35 cases with "narrow" clefts, 50% had ear pathology, and 49% had normal ears. He thus obtained no evidence of any relationship between frequency of middle ear disorders and the width of the cleft.

Except for the results of Masters *et al.* (1960), there is no evidence to support a hypothesis that degree of cleft is related to the incidence of hearing loss and aural pathology. It should be acknowledged, however, that subjectivity is involved in evaluating "degree" of cleft; and it is still possible that the greater the extent to which such an anomaly involves structures which relate to Eustachian tube function (discussed in Section III, G) the more likely it is that hearing will be affected. Present evidence, however, does not support a hypothesis that "degree" of cleft as such and degree of involvement of Eustachian tube function are related.

D. SEX

No difference between sexes has been found in the incidence of hearing loss and aural pathology (Skolnik, 1958; Goetzinger *et al.*, 1960; Spriestersbach *et al.*, 1962).

E. TYPE OF PHYSICAL MANAGEMENT AND AGE AT SURGERY

Skolnik (1958) evaluated the relationship between ear pathology and closure of the palate by surgery or prosthesis for two groups, 90 preschool children and 133 school-age children. Ear pathology was noted in only 27% of the entire preschool group as compared to 68% of the entire school-age group, a finding which is explained, at least in part, by a higher percentage of postoperative cases in the older group. Among 52 cases in the school-age group whose palates were short, tight, and scarred, 79% had ear pathology and 21% had normal ears. Among 32 cases in this same group considered to have good surgical repair, a smaller proportion, 53%, had aural pathology and a larger proportion, 47%, had normal ears.

Skolnik, in evaluating the effects of palatal surgery on ear pathology, also noted that of the 41 cases in the school-age group who had palatal closure before the age of 1 year 73% had ear pathology and 27% had normal ears. Among those children whose palates were closed after 2 years of age 75% had ear pathology and 25% had normal ears. Thus, the age at which the palatal surgery was performed did not appear to be related to the ear pathology. He stated that surgical closure of the palate appears to be an extremely important factor in the pathogenesis of middle ear disorders, the mechanism for which the disorders occur seeming to be related to a process of atrophy, scarring, and sclerosis of tubal muscles after surgery. He supported this inference by reference to the higher incidence of ear pathology among cases with a scarred, tight palate than among cases with good operative results.

Skolnik also stated that "the inadequacy of tubal musculature after surgery should be considered in the evaluation of a surgical repair of the palate; furthermore, the opinion that early closure of the palate avoids secondary atrophy of palatal muscles and prevents otitis media, is not supported by this study." He questioned the wisdom of surgery at an early age in many cases because of "dangers of early closure in relation to inter-ference with centers of bone growth, and consequent serious disturbances of development of the bones of the jaw and face, and the high incidence of middle ear pathology, factors which are probably directly or indirectly related to each other." Skolnik thus implied that the important factor is not surgery as such but the degree to which such surgery restores or maintains good tubal function. He also maintained that even with a good surgical result, that is, good velopharyngeal competency, there is a high probability for Eustachian tube dysfunction due to the division, in many cases, of the hamular process, which results in releasing tension of the tensor veli palatini (see Section III, G). He also pointed out that a pushback or pharyngoplasty may possibly result in impairment of the neuromuscular mechanism involved in Eustachian tube function. He would not recommend palatal surgery before the age of 2.

On the basis of data for 24 cases fitted with a prosthetic appliance Skolnik reached no definite conclusions with respect to any relationship between ear pathology and cleft palate prosthesis. He noted from clinical experience, however, that inflammation of the upper airways, lymphoid hyperplasia, and middle ear pathology often accompanied the use of a prosthesis and probably were usually caused by a poorly fitting appliance or by poor hygiene practices in caring for it. He pointed out that in such instances "there is a disturbance of the physiology of the nose and nasopharynx with consequent dysfunction of the Eustachian tube."

Masters *et al.* (1960) compared the incidence of hearing loss among groups of subjects who underwent the (1) Von Langenbeck procedure for closure, (2) a combined closure and lengthening procedure, and (3) prosthetic management of the cleft. Repair which provided surgical closure without lengthening the existing mucoperiosteal flaps, for example, the Von Langenbeck, was found to result in a "significantly higher incidence of hearing loss" than did those procedures which not only closed the palate but also included the attempt to add more length, for example, pushback and V-Y advancement. They also observed that those children whose palates were closed by prosthetic management had the highest incidence of hearing loss. This difference in the incidence of hearing loss between those whose palates were surgically repaired and those who were fitted with prostheses was explained by a difference in the intactness of the anatomy of the Eustachian tube and its associated musculature, especially the tensor and levator palatini. Also noted were the difficulties of maintaining an "adequate appliance" in the very young child and the fact that the prosthesis does not improve the dynamic mechanism involved in Eustachian tube function. They stated: "We feel that early restoration of a normal insertion of the tensor and levator muscles may prove to be the best prophylactic measure in the prevention of hearing loss." Also stated is the opinion that with surgery delayed beyond 18 months "the incidence of hearing loss appears to rise almost by arithmetic progression as age increases."

Spriestersbach *et al.* (1962) found a significantly higher incidence of hearing loss, for the better ear only, for those children who had been fitted with obturators than for those whose palates had been surgically repaired. The degree of loss, however, was not significantly different between the two management groups. Differences between those children whose palates were unrepaired and those whose palates had been surgically repaired were also not significant. On the basis of these findings they questioned the finding by Masters *et al.* (1960) of a higher incidence of hearing loss among those fitted with obturators with the explanation that the higher incidence is due to a lack of intactness of the levator and tensor palatini.

Spriestersbach *et al.* also pointed out other possible sources of bias in relating type of management to hearing losses. They suggested that in some centers surgical repair is carried out at an earlier age than is the fitting of an obturator, and it is possible that children receiving surgery at such centers would have been evaluated earlier in age than those receiving obturators. However, it was noted in their study that although no differences were found among management groups with respect to ages at the time of testing, those children who were "typically" selected for obturators rather than surgery might be those with clefts which were wider and which thus were difficult to repair surgically. Masters *et al.* (1960) also implied that such a factor was operating in the selection of their patients.

Holborow (1962b) has suggested that some means be found to anchor the tensor palatini to the hamulus before its tendon is cut. He recognizes that in some cases there would not be enough tissue available to close the palate without a considerable shifting of the tensor and levator and that the tensor thus might have to be sacrificed, but he cautions that the importance of the tensor to hearing should not be minimized. While there remains the possibility that the incidence in ear disease levels off at least after age 5, perhaps because the levator plays a more important role in Eustachian tube opening at this age than at younger ages, "damage to the tensor, especially in early childhood, must be recognized to be a potential source of deafness. Even temporary Eustachian malfunction may lead to permanent middle-ear changes."

Holborow (1962a) also has appeared to favor early surgery on the basis that an anchorage for the tensor tendon sometimes may be provided. Absence of a firm anchorage, he states, may prevent this muscle from exerting any force upon the lateral lamina of the Eustachian tube cartilage.

Graham and Lierle (1962) have reported that children with clefts who are followed otologically from infancy and who have a pharyngeal flap palatoplasty after the age of 5 years will have no otological effects from such surgery.

Loeb (1964) reported that the incidence of hearing loss in those children with clefts who wear prostheses is higher than in those with other forms of treatment. However, Graham et al. (1962) have reported that in no case among 54 children with clefts which were obturated did the hearing become worse and that in several cases the hearing improved, in some instances to normal levels even in the presence of abnormal tympanic membranes. They also noted that the insertion of an obturator did not result in a normal restoration of the palatal mechanism and that many of the patients selected for obturators had deficient soft tissue. (As has been noted above, however, no relationship between the width of the cleft and the incidence of hearing loss has been demonstrated.) They found no evidence that patients fitted with obturators developed ear disease for the first time following the insertion of the obturator; they also found no evidence for any of these that hearing loss increased after the insertion of an obturator when there had been consistent otological treatment from infancy. They suggest that when there is a problem of reflux of saliva, food, or fluid into the nose and up the Eustachian tube (see Section III, L), the obturator can act as a static mass which, when combined with the muscular movement of the pharyngeal wall during speech, provides a fairly effective seal against gross escape of material from the oropharynx into the nasopharynx. They thus maintain that the obturator acts in much the same way as early surgical closure in the prevention of or decrease in ear infection. Skolnik (1958), however, points out that an ill-fitting prosthesis or one for which there is poor hygiene may result in inadequate drainage of secretion from the nasopharynx, pharyngitis, or hyperplasia of lymphoid tissue.

Gannon (1950) found no relationship between the age of the first palatal operation and the degree of hearing loss. Holmes and Reed (1955) found no relationship between the age of closure and the incidence of loss. Halfond and Ballenger (1956b) found no difference between hearing-loss and no-hearing-loss children with clefts either in the age of the first or in the age of last palatal operation. They stated that early surgery does not necessarily preclude the possibility of middle ear pathology and hearing loss. They felt that, since a palatal operation may adversely affect hearing acuity, use of a palatal prosthesis might be advisable until that time when surgery could be performed with minimal risk of damage to the structures involved in Eustachian tube function.

Spriestersbach *et al.* (1962) found a higher incidence of hearing loss and a higher mean hearing threshold for children whose soft palates were closed between 30 and 48 months than for children whose clefts were repaired before or after these ages. This difference was statistically significant only for the better ear. The importance of this finding, however, was discounted in view of the fact that the 30- to 48-month-old group was significantly younger at the time of testing than either of the other two groups.

In summary, then, the effect of surgery, in general, upon hearing acuity or upon incidence of hearing loss has not been clearly established. As pointed out previously (Masters *et al.*, 1960), restoration of Eustachian tube muscle function by early surgery designed to lengthen the palate and close the cleft may be important in the prevention of hearing loss. Another reason for early surgery is that an anchorage for the tensor may sometimes be provided (Holborow, 1962b). Some investigators (Gannon, 1950; Holmes and Reed, 1955; Halfond and Ballenger, 1956b), however, have found no evidence that age of surgery makes a difference in the incidence of hearing loss and aural pathology. On the other hand, one investigator (Skolnik, 1958), although his findings do not establish early surgery as a cause of hearing loss, has noted an increase in the incidence of ear pathology following surgical closure of the palate, especially among those cases for whom a poor result was obtained, and has advised against surgery before the age of 2.

That Eustachian tube function should be maintained or restored, if possible, is generally recognized. The best procedure to accomplish this end, however, is apparently still a controversial issue. Factors other than good Eustachian tube function undoubtedly must be considered in each individual case; but considerable evidence does indicate the importance of the improvement of surgical techniques for, and of more surgical attention to, maintaining or restoring good Eustachian tube function. The best age at which surgical procedures should be employed remains in question.

The insertion of an obturator has not been shown to be a cause of hearing loss. The evidence is more reasonably interpreted as indicating that those clefts which are obturated are those not best managed by surgery and which, furthermore, are also likely to be associated with more deviations of those structures important to good Eustachian tube function than are those which are not obturated.

F. ASSOCIATED CONGENITAL ANOMALIES

Snodgrasse (1954) reported finding "hearing deficiencies" in 45.9% of 40 cleft lip and cleft palate patients who had one or more additional "abnormalities." Usually the hearing loss was associated with the more severe types of clefts. Skolnik (1958), however, noted that only 62, or 15%, of 401 cases with cleft palate had other congenital anomalies and only 8, or 2%, had anomalies of the ear. For those subjects with cleft palate only, Spriestersbach et al. (1962), in studying incidence of hearing loss as a function of cleft type, found that the relative incidence of hearing loss was greater and that the mean threshold was higher for those with than for those without other associated anomalies. For children with clefts of both the lip and palate the difference in the incidence of hearing loss between those with and those without other congenital anomalies was not significant.

Whether other congenital anomalies associated with cleft palate are related to the incidence of hearing loss and aural pathology is not clear; nor, if there is any relationship, is it possible to infer what the implications might be. The study of such anomalies is complicated by special problems, and further research in this area appears indicated. One reasonable conclusion, however, is that the incidence of congenital anomalies of the ear itself is very low, too low to account in any important extent for the high incidence of hearing loss in the cleft palate population.

G. Eustachian Tube and Palatal Muscle Function

1. Normal Function

For an understanding of the possible physiopathology of the Eustachian tube in the cleft palate individual, it is helpful first to consider the anatomy and physiology of a normal Eustachian tube and its related palatal structures. Skolnik (1958) has summarized the anatomy and physiology of a normal velum as follows:

> The soft palate is a muscular hinge which is attached anteriorly at the posterior border of the hard palate by means of an aponeurotic structure and moves freely posteriorly. The muscles enter from the sides and interlace in the midline, each pair forming a sling arching either upward or downward. The musculus uvulae fastens longitudinally all of these muscles in the midline without forming a real raphe. Three pairs of muscles arch upward; the levator palati, the tensor palati and the pterygopharyngeus of the superior constrictor muscle of the pharynx. The levator veli palatini arises from the apex of the petrous bone and from the medial lamina of the cartilage of the auditory tube, enters the velum with its fibers spreading downward and medialward, and blending with those of the opposite side. The tensor veli palatini arises from the scaphoid fossa and the spina angularis of the sphenoid and from the lateral wall of the cartilage of the auditory tube; its tendon, after winding around the pterygoid hamulus, is inserted into the palatine aponeurosis and the posterior border of the palatine bone. The pterygopharyngeus muscle arises from the pharyngeal raphe approximately 1.5 centimeters below the pharyngeal tubercle of the occipital bone. It runs outward toward the pterygoid plate of the sphenoid bone, one part being inserted on it, and the hamular process and the remaining fibers running medially to be inserted into the palatal aponeurosis. Two pairs

of muscles arch downward: the glossopalatinus in front forms the anterior pillars and the pharyngopalatinus behind forms the posterior pillars. The glossopalatinus arises from the anterior surface of the soft palate, where it is continuous with the muscle of the opposite side and is inserted into the side of the tongue. The pharyngopalatinus arises from the soft palate and divides into two fasciculi. The anterior fasciculus is inserted into the posterior border of the thyroid cartilage and into the lateral and posterior wall of the pharynx. The posterior fasciculus joins the opposite muscle in the midline. An important muscular bundle connected with the latter fasciculus is the salpingopharyngeus muscle, which forms the salpingopharyngeal fold. It arises from the inferior part of the auditory tube and blends with the posterior fasciculus of the pharyngopalatinus.

Podvinec (1952) has stated that the muscles of the soft palate do not work individually but together. Among their important functions is that of opening the Eustachian tube during swallowing and yawning.

Rich (1920), on the basis of results of a comprehensive study of the function of the Eustachian tube in dogs, concluded that the Eustachian tube is usually closed and is opened during swallowing, yawning, and sneezing reflexes. He found no evidence of an independent reflex. The tubes were not opened by respiratory movements, either quiet or forced, by mouth breathing or by a mere elevation of the velum resulting from contraction of the levator palatini. Although an important function of the Eustachian tube is known to be equalization of the atmospheric pressure on the two sides of the tympanic membrane, tensing the eardrum itself did not open the tube.

Rich also concluded that contractions of the levator palatini, the palatopharyngeus, the internal pterygoid, and the superior constrictor muscles of the pharynx had no effect on the opening of the Eustachian tube and that the tensor palatini was the only muscle functionally related to it. He found no constrictor muscle in the tube itself. After the tube opened relaxation of the tensor muscle returned the tube to its normal resting, that is, closed position. That normal tensor function is essential for Eustachian tube opening has also been shown by Holborow (1962b).

Perlman (1951a,b) has shown that in phonation only the posterior lip of the torus moves as the result of action of the levator and salpingopharyngeus. In swallowing, according to Perlman, both the anterior and posterior lips of the torus actively move and the Eustachian tube opens considerably more than it does on phonation. The opening of the tube, however, is brought about not through simultaneous muscle movements but through a series of movements. The initial or passive movement of the posterior portion of the tube comes about through contraction of the salpingopharyngeus and levator muscles, but the final and active movement of the lateral portion of the tube follows as a result of a contraction of the tensor muscle which displaces the tube anteriorly, bringing about a complete opening.

The Eustachian tube is shorter and its orifice relatively larger in the infant than in the adult. In the infant the course of the tube is straight and rests on a level with the hard palate; in the adult it is forward, inward, and downward, and it is situated high up in the epipharynx on a level with the inferior turbinate (Ersner and Alexander, 1960). Holborow (1962b) has also suggested that the tensor is relatively more important in early life than in adulthood, when the levator may play a more important role in opening the Eustachian tube than it does in early life.

2. *Function in Clefts*

For individuals with cleft palate, palatal muscle function may not be normal in relation to the Eustachian tube. Holdsworth (1963) has said that "the tensors and levators are often underdeveloped and shortened in individuals with cleft palates.... In conjunction with a possible increase in the distance between the pterygoid hamuli, this shortening of the tensors produces such tension in the palatal aponeurosis that suture of the two parts of the soft palate is well-nigh impossible unless it be abolished, either by section of the tendons or their displacement following fracture of the hamuli. The levator sling is broken by the cleft, and, acting individually, each muscle can achieve little elevation of the palate."

Skolnik (1958), citing Veau, states that in the cleft palate fetus the palatal and pharyngeal muscles have a "normal volume." With increasing age atrophy takes place because of anomalies and muscular inactivity, and the opening of the Eustachian tube becomes more and more difficult. Poor surgery may hasten this atrophy. Skolnik also states that even in "good" surgery, that is, surgery which results in good velopharyngeal closure, the probability of impaired Eustachian tube function is still high. He notes that:

> The division of the hamular process, advocated by so many surgeons, will release the tension of the tensor veli palatini and permit medial displacement of the velar tags restoring the velopharyngeal closure; however, the function of the tensor will be altered into an elevator, and no further lateral displacement of the lateral wall of the tube will be possible. If a pushback or pharyngoplasty procedure is performed, the change of environment for palatal and pharyngeal muscles may result in a relative inactivity of the neuromuscular mechanism. On the other hand the action of the superior constrictor should be noted. When compensatory hypertrophy of pharyngeal muscles develop and a considerable Passavant's ridge is seen, the medial displacement of the tubal cartilage and salpingeal folds unassociated with the anterior and outward shift of the tube impairs the opening of the Eustachian tube.

Wagner (1941) has attributed the high incidence of hearing loss in the cleft palate population to the "irregularities in and stoppage of the Eustachian tube due to the functional failure of the levator and tensor palati muscles." Holmes and Reed (1955), however, found no relationship between hearing and degree of tightness or flexibility of the postoperative palate.

Halfond and Ballenger (1956b), studying 69 subjects with cleft lip and palate, found a greater number of small Eustachian tube orifices among those having significant hearing loss than among those with nonsignificant loss. Among the hearing-loss subjects they found also a greater number of "abnormal pneumophonic readings," evidence suggesting the presence of tubal stenosis. There was no evidence, however, of tubal scarring as a result of palatal surgery. Neither group had unhealthy, inadequate, or tense pharyngeal mucous membrane. From intraoral examinations they noted no difference between the two groups with regard to the frequency of immobile soft palates or decreased pharyngeal mobility.

Miller (1959) stated that Eustachian tube disturbance could be caused by "mutilating" palatal surgery which presumably resulted in poor palatal function. Skolnik (1958) noted that, among 401 subjects with clefts, those with good palatal closure, which is assumed to include good velar activity, had a lower incidence of hearing loss than those without good palatal closure. Masters et al. (1960) stated that the pathogenesis of hearing loss in the cleft palate population is primarily related to problems of Eustachian tube physiology. These problems they have attributed to three possible types of causes: mechanical, infectious, and dynamic. The mechanical problem, in their opinion, is the result of abnormal hypertrophy of adenoid pads. They found, however, that a selective adenoidectomy or "lateral bandectomy" to remove the obstruction does not, in general, result in effective treatment of the conductive hearing loss associated with congenital clefts of the palate (see Section III, H). With regard to infection, amounts of flora from cultures taken in the nasopharynx and Eustachian tube orifice of children with cleft palate were not found abnormal in comparison to amounts from cultures taken in the nasopharynx of children without cleft palate (see Section III, L). The dynamic factor, which they considered the most important, includes abnormal action of the tensor and levator muscles.

Tangen (1960) attributed the high incidence of secretory otitis media in cleft palate children primarily to altered Eustachian tube function, secondary to palatal muscle dysfunction which may result either from scarring and atrophy or from surgical repair of the palate.

Holborow (1962a,b) discussed possible causes for malfunction of the tensor muscle, suggesting poor development of the tensor or a "general hypoplasia" of the muscles of the soft palate. Also suggested was the possibility that before surgical closure of the cleft there may be a lack of firm anchorage for exertion of force by the tensor upon the lateral lamina of the Eustachian tube cartilage. Such a condition is corrected by the union of the two halves of the palate, and, according to this investigator, early surgery is indicated. Another possible cause, he suggested, is damage during surgery: damage by fracturing of the hamulus or by cutting the tendon of the tensor, for example, by the Von Langenbeck operation; damage to the nerve supply of the tensor (a branch of the trigeminal via the otic ganglion) by an incision lateral to the pterygoid plate; damage by scarring or fibrosis of muscle; or damage by a circumpharyngeal suture, which permits the muscles to heal in a contracted position, impeding the actions of both tensors and levators.

Holborow also pointed out that not all children who have a fractured hamulus or a cut tendon have a hearing loss. He accounted for this by assuming that scar tissue may form around the hamular region to provide some anchorage for the muscle; that the hamulus may not be fractured enough to eliminate all functions of the tensor; or that in later childhood it becomes possible in some cases for the levator alone to open the tube.

Holborow (1962b) also cited a possible relationship of Eustachian tube dysfunction both to a lack of pneumatization and to middle ear pathological changes in children with cleft palate.

Sataloff and Fraser (1952) observed that middle ear pathological change in their cleft palate patients was due not so much to the presence of infection in the ear as to the differences in air pressure between the middle ear and the atmosphere.

Skolnik (1958) found no movement of the tympanic membrane with respiration, a movement which might be expected when the Eustachian tubes are consistently open. On the bases of this finding and of observations of tympanic membrane pathology, along with improvement of hearing with inflation, he concluded that the Eustachian tube was consistently closed.

Poor Eustachian tube function leading to chronic negative ear pressure, according to Tangen (1960), may be a factor in the development of limited or absent pneumatization. On x-ray examination of children with cleft palate he noted that 77% of 65 subjects had limited or no pneumatization of the mastoid area. Middle ear pathology rarely was found in those who had well-developed pneumatization.

Some authors (Glover, 1961; Koepp-Baker, 1957; Fletcher, 1957) have indicated that the competency of velopharyngeal mechanism, which involves muscles also involved in Eustachian tube function, may be related to hearing loss. If it can be assumed that the ability to impound oral pressure is related to velopharyngeal competency (Spriestersbach and Powers, 1959), and also that velopharyngeal competency is related to hearing loss, it follows that oral breath pressure ratios (derived by dividing the wet spirometer or manometer reading obtained with the nostrils open by the reading obtained with the nostrils occluded) should be related to the incidence of hearing loss. Spriestersbach *et al.* (1962), however, with ratios obtained for 113 children with cleft palate, found no difference in the incidence of hearing loss between those who had a ratio of .90 or more and those who had a ratio of .89 or less.

Miller (1965) has noted in subjects without clefts that Eustachian tube function in those with chronic suppurative otitis media is significantly poorer than in those with normal ears. However, within the group of pathological ears there was considerable variation from normal to complete absence of tubal function. Miller also stated, however, that poor tubal function was most often related to a thickened and inflamed mucous membrane lining of the tympanic cavity. Where such a condition existed the probability for an improvement in tubal function with a reduction of the inflammation was high. On the other hand, such probability for improvement was low when the deficiency in tubal function existed in the presence of normal tympanic mucosa.

In children with clefts there are likely to be factors other than tympanic mucosal inflammation which contribute to Eustachian tube dysfunction. Donaldson (1966) has stated that when Eustachian tube dysfunction is not caused by infection the middle ear can be artificially aerated. He described good results from the use of polyethylene and Silastic tubes which were inserted through the tympanic membrane following myringotomy.

Eustachian tube and related palatal muscle dysfunction, then, appear to be very important as a cause of the higher incidence of hearing loss among those with cleft palate than among those without. Eustachian tube dysfunction without concurrent infection can lead to a negative pressure, that is, negative by comparison to atmospheric pressure in the middle ear; such negative pressure, as might be expected, can lead to a retraction of the tympanic membrane and thus very possibly also to a loss of hearing. The partial vacuum in the middle ear appears eventually to increase the probability for poor pneumatization of the mastoid areas (Tangen, 1960) and also the probability of secretion of fluid from the lining of the middle ear. At the same time poor Eustachian tube function provides for inadequate drainage of the middle ear. All of these conditions can lead to pathological changes and to consequent hearing loss.

H. ADENOIDS AND TONSILS

Holmes and Reed (1955) noted no relationship between ear pathology and the presence of diseased tonsils or adenoids. Halfond and Ballenger (1956b) found no difference between hearing-loss and no-hearing-loss cleft palate groups in the incidence of adenoid pathology. Miller (1959), on the other hand, lists lymphoid hyperplasia in the nasopharynx as one of the probable causes of hearing loss. Halfond and Ballenger (1956b), however, found a significantly greater frequency of tonsillar pathology among those with hearing loss than among those without. These two groups were not significantly different in age of adenotonsillectomy. The only foci for infection found among their subjects were in the tonsils, and they concluded that the removal of diseased tonsils should routinely be seriously considered. In combination with Eustachian tube dysfunction, such infection, in their opinion, could lead to increased middle ear pathology.

Koepp-Baker (1957), however, has stated that, since lymphoid tissue may play an important role in velopharyngeal closure and consequently in speech production, many otolaryngologists recommend only partial removal of this tissue, that is, specifically, the tissue around the region of the Eustachian meatuses.

Skolnik (1958) noted, among 48 school-age children with clefts accompanied by hypertrophied tonsils and adenoids, that 84% had ear pathology and 16% had normal ears. For another group, 63 school-age children with operated or unoperated clefts and with "small tonsils and scanty amount of adenoid tissue," he reported that 54% had ear pathology and 46% had normal ears. Skolnik recognizes not only the importance of tonsil and adenoid hypertrophy as a cause of otitis media but also the need of adequate velopharyngeal closure for good speech, and he thus recommends immediate but conservative treatment consistent with the patient's overall problems and health.

Tangen (1960) found that 41.5% of 65 cleft palate subjects had hypertrophied adenoids; these he considered to be of etiological importance in Eustachian tube swelling and consequent dysfunction. Of those children who had hypertrophied adenoids, 81.5% had pathological changes in their middle ears, and, of those who had normal appearing adenoids, 31.3% had pathological changes in their middle ears.

The question of the proper treatment of diseased or hypertrophied adenoids and tonsils in a child with a cleft is controversial. Some (Sataloff and Fraser, 1952; Halfond and Ballenger, 1956b; Whaley, 1957; Skolnik, 1958; Miller, 1959; Graham, 1963; Graham and Lierle, 1962; Loeb, 1964; Chalet, 1965) are of the opinion that the benefit to hearing of treatment by an adenoidectomy (with or without a tonsillectomy) will outweigh, in the general welfare of the patient, any detriment to speech. Others (Koepp-Baker, 1957; Drettner, 1960; Glover, 1961; Holborow, 1962b) recommend considerable caution in the making of any decision to remove adenoids, believing the resultant bad effect of removal of adenoids upon speech to be more importantly detrimental than the bad effect of their presence upon hearing.

According to Sataloff and Fraser (1952) tonsils should not be removed until age 6; adenoids, since they are most easily removed before palatal repair or during first palatal repair, should be removed as early in infancy as possible, especially since early removal reduces the probability of middle ear infection and of permanent hearing loss. In the opinion of Glover (1961), however, an adenoidectomy will have, in many cases, a markedly adverse effect on the speech of a child with a cleft palate. He states that most children with clefts have repeated middle ear infections from the ages of 2 to 5 years whether the palate is repaired or not and that most middle ear infections can be "ridden through safely" without adenoidectomy until adequate palatal function takes place in "the normal course of events." At this time, he says, the infection usually subsides and "rarely will serious, permanent deafness result." He also believes that incompetent velopharyngeal closure "favors regurgitation of infectious material via the Eustachian tube to the middle ear" and that removal of adenoids may contribute to this possibility. Spriestersbach *et al.* (1962), however, as mentioned previously, found for children with clefts no evidence that pressure ratios (indirect measures of velopharyngeal competency) are related to incidence of hearing loss.

The present authors believe that some sort of compromise between extreme positions is in order. Koepp-Baker (1957) has recommended "judicious" removal of adenoids but does not elaborate. Masters *et al.* (1960) have noted that "selective" adenoidectomy does not appear to result in any important changes in hearing acuity. It is known that adenoids, because they may be foci for repeated or persistent infections in the nose and paranasal sinuses, sometimes adversely affect the function of the middle ear, either directly or indirectly (Kos, 1956). It is also known that an adenoidal pad sometimes is important to velopharyngeal closure and that its removal may have serious consequences for speech production. Probably the most important consideration, however, is the danger of hearing loss which may result from the presence of diseased or hypertrophied adenoids. Not only this danger of hearing loss and the possibility of permanent damage to the ear, but also the importance of hearing in the acquisition of speech, should be factors carefully weighed and considered with reference to any decision as to whether adenoids should or should not be removed. Leaving the adenoids intact can result in a severe enough hearing loss that speech may be impaired, especially if the loss is present during preschool years. Tonsils also may serve as foci for infection. The present trend toward avoiding, if possible, tonsillectomy and adenoidectomy for the child with a cleft palate creates a need for increasing otological supervision.

I. NASAL OBSTRUCTION, SWOLLEN TURBINATES, AND SINUSES

There is some evidence, to be discussed later, that the nose may be less resistant to infection when improperly ventilated, and it is known that nasal infection can spread to the Eustachian tube and subsequently to the middle ear. Observation of such spread of infection in persons with cleft palate who also have deflected nasal septa has led to a hypothesis that the relatively high incidence of nasal obstruction among those with cleft palate is one of the factors related to the relatively high incidence of hearing loss and ear pathology in the same population (Casteel, 1960). If it may be assumed that reduced nasal ventilation is causally related to nasal infection, then, of course, the hypothesis is a reasonable one.

Turbinates which are enlarged may be inefficient in their function of heating and humidifying the nasal cavity and thus may be causally related to infection. Maxillary and other sinuses can also be sources of infection. A septal bulge, for example, impacted against a middle turbinate, may close off the anterior series of sinuses and thus promote infection. Also suggested as causes of hearing loss are such conditions as surgical adhesions, deformity of the tip of the nose, and shortening of the columella (Casteel, 1960).

Phillips (cited in Casteel, 1960) has stated a belief that the most important cause of hearing loss is pathology of the nasal septum and sinuses. He found such pathology frequently in cases with clefts of lip and palate but not in cases with clefts of the lip or palate only.

Halfond and Ballenger (1956b), however, found no difference between hearing-loss and no-hearing-loss cleft palate groups in the incidence of septal deviations nor in incidence of oversized anterior and posterior aspects of inferior turbinates, with incidence for the latter comparison high in each group.

Skolnik (1958) found ear pathology for 75% of 41 school-age children with "complete unilateral or bilateral obstruction of the nasal airway on an anatomical, catarrhal or vasomotor basis" and for only 52% of 56 school-age children with "adequate bilateral nasal airway."

Drettner (1960), who studied 63 individuals with clefts of the lip and palate and of the palate only, aged 5 to 53 years, reported tympanic membrane "changes" in 56% of the patients, auditory impairment (loss of 15 dB or more in the speech frequency range) in 49%, and a narrowing of the nasal airway in 45%. The incidences of both aural pathology and nasal obstruction were significantly higher in the cleft lip-and-palate group than in the palate-only group. Although he found no statistically significant relationship between aural pathology (defined as hearing loss or tympanic membrane change) and nasal obstruction he concluded that it was "possible that nasal obstruction facilitates the occurrence of otitis."

Casteel (1960) observed 41 children, aged 4 to 18 years, who had clefts of the palate only and also unilateral nasal obstruction. Degree of nasal obstruction was rated on a 1 (normal) to 5 (severely obstructed) scale by subjective evaluation of five factors: deformity of the tip of the nose, shortening of the columella, deviation of the septum, size of the turbinates, and the presence of infections. The percentage of cases with normal hearing (defined as a hearing loss of no more than 0 to 9 dB in the speech frequency range), was found to increase with a decrease in degree of obstruction. The septum seemed to be the most frequent contributor to obstruction and the floor of the nose the least frequent. The total number of ear pathologies on the obstructed side was greater than on the unobstructed side. Hearing loss, however, occurred more frequently on the unobstructed side than on the obstructed side.

The relatively high incidence of nasal obstruction among persons with cleft palate thus appears to be one of the causal factors in the higher incidence of hearing loss among those with cleft palate than among those without. The degree to which such obstruction contributes to hearing loss, however, is not known.

J. ALLERGY

Halfond and Ballenger (1956b) make reference to the possibility that "allergic swellings" are sometimes related, at least indirectly, to hearing loss. Tangen (1960), although he found that 16.9% of 65 children with clefts had allergies according to their otological histories, has stated that allergy is possibly, not definitely, an etiological factor in ear disease.

K. AGE

Skolnik (1958) found middle ear pathology for children with cleft palate is 6% below 1 year of age, 27% between ages 1 and 4 years, and 67 to 69% between ages 5 and 13 years. A gradual increase in ear disease was noted up to school age, the incidence at this time reaching a plateau maintained into adult life.

Results of a study of cleft palate children by Linthicum et al. (1959) indicate some mean improvement in hearing acuity with age. Drettner (1960) noted for 43 patients 10 years of age or older that 26% had tympanic membrane changes or auditory impairment in contrast to 70% for 20 patients under 10 years of age. He concluded that "aural pathology usually appears in childhood."

Tangen (1960) noted a relationship between type of ear pathology and age, finding secretory otitis only in those children under the age of 10 years and finding chronic otitis more frequently in children over 10. He suggested that the latter finding possibly might be explained by normal regression of lymphoid tissue.

Stool and Randall (1967) examined with magnification the middle ears of 25 infants with clefts aged 9 days to 12 months. The examinations were conducted after the babies had had myringotomies and while they were under general anesthesia. In 47 of these ears they extracted "appreciable amounts of mucoid material." They advised that such examinations and appropriate careful otological care be carried out whenever infants with clefts were undergoing reconstructive surgery to prevent the "sequelae of infantile otitis."

Goetzinger *et al.* (1960), reporting on 42 adults with cleft palate, aged 16 to 75 years, found that with few exceptions the hearing acuity of these subjects fell within normal (hearing loss of no more than 15 dB for the speech frequencies) limits. They also noted a high incidence of previous middle ear pathology in comparison to present incidence, a finding which led to the conclusion that in general "middle ear disease runs its course before adulthood."

Spriestersbach *et al.* (1962), reporting on 163 children with clefts of the palate and lip and of the palate only, found significant differences between two age groups (56 between 33 to 71 months and 107 between 72 and 191 months), both for the better and for the worse ears, in per cent with hearing loss of 20 dB or more over the speech frequencies, the higher incidence of hearing loss occurring among the younger children. They concluded, after additional analysis of results from finer subgroupings by four age levels, that hearing acuity of children with cleft palate does improve with age, and that the incidence of hearing loss is smaller for children over 6 years of age than for those under 6. These findings on hearing loss provide additional support for some of those reported above by other investigators concerned primarily with ear pathology.

Additional evidence that hearing acuity of children with cleft palate improves as they grow older has been provided by Graham (1963) in a report of a longitudinal study of 190 patients, all of whom had had otological attention from the time they were 6 to 8 weeks of age. At the first possible time of reliable test results, that is, ages 4 to 6 years, 28.5% had an average hearing loss in the better ear of 15 dB or more; in comparison, by test results obtained at the age of 8 or more years, only 9.7% had this much loss in the better ear. A similar difference was observed between the same younger and older ages for the worse ears. Only 4% had a decrease in hearing level between the two tests. An important inference is made in Graham's statement that "otologic anomalies and hearing losses do appear to be reversible when individuals with cleft palates are afforded systematic otologic care from infancy until eight to ten years of age." For the subjects of this study, according to Graham, most of the changes in hearing acuity, particularly changes in the direction of better hearing, took place before the age of 8 years. For similar circumstances, especially in view of the fairly large number of subjects, a parallel generalization, that is, a generalization with reference to changes in hearing acuity for all children with cleft palate, is reasonable or, at least, tenable.

As Graham (1963) and others have pointed out, the importance of good otological care should not be overlooked in interpreting findings on changes in the incidence of hearing loss and aural pathology with age. These findings undoubtedly depend to a great extent upon other factors which change with age, such as the following: the anatomical relationship of the Eustachian tube and the nasopharynx; incidence of surgery or other palatal management; degree of pneumatization of the temporal bone; susceptibility to upper respiratory infections, which decreases with age; incidence of adenotonsillectomies; condition of the nasal airway, which is likely to improve with age. Some of these factors, or variables, are influenced by good otological care (or lack of it); and a child who receives good otological care from infancy certainly is less likely, because of this care, to develop a hearing loss, or, at least, as severe a loss as he might have without it.

L. REFLUX OF FOOD AND OTHER MATTER

The "mere presence" of a palatal cleft, according to Gannon (1950), makes the middle ear more susceptible, by way of the Eustachian tube, to an infection which has originated in the nasopharynx. Holmes and Reed (1955) have stated that the incidence of hearing loss is relatively high among those with cleft palate especially because of the opening between the nasopharynx and the mouth. Miller (1959) with particular reference to "exposure" of the Eustachian tube orifice, has made the same point. Masters et al. (1960), however, reported finding at the time of palatal repair that amounts of flora in the cultures taken from the nasopharynx and Eustachian tube orifice of children with cleft palate were not higher than "normal."

M. UPPER RESPIRATORY INFECTIONS

Koepp-Baker (1957) has reported the belief of many clinicians in the statement that upper respiratory infections occur more often among children with cleft palate than among those without. Holmes and Reed (1955), however, have noted that closure of the palate appears to have little effect upon the number of attacks of upper respiratory infections. Halfond and Ballenger (1956b), with reference to frequency of these attacks in persons with cleft palate, have reported finding no evidence of a difference between those with a hearing loss and those with no hearing loss. Tangen (1960) has stated that upper respiratory infections with ear complaints were reported in the histories of 44.6% of his patients. In addition, upon physical examination, he found ear pathology among all children with cleft palate who, at the time of the examination, also had acute upper respiratory infections.

Incidence of upper respiratory infections, including colds, is high among school-age children without cleft palate (Eagles et al., 1963) as well as among children with cleft palate; and there cannot be, on the basis of available information, any definite conclusion that these infections are a contributing cause of the high incidence of hearing loss among children with cleft palate. To be accepted at present, however, is the assumption that repeated upper respiratory infections can be an important factor in the etiology of hearing loss, particularly for the child with a cleft palate; for this reason alone, then, careful and systematic otological supervision of him seems very important.

IV. Discussion and Implications for Management

Making definite conclusions based upon results of a number of research studies employing different methodologies and definitions presents problems. To evaluate and to find relationships among findings when, for example, hearing loss is defined variously, if at all, becomes difficult or sometimes impossible. For the purpose of making inferences it is important to know in any case, but especially when several sources are being considered, whether reported data or findings are for the better ear, the worse ear, or both; what type of auditory assessment was employed; what frequencies were tested when pure tone audiometry was employed; what the conditions of testing were; and any other relevant information on factors which might vary from one study to another.

No single criterion for the determination of hearing loss is, of course, adequate for all situations. The criterion, as has been pointed out by Spriestersbach *et al.* (1962), should depend upon the purpose for which the information is desired. The criterion most useful to the educator who is interested in a child's classroom problems is different from the one most useful to the otologist who is interested in the health of a child's ear. For interpretation of reported findings a specific definition of the criterion thus is needed. This is especially true for comparisons among findings from several sources, and most particularly when different physical management philosophies are involved. Incidence data on hearing loss, for example, can be meaningful only with reference to specific definition of the criterion and within relevant context.

Reports of incidence of hearing loss among preschool-age children are subject to relatively more error than such reports for older children. Age is not, of course, the only factor which affects reliability of hearing test results, but on the average, reliability of results for children becomes lower with younger ages. An important consideration, then, in the evaluation of these incidence data for young children, is the fact that it is possible for results to be unduly influenced by unreliability, which, most importantly, may act to obscure true differences between groups. On the other hand, a biasing influence may act either to obscure a true difference or to result in an observed and possibly large difference which is invalid for the purpose of generalization. A case in point is what may result from discarding those data judged to be unreliable, a procedure which, if some selective factor operates, can destroy in a biasing fashion the "representativeness" of the sample or samples.

Hearing loss incidence data in general are most meaningfully evaluated with reference to comparable data obtained for a well-matched, control sample. Results of screening audiometry, although adequate for evaluating differences between the percentages of those testing above or below a given cut-off score, are not useful for evaluations with reference to "normal" and "impaired" hearing. Such evaluations are best made with reference to a control sample. The average hearing acuity of otoscopically normal, school-age children, according to recent evidence (Eagles *et al.*, 1963), is better than would be indicated by the American Standard norm used generally for audiometric zero in the United States (prior to 1965; see footnote 1 on page 169), and to set a certain cut-off score above which or below which hearing is "normal" or "impaired" is at least to some extent unrealistic. As Eagles has pointed out, too few children would be classified, according to the ASA standard, as having "impaired" hearing. It seems reasonable to assume that similar misevaluations could occur in classifying as "normal" or "impaired" the hearing levels of children with cleft palate. It also seems reasonable to assume that the use of the new ISO (1964) reference standard for audiometric zero will result in fewer such misevaluations for children either with or without clefts. In this connection also, using "air-bone gap" as a criterion, at least for a medically significant hearing loss, rather than the more traditional screening by air conduction only, has been suggested recently by Sweitzer *et al.* (1967).

Neither a history of ear pathology nor a history of physical symptoms or "ear complaints," according to fairly definite evidence, is necessarily indicative of hearing loss. Eagles *et al.* (1963) have reported finding many children with "otoscopic evidence of disease" who also had hearing as acute as that of children considered otoscopically normal. For ears of children with cleft palate Graham (1963) has reported finding no hearing loss of 15 dB or more for 65% of those considered deviant by otological examination and also, for the same ears, finding such a loss for 20.6% of those not considered deviant by otological examination. Relevant to the point to be made is a statement by Sataloff and Fraser (1952) that middle ear "pathology" often is caused by a pressure differential between the middle ear and the atmosphere. With reference to hearing, no assumptions should be made, obviously, solely on the basis of presence or absence of ear pathology noted by otological examination, and, vice versa, ear pathology cannot be diagnosed solely by presence or absence of hearing loss.

Quite a number of different factors, then, as indicated by the above review of the literature, may possibly have some effect upon data for incidence of hearing loss. Any factor which might bear such an influence should, of course, be evaluated and considered whenever relevant in the interpretation and use of these data. Those which appear to be important, depending upon various circumstances, are the following: frequency of earaches and ear discharge; cleft type; degree of cleft; age at surgery; frequency of upper respiratory infections; any influence upon frequency and effects of tonsil and adenoid hypertrophy; age at testing or otological examination; any influence upon the effects of nasal and sinus abnormalities; management procedures; Eustachian tube function or dysfunction; frequency of associated anomalies, velopharyngeal closure or lack of it; and frequency of respiratory allergies.

Interpretation and evaluation of data on aural and related pathologies, particularly for comparisons between groups, may often be difficult because of, as with hearing loss, problems of definition. A closely related problem of interpretation is the difficulty, or impossibility, of weighing differences among observers when their evaluations are to some extent subjective: for example, a condition which might, after otoscopic examination, be labeled as abnormal by one observer might not be so labeled by another. Stool and Randall (1967), for example, point out that the infant eardrum is very difficult to view in appropriate detail without magnification and thus "subtle signs of pathology are easily missed." An additional complication often arises when data have been obtained from histories or *ex post facto*, that is, by a method involving the inevitable inaccuracies resulting from such factors as vagueness of memory and sociological influences.

Fairly specific conditions and events which in varying degrees are associated particularly with the abnormality of cleft palate can be said, in spite of conflicting evidence and disagreement of opinions, to account reasonably for the high incidence of hearing loss and aural pathology among children with cleft palate. The most important of these predisposing factors which operate to cause the high incidence of hearing loss, according to an evaluation of presently available evidence, is a high incidence of Eustachian tube dysfunction among those with cleft palate. If this evaluation is correct, then particular attention and care, with perhaps more emphasis in the total management of the child with a cleft palate than has usually been the case in the past, should be given toward prevention of such dysfunction and toward the alleviation of it. Surgery for the prime purpose of closing the palate or of improving velopharyngeal closure for speech production apparently has not in most instances resulted in improved Eustachian tube function.

In addition to the specifically related factors already discussed, others of a more general nature, according to Skolnik (1958), may be of some importance in the etiology of hearing loss, these less obvious possibilities including such factors as prematurity, malnutrition, dehydration, improper feeding methods, and acute exanthemata. Upon consideration of all possible factors, and even with no evidence to establish any of these of a more general nature as a direct cause of hearing loss, as pointed out by Halfond and Ballenger (1956b), it is possible that any one, or any combination, of them could be of some importance to the best management procedures for hearing loss and its prevention. Their relative importance, of course, might be expected to vary from one individual case to another.

Emphasis should undoubtedly be given to careful, frequent, and consistent otological care of children with cleft palate from infancy until the age of at least 8 to 10 years. Because of the multidimensionality and complexity of their problems, individuals with cleft of the palate have in recent years been managed more and more by team approach, and the inclusion on this team of an otologist is important. The high incidence of hearing loss among individuals with cleft palate, as well as in many instances the severity of loss, can be considerably reduced both by his participation in physical management procedures and by his contributions to relevant research. Moreover, as Hayes (1965) has pointed out, if normal hearing cannot be medically or surgically restored to a child with a cleft, then his speech and language acquisition and production may be affected and appropriate rehabilitative measures (e.g., amplication and auditory training) must be considered.

Among various needs for additional or continued research which are important for the eventual provision of the best audiological and otological care consistent with the best care in all aspects of management procedures is the obtaining of additional and complete information on the following: improvement of surgical techniques for provision of or maintenance of good Eustachian tube function, this improvement, of course, to be evaluated with reference to general welfare and particularly with reference to other surgical techniques such as those employed for closing the palate and for making possible adequate velopharyngeal closure; the effects, with reference to hearing loss, of consistent and of the best available otological care for children with cleft palate when this care extends from birth to the age of at least 8 or 10 years; and differences among the various subclassifications of persons with cleft palate with reference to hearing loss and its management or prevention.

Audiological and otological considerations with reference to the best possible management of persons with cleft palate obviously involve questions to which there are no specific answers at the present time, and additional research, particularly research with an experimental approach, is necessary if these much-needed answers are to be found.

Research in this area is complicated not only because of the complexity of audiological and otological considerations, but also because of the complexity of other management considerations important to general welfare, and particularly because best management by one consideration alone possibly may conflict with best management by some other consideration alone. Good otological care for the preservation of hearing acuity, for example, conceivably might conflict with the best surgical procedure for accomplishing velopharyngeal closure. Important, then, is the taking into account of all management considerations, the weighing of them, and also the weighing of the effects of possible procedures, both in relation to each other and in relation to the general welfare of the patient. The results of systematic, long-term audiological testing and otological examinations, properly classified and analyzed, should result in knowledge which will improve the effectiveness of these management decisions.

REFERENCES

Berry, Mildred F., and Eisenson, J. (1956). "Speech Disorders: Principles and Practices of Therapy." Appleton, New York.

Casteel, R. L. (1960). An Investigation of Hearing Acuity of Cleft Palate Children Having Unilateral Nasal Obstruction. M. A. Thesis, Univ. of Washington, Seattle, Washington.

Chalet, N. I. (1965). Tonsillectomy, adenoidectomy and the cleft palate clinic. *Laryngoscope* **75**, 408.

Counihan, D. T. (1956). A Clinical Study of the Speech Efficiency and Structural Adequacy of Operated Adolescent and Adult Cleft Palate Persons. Ph. D. Thesis, Northwestern Univ., Chicago, Illinois.

Davis, H., and Silverman, S. R., eds. (1960). "Hearing and Deafness." Holt, New York.

Donaldson, J. A. (1966). The role of artificial Eustachian tube in cleft palate patients. *Cleft Palate J.* **3**, 61.

Drettner, B. (1960). The nasal airway and hearing in patients with cleft palate. *Acta Otolaryngol.* **52**, 131.

Eagles, E. L., Wishik, S. M., Doerfler, L. G., Melnick, W., and Levine, H. S. (1963). Hearing sensitivity and related factors in children. *Laryngoscope* **73**, 1.

Ersner, M. S., and Alexander, M. H. (1960). *In* "Otolaryngology" (G. M. Coates and H. P. Schenck, eds.), Vol. I, Chapter 10. W. F. Prior, Hagerstown, Maryland.

Fletcher, S. G. (1957). A Cinefluorographic Study of the Movements of the Posterior Wall of the Pharynx During Speech Deglutition. M. S. Thesis, Univ. of Utah, Salt Lake City, Utah.

Gaines, F. P. (1940). Frequency and effect of hearing losses in cleft palate cases. *J. Speech Disorders* **5**, 141.

Gannon, J. (1950). A Study of the Effect of Certain Surgical Variables on the Auditory Acuity of Fifty Cleft Palate Children. M. A. Thesis, Univ. of Washington, Seattle, Washington.

Glover, D. M. (1961). A long range evaluation of cleft palate repair. *Plastic Reconstruc. Surg.* **27**, 19.

Goetzinger, C. P., Embrey, J. E., Brooks, R. S., and Proud, G. O. (1960). Auditory assessment of cleft palate adults. *Acta Oto-Laryngol.* **52**, 551.

Graham, M. D. (1963). A longitudinal study of ear disease and hearing loss in patients with cleft lips and palates. *Trans. Am. Acad. Ophthalmol. Otolaryngol.* **67**, 213.

Graham, M. D., and Lierle, D. M. (1962). Posterior pharyngeal flap palatoplasty and its relationship to ear disease and hearing loss. *Laryngoscope* **72**, 1750.

Graham, M. D., Schweiger, J. W., and Olin, W. H. (1962). Hearing loss and ear disease in cleft palate patients with obturators. *Plastic. Reconstruc. Surg.* **30**, 348.

Halfond, M. M., and Ballenger, J. J. (1956a). An audiologic and otorhinologic study of cleft-lip and cleft-palate cases. I. Audiologic evaluation. *Arch Otolaryngol.* **64**, 58.

Halfond, M. M., and Ballenger, J. J. (1956b). An audiologic and otorhinologic study of cleft-lip and cleft-palate cases. II. Otorhinologic evaluation. *Arch. Otolaryngol.* **64**, 335.

Hayes, C. S. (1965). Audiologic problems associated with cleft palate. In "Proceedings of the Conference: Communicative Problems in Cleft Palate." *ASHA Rept. No. 1.*

Hearing Conservation: The Incidence of Hearing Loss (1962). *J. Iowa Med. Soc.* **52**, 431.

Holborow, C. A. (1962a). Conductive deafness associated with the cleft-palate deformity. *Proc. Roy. Soc. Med.* **55**, 305.

Holborow, C. A. (1962b). Deafness associated with cleft palate. *J. Laryngol. Otol.* **76**, 762.

Holdsworth, W. G. (1963). "Cleft Lip and Palate," 3rd ed., Grune & Stratton, New York.

Holmes, E. M., and Reed, G. F. (1955). Hearing and deafness in cleft-palate patients. *Arch. Otolaryngol.* **62**, 620.

Koepp-Baker, H. (1957). *In* "Handbook of Speech Pathology" (L. E. Travis, ed.), Chapter 19. Appleton, New York.

Kos, C. M. (1956). Relation of adenoids and sinusitis to otologic disease. *Texas State J. Med.* **52**, 352.

Linthicum, F. H., Body, H., and Keaster, Jacqueline (1959). Incidence of middle ear disease in children with cleft palate. *Cleft Palate Bull.* **9**, *No. 1*, 23.

Lis, E. F., Pruzansky, S., Koepp-Baker, H., and Kobes, H. R. (1956). Cleft lip and cleft palate. *Ped. Clin. N. Am.* **3**, 995.

Loeb, W. J. (1964). Speech, hearing, and the cleft palate. *Arch. Otolaryngol.* **79**, 20.

Masters, F. W., Bingham, H. G., and Robinson, D. W. (1960). The prevention and treatment of hearing loss in the cleft palate child. *Plastic Reconstruc. Surg.* **25**, 503.

Means, Beverly J., and Irwin, J. V. (1954). An analysis of certain measures of intelligence and hearing in a sample of the Wisconsin cleft palate population. *Cleft Palate Bull.* **4**, *No. 2*, 4.

Miller, G. F. (1965). Eustachian tube function in normal and diseased ears. *Arch. Otolaryngol.* **81**, 41.

Miller, M. H. (1956). Hearing losses in cleft palate cases. *Laryngoscope* **66**, 1492.

Miller, M. H. (1959). Hearing problems associated with cleft palate. *Ann. Otol. Rhinol. Laryngol.* **68**, 90.

Perlman, H. B. (1951a). Mouth of the Eustachian tube: Action during swallowing and phonation. *Arch. Otolaryngol.* **53**, 353.

Perlman, H. B. (1951b). Observations of the Eustachian tube. *Arch Otolaryngol.* **53**, 370.

Podvinec, S. (1952). The physiology and pathology of the soft palate. *J. Laryngol. Otol.* **66**, 452.

Rich, A. R. (1920). A physiological study of the Eustachian tube and its related muscles. *Johns Hopkins Hosp. Bull.* **31**, 206.

Sataloff, J., and Fraser, M. (1952). Hearing loss in children with cleft palates. *Arch. Otolaryngol.* **55**, 61.

Skolnik, E. M. (1958). Otologic evaluation in cleft palate patients. *Laryngoscope* **68**, 1908.

Snodgrasse, R. M. (1954). Heredity and cephalo-facial growth in cleft lip and/or cleft palate patients. *Cleft Palate Bull. Monogr. Suppl.* **1**, 1.

Spriestersbach, D. C., and Powers, G. R. (1959). Articulation skills, velopharyngeal closure, and oral breath pressure of children with cleft palates. *J. Speech Hearing Res.* **2**, 318.

Spriestersbach, D. C., Lierle, D. M., Moll, K. L., and Prather, W. F. (1962). Hearing loss in children with cleft palates. *Plastic Reconstruc. Surg.* **30**, 336.

Stool, S. E., and Randall, P. (1967). Unexpected ear disease in infants with cleft palate. *Cleft Palate J.* **4**, 99.

Sweitzer, R. S., Melrose, J., and Morris, H. L. (1967). The air-bone gap as a criterion for identification of hearing losses. *Cleft Palate J.* In press.

Tangen, G. V. (1960). An Otologic Evaluation of Cleft Palate Children. M. S. Thesis, Univ. of Minnesota, Minneapolis, Minnesota.

Wagner, J. A. (1941). A Survey of the Hearing and Intelligence of Fifty Cleft Palate Children. M. A. Thesis, Univ. of Washington Seattle, Washington.

Whaley, J. B. (1957). The otolaryngologist's role in the care of the cleft palate patient. *J. Can. Dental Assoc.* **23**, 574.

VI

Psychosocial Aspects of Cleft Palate

Leonard D. Goodstein

I. Introduction 201
  A. General 201
  B. Cleft Lip and Palate 202
II. The Parents of a Child with a Cleft Lip or Palate 203
  A. Learning about the Defect 203
  B. The Immediate Concerns of the Parents 203
  C. The Psychological Adjustment of the Parents 207
III. The Psychosocial Development of the Child with Cleft Palate 209
  A. General 209
  B. Intelligence 209
  C. Social Competence 212
IV. The Personality and Adjustment of the Child with Cleft Palate 213
V. The Psychosocial Problems of the Adolescent and Adult with Cleft Palate 217
VI. Some Methodological Considerations in Cleft Palate Research 218
  A. General 218
  B. Heterogeneity of Samples 218
  C. Representativeness of Samples 219
  D. Retrospective Reports 220
VII. Recapitulation 220
  References 222

I. Introduction

A. GENERAL

In both the clinical and research literature on physical disabilities and handicaps there is general agreement that the social and psychological problems of the disabled person are of major importance (Barker *et al.*,

1953; MacGregor *et al.*, 1953; Meyerson, 1948). Indeed, from a (re)-habilitation point of view, these psychosocial problems of the patient may transcend in importance the actual physical disability or handicap. That such psychosocial problems arise in persons with physical disability should not be surprising in view of the generally negative response to atypical physical functioning and the highly positive values placed in our culture upon adequate physical functioning.

B. CLEFT LIP AND PALATE

In view of the obvious nature of the disability the psychosocial consequences of a cleft lip and/or palate should be especially significant. The high value placed by our society upon physical attractiveness, especially facial attractiveness, would make the disability of a cleft lip especially potent; and the premium placed upon verbal communication and adequate speech would further suggest that the speech handicap of the individual with a cleft palate has profound psychosocial sequelae. The individual with both of these disabilities would have to contend with problems arising both from cosmetic and communication difficulties. While the severity of the cleft will obviously be an important consideration in determining both the degree of the actual handicap and its psychosocial consequences, the presumed plight of the person with a cleft lip and palate is invariably pictured as dire. The professional texts which describe the problem of cleft palate and the published clinical observations agree in characterizing the typical individual with such a disability as having a serious personality disturbance, all-pervasive inferiority of behavior, and deep personality difficulties (Backus, 1950; Kahn, 1956; Tisza *et al.*, 1958; Johnson *et al.*, 1967).

The purpose of the present chapter is to survey and to evaluate, in a developmental framework, the information, particularly the quantified research evidence, on the psychosocial aspects of the adjustment of individuals with cleft lip and palate. Before considering the published research findings it is important to note that these studies rarely involve homogeneous samples of persons with cleft lip and palate. While the authors all too often discuss their results as though they were obtained from a rather homogeneous group of individuals, the most casual perusal of the description of the sample studied often indicates a wide range of subject age, a wide range of clefts both in type and severity, a variety of attempts at treatment, and so on. Only rarely have the authors attempted to reduce this heterogeneity by identifying and investigating some of these within-group characteristics, a procedure which should be very helpful in shedding light on the psychosocial factors under scrutiny.

II. The Parents of a Child with a Cleft Lip or Palate

As Spriestersbach (1961a) has noted, the great majority of prospective parents look forward with confidence to having a "perfect baby," one free from mars, blemishes, or deformities. The birth of a baby with a cleft lip and/or palate comes as a psychological shock when the parent learns that the dream of the perfect baby has not been realized. Kinnis (1954) has emphasized the importance of the emotional difficulties of the mother of a child with a cleft palate and the special needs of this mother for emotional support. One relevant question has to do with the time when the mother learns that her child is defective and a second with the sources of concern of the parent about her child.

A. Learning about the Defect

Spriestersbach (1961b) has reported that 75% of the mothers of infants with cleft lip-only and 75% of the mothers of infants with both cleft lip and palate discovered "at birth" that their children were defective; an additional 20% in each group discovered the defect at 1 day postpartum. In sharp contrast, only 8% of the mothers whose infants had cleft palate-only discovered the defect at birth with an additional 14% learning of the defect 1 day postpartum. Thus 22% of the mothers of the palate-only group knew of the defect within 1 day after the birth of the child in contrast to 95% of the mothers of the lip-only and the lip-and-palate groups. It may be presumed that the rather late discovery of the defect in the palate-only group (29% learned of the defect 1 week or more after the birth of the child) further complicates the psychological reaction to the child's deformity, since this reaction comes after some psychological adjustment to the child has already been made. These delays in reporting the defect in the palate-only group occur partially because of concern for the mother's health or psychological condition and partially because of inadequate postnatal examination. Delays may also arise because of the greater concern of the medical staff for a more immediate health problem which is threatening the survival of the infant (for example, a congenital heart defect), such conditions occurring more frequently in the palate-only group than in the other two groups (Spriestersbach et al., 1962b).

B. The Immediate Concerns of the Parents

In view of the potentially serious consequences of cleft lip and palate, with facial disfigurement and the strong likelihood of later communication difficulties, the knowledge about the child's defect is likely to arouse considerable consternation, shock, and despair in the informed parents. Westlake

(1953) has suggested that, in view of the cosmetic appearance and the communication difficulties of the child with cleft palate and the presumed effects of these difficulties upon others, the parents of such children "cannot help feeling a tremendous anxiety" (p. 167). Westlake, although he presents no evidence upon this point, does, quite correctly, indicate the importance of including the parents in any total rehabilitation effort.

Unfortunately, researchers who have studied parental reaction to the birth of a child with cleft lip and/or palate (Weachter, 1959; Spriestersbach, 1961b) have had, of necessity, to rely upon retrospective reports of parental reactions garnered through interviews with these parents. While the data presented in these studies appear to have good face validity, it is difficult to know how the reports of these parents about their early reactions may be colored by the more recent developments and problems they have encountered. These studies, nevertheless, are suggestive of a strong psychological impact upon parents from learning that they do have a defective child.

Tisza and Gumpertz (1962) have reported that their interviews with and observations of an unspecified group of mothers of children with cleft palate have led them to conclude that these mothers "react with strong feelings of hurt, disappointment, and helpless resentment to the revelation that they have a congenitally deformed child" (p. 86). The mothers are reported as initially preoccupied with the question of why the child has been so afflicted and as overwhelmed by feelings of shame and guilt. Next in importance to the initial reaction, the reports of these mothers indicate anxieties during the early childhood period related to (1) the anxieties over the difficulties involved in feeding these children; (2) the concern over the eruption of teeth which are irregularly spaced; (3) the anxiety over the inadequacy of the child's vocalization; (4) the concern over the possibility of intellectual impairment.

Tisza and Gumpertz indicated that the initial negative feelings toward the child are typically buried by the emerging feeling of compassion and maternal love but that the later concerns must be handled by direct consideration by professional personnel of the realities involved in the child's disorder, namely, the nature and extent of the child's difficulty and what can and should be done therapeutically. These authors stressed the need of the mother for emotional support and further pointed out that the mother's concern for the habilitation of her child is motivated not only by reality factors but also by her desire for restitution of her personal sense of adequacy as a mother. It is unfortunate that this well-thought through discussion of some very provocative ideas is not more fully documented or substantiated by quantified, empirical data.

Weachter (1959) has reported that she was able to identify 10 specific major areas of concern, plus a miscellaneous one, from reports of parents of children with cleft palate. In order of frequency of inclusion in the parental reports there were concerns over (1) the child's appearance; (2) the desirability of immediate surgery; (3) speech development; (4) feeding; (5) reaction of the spouse; (6) reaction of siblings; (7) reactions of friends and family; (8) intellectual development; (9) financial problems; and (10) recurrence of the defect in other, yet unborn, children.

The first of these aforementioned concerns, that is, concern over the child's appearance, was reported to have been evidenced by verbal expressions of dismay, shame, and guilt and by attempts to conceal the child's face from nonprofessional persons. The obvious nature of the cosmetic impairment and the consequences of this impairment upon the acceptance of the child was the most frequently recalled area of concern for these parents.

The second concern involved the parents' desire to be able to do "something" to remedy the defect, and the question of immediate surgery was typically raised. It appears that not immediately doing something, in particular not considering immediate surgery, serves to intensify the concern and guilt of the parent. Pressures by the parent for prompt surgical intervention would appear to be an especially important area for counseling assistance by professionally competent personnel, especially with the increasing emphasis upon infant orthodontics. Kahn (1956) has emphasized the potential emotional complications following all pediatrical surgery, including cleft lip and palate repair, and has stressed the importance of minimizing emotional trauma by presurgical counseling with both parents and children who are old enough to benefit by such counseling.

Another area of concern was indicated by the parents' recognition that verbal communication difficulties might result from the cleft. This concern over speech is reported by Weachter to be frequently exaggerated; for example, parents sometimes fear that the child will not be able to speak at all. Here again is an area which appears to require counseling help.

The sucking and swallowing problems associated with feeding these children with cleft lip and palate comprised another area of concern. Indeed, these very feeding difficulties have sometimes led to the actual discovery of the cleft palate in the palate-only group. Since the parents are concerned with how to handle the immediate feeding problems and also with the implications of these problems for the future, they often require professional counseling assistance in this area.

Parents also expressed concern over the possible reaction of the husband or wife to the traumatic news and over the direct impact the child's defect might have upon the marriage. Such concerns appear to Weachter to be especially obvious and important when marital difficulties are present prior to the infant's birth.

The parents of these children were frequently concerned about how the infant would be accepted by his siblings. The age and number of such siblings and their previously expressed attitudes toward a new infant, especially if there appears to be some possibility of sibling rivalry, all apparently are likely to enter into the nature and extent of the parental concern.

The question of the reaction of close friends and family also was a frequent source of strong concern. How could these friends and family be informed and what would be their reactions to the child and his handicap? Parents, according to Weachter, seem to be especially concerned about protecting themselves and their infant from expressions of distaste, repugnance, or dismay from others. In this connection Palmer (1960) has suggested that overprotection is a "natural" concomitant of the handling of the speech-handicapped child.

Parents often were concerned about whether the cleft would impair the intellectual development of the child. Here is still another area in which significant contributions can be made by professional counseling help.

Worry over financial problems was frequently mentioned as another problem area. Parents in general recognize that the child with such a handicap will require extensive and often expensive medical, surgical, and other professional services, and they often express considerable concern over their limited financial resources to secure the needed services.

The likelihood of the recurrence of the defect in other children, yet to be born, was ranked the last of the ten areas of concern reported by Weachter. Parents are likely to consider the possibility that such defects may run in families and thus become quite concerned as to whether this consideration should preclude their having any additional children. Here, too, is an area in which professional counseling would appear to be helpful.

The Weachter study, although useful in identifying some of the concerns of the parents of children with cleft palate, leaves several unanswered questions. The data were not analyzed quantitatively; the reliability of the categorical analysis of the parental concerns was not reported; and the responses of the parents of the children with cleft palate-only were not differentiated from those of children with both cleft lip and palate. Spriestersbach (1961a), in a preliminary report of the results of a large-scale study at the University of Iowa of the psychosocial factors involved in cleft palate disorders, has suggested that the initial concerns of parents of children with cleft palate-only are less profound than those of parents of children with both cleft lip and palate and, further, in each subgroup of parents the nature of the concerns of the mothers and of the fathers was not the same. It should be noted that these two studies, since the Weachter study was based partially upon the then-available Iowa material, are not dealing with completely different populations.

It thus would appear that the birth into a family of a child with a cleft lip and/or palate is undoubtedly an anxiety-arousing circumstance. The parents of such children are understandably very concerned about the nature of the defect and its implications for survival and later adjustment. While definitive research is still required in the analysis and quantification of these concerns, and it is expected that the final report of the University of Iowa group will fill some of this void, it is at the same time clear that the initial anxieties and concerns of these distressed parents indicate an imperative need for prompt professional counseling help. Professional workers who deal with the emotional problems of the parents of such handicapped children will find McDonald's (1962) recent and readable volume valuable both as a personal reference and as a bibliotherapeutic aid, although it should be restricted in this latter use to better-educated and more literate parents.

The desire and the need for direct information and counseling, especially during the first year of the child's life, and preferably from highly trained specialists rather than from tape recordings or from printed matter, have also been indicated by the results of a questionnaire study of 43 parents of children with cleft palate (Bradley, 1960). Hill (1956), who employed both interviews and a specifically devised objective test in a study of 70 parents of children with cleft palate, has also demonstrated this need. He found a statistically significant relationship between the amount of information which the parents have received and the favorability of their attitudes toward the children.

C. THE PSYCHOLOGICAL ADJUSTMENT OF THE PARENTS

In light of the initial anxieties and concerns of parents of children with cleft lip and palate, the adequacy of their later psychological adjustment may be questioned. To evaluate this later personality and adjustment Goodstein (1960a) administered the Minnesota Multiphasic Personality Inventory (MMPI), an objective paper-and-pencil personality inventory, to 170 mothers and 157 fathers of children with cleft lip and/or palate and compared their responses with those obtained from a control group of 100 mothers and fathers of physically normal children. The most striking aspect of the results of this study is the failure to demonstrate any obvious differences in the MMPI scores between the parents of the children with cleft palate and the parents of the children without. Although certain rather small differences between the two groups are statistically significant, the overall impression left by the results is that if any important personality differences exist between these two groups, these differences are not reflected in MMPI responses. As might be expected there is some indication that the parents of children with cleft lip and palate are more anxious and concerned than the parents of children without; these differences, however, are rather small and the overlap in the distribution of the two sets of scores is substantial. It thus would appear that, despite some genuine concern and apprehension on the part of the parents of the children with the handicap, there is no substantial or important difference between the two groups in personality structure or general level of adjustment.

In a further analysis of the MMPI data, Goodstein (1960b) attempted to relate the level of adjustment, as measured by the MMPI, of the parents of the children with cleft palate and lip to certain other clinical data, that is, age of the child, type of cleft, social adjustment of the child, and adequacy of overall child handling. He reported that his results demonstrate no relationship between parental adjustment and the type of cleft, or the rated social adjustment of the child, or the rated adequacy of the parents' handling of the child. It was found, however, that parents of the older handicapped children are rated as more poorly adjusted than parents of the younger ones, and this finding appears to be independent of parental age per se. The author interpreted these findings as indicating that the effects on adjustment, as measured by the MMPI, of having a child with this type of physical handicap are not immediately evidenced but that these effects develop with time. It should be noted, however, that the observed particular differences in adjustment were rather small and should be regarded as of little help either in understanding the parents of children with cleft palate or in making any practical decisions about how to have them take part in a treatment program.

The current failure to identify, within the group of parents of children with cleft palate, personality or adjustment measures that are associated with the adequacy of techniques of child handling should not obscure the potential importance of developing such measures. Moffat (1951), McWilliams (1956), and Carr (1959) all highlight the importance of parental attitudinal factors in nurturing the handicapped child toward a fuller psychological development. In planning and executing remedial programs for these children, it is important to identify those parents who, because of their own needs, can benefit by special counseling help, or who, because of their own psychological inadequacies, are unable to provide emotional support for their children. It should be noted, however, that the present evidence suggests that most of these parents, despite the presence in the children of a rather obvious physical disability, are generally well adjusted and able to provide adequate support for their developing children.

III. The Psychosocial Development of the Child with Cleft Palate

A. GENERAL

The most casual study of the early development of typical children with cleft palate provides considerable anecdotal support for the contention that they have serious developmental problems. The difficulties encountered in feeding, the frequent infections, the frequent presence of other congenital anomalies such as a club foot or a congenital heart defect (Spriestersbach et al., 1962b), the frequently severe hearing losses (Spriestersbach et al., 1962a), and the many difficulties associated with the medical management of the cleft itself, often involving long periods of hospitalization, all lead to the impression that these children are badly impaired in their general and intellectual development.

Unfortunately, there is no direct research evidence concerning the nature and extent of the general impairment of physical development in these children. Hospital and medical records are not maintained in such a fashion as to permit the ready identification of a group with cleft palate so that developmental status at various ages could easily be compared with some matched control group. Spriestersbach and his colleagues at the University of Iowa have attempted to investigate some aspects of this problem by obtaining, through carefully standardized and coded clinical interviews with the parents, retrospective accounts of the development of children with cleft palate. The publication of their final report should shed considerable light on this problem. In a preliminary report of these findings, Spriestersbach (1961b) has reported that, in comparison to the parents of physically healthy children, these mothers rated the physical development of their children less favorably and were also more defensive in reporting behavior problems such as teasing, overt aggression, and so on. These preliminary reports are only suggestive of the specific results of the entire study and little can yet be said of the extent of the developmental difficulties encountered by the parents of the child with cleft palate.

B. INTELLIGENCE

The developmental difficulties noted above are commonly regarded as important etiological factors in intellectual retardation. Furthermore, the poor quality of the speech produced by these children (see Spriestersbach et al., 1956, 1961) would presumably lead to fewer rewards for speaking and a consequent retardation in the development both of language skills and intelligence. Morris (1962) analyzed 50 responses of connected speech obtained from each of 107 children with cleft palate, aged 3 through 8. He found, by comparison of his results with established norms, that these children were retarded in the mean length of responses, the structural complexity of responses, the number of different words used, and articulation test scores. He found no significant differences between children with cleft lip and palate and children with cleft palate-only. These results are in essential agreement with those reported earlier. (Spriestersbach *et al.*, 1958).

A number of investigators have attempted to assess the nature and degree of the intellectual impairment suffered by individuals with cleft palate. Although Wolstad (1932) concluded in an early paper that the intelligence of persons with cleft palate is "definitely not subnormal," he offered no evidence for his conclusion. Billig (1951) reported that the Intelligence Quotients (IQ's) of 60 children with cleft palate, ages 2 months to 17 years, ranged from 64 to 130 with a median of 97 and a mean of 94. Billig's results require caution in their interpretation as they are based upon eight different intelligence tests, each with somewhat different normative characteristics. Irwin and Means (1954) reported that the results of the administration of the Revised Stanford-Binet Intelligence Test to 225 children with cleft lip and palate indicated that the "norm-distribution was shifted 10 IQ points to the lower end of the IQ scale" (p. 4). May and Munson (1955) reported a mean IQ of 96 for 151 persons with the same handicap and of unspecified age. These results are, however, based upon two different intelligence tests. Lewis (1961) reported a mean IQ of 94 for a sample of 548 children, aged 4 through 16, with cleft lip and palate based upon the administration of Form L of the Revised Stanford-Binet Intelligence Test. These four studies, however, all failed to include any matched control group, each investigator comparing his obtained results with published test norms.

In a more carefully controlled study Goodstein (1961) reported the results of the administration of the Wechsler Intelligence Scale for Children (WISC) to a group of 105 children, aged 5 through 16, all with cleft lip and/or palate, and a control group of 95 children without known physical defects, matched to the experimental group on the basis of the children's age, sex, and birth order and also on the basis of family size, rural-urban background, and religious affiliation. The mean Full Scale WISC IQ was 94 for the experimental children and 104 for the control children. The intellectual impairment of the experimental children was more substantial in the area of verbal skills than in the area of manipulative skills; the mean differences between the two groups were 11 points in the mean Verbal IQ and only 7 points in the mean Performance IQ, with both differences in favor of the control group.

Goodstein further reported that, in contrast to only 13% of the matched control group, 40% of the children with clefts had a Full Scale IQ of less than 90 and that they thus could be classified Dull Normal or lower in general intellectual ability. He pointed out (p. 292) that, although, according to the established norms, 25% of a random sample can be expected to have such

IQ's, in this study the carefully matched control group provided the more legitimate base rate for comparison. Lewis (1961) has reported that only 25% of her group with cleft palate had an IQ of less than 90. These two studies, however, cannot easily be compared since they used different measuring instruments with somewhat different normative characteristics and since Lewis did not report any matched control group data. She did report, however, that she had obtained greater than a 10-point difference in mean IQ between 100 children with cleft palate and their unaffected siblings, with the siblings receiving the higher mean IQ of 105. The mean IQ for the impaired group might thus be "expected to be closer to 105 than to 100," which raises some question about the possibility of misinterpretation of her results.

Ruess (1965) compared 49 pairs of siblings aged 7 to 12 years, one of whom had a cleft, on the WISC and several other measures of "secondary language," including tests of oral readings, reading comprehension, reading vocabulary, and spelling. He reported a mean Full Scale WISC IQ of 99, a mean Verbal IQ of 97, and a mean Performance IQ of 101 for the children with clefts. The means for the normal siblings, in contrast to the 10-point differential reported by Lewis, were 3 IQ points higher in all three instances. The description of the physical condition and medical treatment previously received by these children with clefts suggests that they had received more complete habilitative services than is ordinarily the case which, in some measure, may account for the relative lack of impairment in these cases. Ruess further reported that there were no discernible differences between the children with clefts and their unaffected siblings on the four measures of language achievement or in general progress or social adaptation in school. The findings reported by Ruess are the most clear-cut evidence that children with clefts can become very much like their normal siblings in intelligence and school achievement, provided adequate habilitative services are promptly and continually available.

Smith and McWilliams (1966) compared on various measures of creativity a group of 22 children with cleft of the lip and palate, aged 10 to 11 years, with 22 children without cleft palate matched on the basis of race, sex, socioeconomic status, and IQ. The children with clefts were significantly less creative on two of the seven indices of verbal creativity and four of the seven indices of nonverbal creativity as well as on the overall index of creativity. Smith and McWilliams tend to regard the overprotective, rejecting, and overstriving attitudes of the parents of the children with clefts as responsible for this defect in creativity. This argument would have been strengthened if they had shown a comparable deficit in creative thinking in a group of children with other physical handicaps whose parents are regarded as holding similar attitudes. Nevertheless, their conclusion that there is a need for careful attention to parental attitudes in the habilitation of children with clefts should not be dismissed or overlooked.

Following a further analysis of differences in intelligence within the group with cleft palate, Goodstein (1961) concluded that those children with cleft palate only, according to the obtained scores, were significantly more impaired intellectually than were children with both cleft lip and palate. He proposed a possible explanation of these results by reference to the differential frequency of congenital anomolies in the two groups, with the cause seen as higher incidence of anomolies among children with cleft palate only. Lewis (1961) reported rather similar results for her sample with those children with multiple anomolies having a mean IQ 10 points lower than the mean IQ of those with cleft only.

Despite the differences in methodology and procedure in the studies discussed above, the seven studies of the intelligence of children with cleft palate in general yielded strikingly similar results with the reports of mean IQ ranging only from 94 to 99. The findings of these studies do suggest a generally mild to moderate degree of intellectual impairment, with the distribution of IQ for the group of children with cleft palate displaced to the lower end of the entire distribution. Such intellectual impairment appears to be more pronounced in the verbal area than in the performance area and raises important practical questions in the development of therapeutic and educational plans for children with cleft palate. Children with Dull Normal or lower intelligence levels (IQ < 90) will experience some difficulty in quickly assimilating ordinary educational matter and can be expected to be somewhat retarded educationally. The probability of intellectual impairment in children with cleft palate strongly suggests the importance of including a rather complete intellectual assessment in the planning of any total habilitative program for them, particularly in view of the tendency of some of their parents to have unrealistically high academic or professional goals for these children.

C. SOCIAL COMPETENCE

In an effort to evaluate the development of social competence in children with cleft palate, Goodstein (1961) had trained clinicians interview 139 mothers of children with cleft palate and then, according to the information obtained in the interview, complete the Vineland Social Maturity Scale (VSMS). The interviewer attempted to secure as much detail as possible about the child's "actual and habitual performance" in several areas of social competence including eating, dressing, and so on; he then rated the child's reported performance by means of an objectified and standardized schedule of typical development. Identical data were also obtained from a control group of 174 mothers of physically healthy children who had been matched to the children with cleft palate on the basis of age, sex, and birth order as well as a number of social class variables. The results of the comparison of the obtained mean Social Quotients (SQ: a score obtained for each protocol in the same manner as an age-scale IQ) indicated a highly significant difference in social competence in favor of the control children. This difference was more pronounced for the younger children (from newborns through 5 years of age) than for the older children (from age 5 years through 16). The mean SQ of the younger children with cleft palate was 11.8 points below that of the younger controls while the mean SQ of the older children with cleft palate was only 3.7 SQ points lower than that of the older controls. Younger children with cleft palate thus are expected to be somewhat retarded in their development of social competence as compared to a matched control group, but this retardation will in general be almost eliminated in the older children. The author hypothesized that, as these children with cleft palate grow and mature, perhaps any overprotective parental attitudes are reduced, especially after the development of reasonably adequate speech. Such an analysis would suggest that Palmer's (1960) contention that overprotective parental attitudes are a concomitant of a speech handicap may need to be amended to include the changes in parental attitude which improvements in speech can accomplish. Without regard to these speculations, it can be noted that children with cleft palate, although they may have a somewhat retarded rate of social development, do seem nevertheless to reach in general an average level of social maturity as they grow older. None of the available evidence tends to support the contention of Harkins and Nitsche (1950) that both children and adults with cleft palate should be regarded as "crippled" by professional and lay workers alike.

IV. Personality and Adjustment of the Child with Cleft Palate

A large number of writers have maintained that, in view of the frequently serious cosmetic and communication problems involved, persons with cleft lip and palate develop rather limited personalities, are shy and retiring, are self-conscious about their appearance, and show signs of emotional maladjustment requiring professional therapeutic help. For example, Backus (1948) unequivocally stated of cleft palate children: "Symptoms of personal and social maladjustment are usually present, both because of defective speech and real or fancied facial deformity" (p. 129).

Further, many personality theorists, particularly those with a fairly classical Freudian orientation, have stressed the importance of the oral activities of childhood, such as sucking, feeding, and chewing, in the development of a healthy mature personality (for example, see Prugh, 1956). Since frequently there is severe impairment of or interference with such activities in children with cleft palate, a consequence of this handicap which might be anticipated would be fairly major personality disturbance and possibly even the development of some unique personality characteristics.

Both Hackbush (1951) and Ruess (1958), however, have concluded that there are no psychological or personality characteristics unique to individuals with cleft lip or palate, although both authors regard such individuals as typically having adjustment difficulties. Hackbush, in a report of an impressionistic study of the projective test results obtained from a group of individuals with clefts, further concluded that these persons were similar in personality to persons with other serious physical handicaps, such as cerebral palsy. Since no empirical data were actually given in either of these reports it is not possible to compare them directly, either with each other or with other published data.

Tisza et al. (1958) have reported the results of an intensive observational study of 11 children (aged 5 to 8) who were seen for evaluation in the Tufts College Cleft Palate Institute. No actual data were presented, no control group was used for the purpose of establishing a base line for their comparisons, and no statistical analyses were reported. These children all appear to have had fairly serious types of clefts, involving considerable disfigurement. The authors noted that "The drive for self-mastery and for mastery of the situation ... was observed in a striking number of the children" (p. 421). They further noted that these children with cleft palate compared to physically normal children characteristically showed higher levels of muscular rigidity, postural tension, motor activity, and distortions in psychomotor tasks. While their interpretations were somewhat guarded, the strong impression left with the careful reader is that these children were rather maladjusted and disturbed, requiring psychiatric care for their emotional problems.

Gluck et al. (1965), using a coding system of behavior pathology, have compared the clinical records of 50 children with cleft palate seen at a cleft palate research center with those of 292 children with behavior problems seen at a child guidance clinic. They have reported that the children with cleft palate had more physical anomalies and chronic illnesses and were regarded as more shy and enuretic than the children from the child guidance clinic. Although the reported evidence is far from clear and they did not report upon any control group, the authors nevertheless concluded that children with cleft palate "do display evidence of psychological maladjustment" (p. 806) which deserves more emphasis and formal study.

Birch (1952), on the other hand, has concluded that, popular and professional opinion to the contrary, there "is no substantial evidence that a cleft palate or cleft lip will usually prevent a child from becoming a healthy and happy and useful citizen" (p. 7). At least four studies support his statement and do indeed include a report of failure to find evidence of maladjustment in individuals with cleft palate.

In the first of these studies Barker (1951) administered the California Test of Personality, a paper-and-pencil self-description inventory, to 26 persons with cleft lip or palate, ranging in age from 8 to 45 years, all of whom were receiving speech therapy at the University of Michigan. Her comparison of the obtained scores with the established norms yielded no statistically significant results, thus providing no evidence of any differences from the general population in maladjustment or emotional disturbance. The smallness of the sample, the wide range of the subject's ages, and the failure to include a control group all, however, tend to raise serious questions about drawing definitive conclusions.

In a more complete study, Sidney (1951) compared a group of 21 children with cleft palate, aged 8 to 17 years, with two separate control groups, matched to the cleft palate group on the basis of sex, age, color, intelligence, and class grade. The social adjustment of each child was evaluated by means of a sociometric questionnaire (a measure of peer group acceptance), the California Test of Personality, the Thematic Apperception Test (a projective test of personality), and a teacher's rating scale of adjustive behavior (ratings of the frequency of such responses as appearing cheerful rather than depressed). In general the three groups obtained rather similar mean scores on these several adjustment indices with no significant differences between the cleft palate group and the first control group reported on any measure. The second control group received significantly higher sociometric acceptance ratings than the cleft palate group but there were no significant differences on the other measures. The author seemingly attributed this single significant difference to sampling errors, and generally concluded that her study failed to provide any clinically significant evidence that children with cleft palate are different in their social adjustment from children without cleft palate. These same results have also been abstracted in a published paper by Sidney and Matthews (1956).

Palmer and Adams (1962) compared the Draw-a-Person and the Draw-a-Face Test results obtained from 20 children with cleft lip or palate, aged 4 to 12, and a matched control group. Each drawing was scored for the "typical" signs of anxiety in the oral area. The results of this study do not support the "hypothesis that children with cleft lips or palates harbor restrictive or disturbing feelings toward their own oral structures" (p. 75). Similar negative results, using the Draw-a-Person Test, have been reported by Ruess (1965) and by Corah and Corah (1963).

In a rather comprehensive study of the personality adjustment of children with cleft palate, Watson (1964), compared a group of 34 boys with cleft lip and palate (1) with a group of 19 boys with chronic physical handicaps not involving speech impairment or facial disfigurement and (2) with a control group of 40 physically healthy boys. All subjects were between 8 and 14 years of age and the three groups were not significantly different in intelligence or educational level. All subjects completed the Rogers Personal Adjustment Inventory, a paper-and-pencil test designed specifically for children of this age range. No statistically significant differences among the means of the three groups of subjects were found with this instrument.

To evaluate within-group differences in the cleft palate group, Watson obtained for each child with cleft palate independent, reliable ratings of articulation defectiveness and of facial disfigurement. These two sets of ratings were each then statistically compared with the personality test scores and in each case found to be unrelated. Watson concluded that the results of his study do not support the contention that boys with cleft palate are more poorly adjusted than their physically normal peers, despite the fact that some of the children in his sample had rather serious communication and cosmetic defects.

Although these were children under continuing medical care, it should not be assumed that they were children with especially severe clefts as they may simply have had very concerned or very cooperative parents. Such concern and interest by these parents may have prevented the children's physical disability from leading to the predicted state of maladjustment. In this connection it should be noted that the families studied by Watson had received considerable counseling help as well as the typical traditional medical care.

Even more striking was Watson's failure to find any relationship between the degree of these defects and personality maladjustment. It is especially noteworthy, particularly in view of the stress previous writers (e.g., MacGregor et al., 1953; Westlake, 1953) have placed upon the adjustive consequences of cosmetic factors, that there was no indication of any relationship between the rated degree of facial disfigurement and personality even for those children with the most extreme ratings of disfigurement. It should be remembered that the cases reported by MacGregor and her associates were not run-of-the-mill cases but were patients seeking plastic surgery for rather severe cosmetic defects. Such a relationship as that reported by MacGregor may indeed exist in very severe cases, and these may not have been adequately sampled in Watson's study. It is unfortunate that Watson was not able also to secure teacher's ratings and sociometric evaluations for his children. Also, since cosmetic factors may be more significant for girls than for boys, the extension of this design to a sample of females with cleft palate seems worthwhile.

These four studies appear to offer rather strong support for Birch's (1952) position that the child with cleft palate is able to adjust to his psychological environment. Further support for this position is found in Sidney's (1951) report that not a single child with cleft palate was included among the over 600 maladjusted children referred during a 3-year period to the Pittsburgh Board of Education for psychological services. The only evidence that these children are emotionally maladjusted or disturbed appears to be rather impressionistic and nonsystematic. Until more convincing evidence is provided, it appears safe to conclude that as a group children with cleft palate are not typically maladjusted or seriously disturbed emotionally, although they may have some problems of social acceptance.

V. The Psychosocial Problems of the Adolescent and Adult with Cleft Palate

None of the several studies discussed above have dealt with either adolescents or adults but have been concerned especially with children who have cleft lip or palate. While several investigators have included some adults in their samples of individuals with cleft palate, the number of such adults has been small and no attempt was made to study the adults separately from the children. While this preoccupation with children partially stems from a proper concern with understanding the significance of handicaps and defects in a developing organism, it also reflects the relative ease of obtaining children as subjects through schools, speech clinics, and medical centers. In this current survey of the literature, it unfortunately was not possible to uncover a single research study of the particular psychosocial problems of adolescents or adults with cleft palate.

It is of course quite possible to extrapolate the findings of psychosocial studies of children with cleft palate to adolescents and adults and thus to conclude that these individuals continue the patterns of relatively successful adjustment of childhood into later maturity. It should be noted, however, that these later years may pose some rather crucial situations that persons with cleft lip and palate might have difficulty resolving. For example, Goodstein (1961) has noted that less than 15% of his sample of children with cleft have Bright Normal or higher intelligence. The typical individual with a cleft palate will be faced with the realization that collegiate training, which requires at least a Bright Normal level of intelligence, is beyond his capacity and that he is ineligible for the occupations that require such training for entry. The psychological impact of accepting these limitations, especially in a society which is placing increasing emphasis on higher education, remains to be evaluated. Watson (1964) has suggested further that cleft lip and palate may be more crucial in determining the level of adjustment in adolescence than in childhood because of the increased importance of cosmetic appearance, especially in the dating, kissing, and marital planning which follow puberty. The suggestion that research in this area is necessary and important seems obvious.

It can be noted, however, that there is some informal observational evidence that adults with cleft palate do not have relatively serious personality difficulties; there are no reports that such persons typically obtain professional psychiatric care or require institutionalization in mental hospitals. Further, many, if not most, of the adults with clefts seen in speech clinics and other rehabilitation centers are married and are steady wage earners. There is no reported evidence that the·unemployment rate among persons with clefts is higher than among others, although presumably the type of job held would be partially limited due to cosmetic, communication, and intellectual considerations.

VI. Some Methodological Considerations in Cleft Palate Research

A. GENERAL

In general, the methodological and conceptual limitations of the above-reported studies are so important that few useful generalizations are clearly apparent from a careful review of their published results. It may be worthwhile at this point to analyze some of these methodological and theoretical problems especially involved in investigating the psychosocial aspects of cleft palate in the hope that such an analysis will be useful to future researchers in this area. Goodstein (1958) has previously discussed some of the methodological and theoretical considerations in investigations of the relationship between functional speech disorders and personality and adjustment, including such issues as the statistical ones involved in such research, the need for cross-validation, the problems of matching control groups, and the difficulties intrinsic in the measurement of personality and adjustment, most of which are equally relevant for research in psychosocial aspects of cleft palate.

B. HETEROGENEITY OF SAMPLES

In the typical study reported above the tendency has been to treat the particular sample studied as a homogeneous one, regardless of the variety of types and severity of the clefts involved and regardless of such other considerations as the age, sex, and socioeconomic status of the subjects. Spriestersbach *et al.* (1961), however, have clearly indicated the usefulness of separating individuals with cleft lip and palate into subgroups based upon the type of cleft involved for the purpose of describing articulation deviations. Investigators have also failed to recognize the importance of studying subgroups of those with cleft palate based upon the socioeconomic status of the family.

It would appear that the psychological significance to parents of having a child with cleft palate may be a function of the socioeconomic status of the parents and their implicit aspirations for their child's educational and professional career. Professional, middle-class parents with aspirations for a profession for their child may be more disheartened by the birth of a child with a cleft palate than lower-class parents who would not ordinarily have such aspirations. The failure of investigators to employ various subgroups of the sample to study the effects of such categorization have sharply reduced the cogency of much of this research.

The differences among subgroups of individuals with cleft palate are, indeed, potentially the most useful, both practically and theoretically, for understanding psychosocial aspects of cleft palate. As Goodstein (1958, p. 381) has noted, between-groups comparisons, demonstrating only that individuals with speech problems, in this case persons with cleft palate, differ from normally speaking persons, yield relatively little information about the operation or relative importance of the social and psychological factors which caused these differences. That persons with cleft palate are different from persons without is usually obvious, and research studies should do more than reiterate these obvious differences.

C. REPRESENTATIVENESS OF SAMPLES

One persistent problem which can be noted in the research reported above is the question of the extent to which the study sample is representative of the population of individuals with cleft palate. Without any concern for the issue of whether the patients are typical of the total population of those with cleft palate, the majority of studies have utilized patients currently being seen in cleft palate rehabilitation centers, speech clinics, and psychological clinics. Serious attention ought to be directed to the identification of those individuals with cleft palate not typically included in such research studies and to how they might differ from the studied sample along such dimensions as severity of cleft and socioeconomic status of the family. It would be possible to utilize the public school for such a study of school-age children with cleft palate, but older and younger individuals would be more difficult to identify. A long-term longitudinal study of such a representative sample would provide answers for many of the unanswered questions posed by the previous research.

D. RETROSPECTIVE REPORTS

As noted above, many of the research studies of psychosocial aspects of cleft palate have had to rely upon the retrospective reports obtained from parents through interviews. Haggard *et al.* (1960) have reported that such retrospective reports, even by parents of physically healthy children, are somewhat unreliable over time, with the recall of anxiety-arousing events less reliable than the recall of so-called "hard facts," such as age of walking. Findings of such studies raise some fairly serious questions about the general usefulness of retrospective reports of emotional reactions and strongly suggest the need for research on such problems at the time the reactions are actually being experienced.

VII. Recapitulation

What generalities may be gleaned from the above-reported empirical evidence which dealt directly with psychosocial factors associated with cleft palates? First, learning that a newborn infant has a cleft palate or lip is a very anxiety-arousing event for the child's parents. All too frequently their prior knowledge and understanding of this defect is minimal and they are beset with a multitude of questions and concerns, ranging from the immediate problems of how to feed the infant to long-range concerns about educational and vocational plans. These concerns can best be seen as the legitimate and normal ones of properly alarmed and responsible individuals about a newly experienced and poorly understood problem with which they now must contend for some time to come. Although their immediate reactions may suggest to others that the psychological adjustment is an abnormal one, it would appear that the unexpected appearance of the defect, its nature and severity, and the lack of knowledge about the problem, both by the parents and by the available hospital personnel, are all potent factors in determining the nature and degree of these reactions of the parents. Since pregnancy and birth are emotionally arousing situations for even the parents of healthy infants, it is quite probable that the birth of a handicapped child accentuates the initial adjustment problems of parenthood. Despite their concerns, however, there is no evidence that in general the parents of children with cleft palate are themselves poorly adjusted in any substantial degree. The great majority of these parents can very well be included as therapeutic agents in any treatment or habilitation plans for their children.

The nature and the severity of these immediate parental concerns strongly indicate the imperative need for prompt professional counseling assistance. Such counseling help should be provided by professional personnel qualified both to answer competently the specific questions raised and to handle the anxiety and emotional reactions which are present. Such counseling assistance apparently has a therapeutic effect both upon the parents themselves and upon their attitudes toward and handling of the child. Chapter VIII deals specifically with the potential contributions of the speech pathologist and other professional personnel to this counseling process.

There appears to be some minimal evidence that the physical and psychological development of children with cleft palate are in general somewhat retarded; at least the rate of development seems slower on the average than in physically normal children. It is not possible to ascertain to what extent this retarded rate of development in the psychological area, particularly in that of self-care, is a function of parental overprotection. This retardation of social competence seems to be substantially reduced in older children with clefts, apparently after the development of adequate speech patterns.

There is substantial agreement in the literature that, as a group, children with cleft palate suffer a moderate degree of intellectual impairment, with the distribution of intelligence test scores obtained from these children displaced to the lower end of the scale and the impairment more pronounced in the verbal area of functioning than in the motor performance area. Children with cleft palate are more likely to be categorized in the Dull Normal and lower levels of intelligence and less likely to be categorized in the Bright Normal and higher levels than are physically normal children from similar family background. The implications of these intellectual limitations are of importance both in understanding the immediate educational attainments of these children and in the future educational-vocational planning for them. It is strongly recommended that each child with a cleft palate be examined, sometime after his fifth year, with an individual intelligence test administered by a trained psychological examiner and that the results of such an appraisal be imparted to the child's parents within a counseling framework.

Despite considerable published popular and professional opinion to the contrary, there is little, if any, clear-cut evidence that children with cleft lip and palate are in general psychologically disturbed or emotionally maladjusted. Without suggesting that these children have no problems and limitations as a function of their physical defects, the total picture portrayed by these research findings is that the child with cleft palate usually makes a reasonable social, psychological, and emotional adjustment both to his handicap and to his total environment. There appears to be good reason to suppose that this state of affairs is a consequence of the firm psychological support and warm affection typically provided by the parents of the child with cleft palate. It would seem that these parents are able to handle their initial anxieties and concerns and to help their children become reasonably happy and contented individuals; and it would seem that proper professional support is an important factor in the development of these desirable responses. Furthermore, there is considerable evidence to indicate that the procedures for the physical management of cleft palates, with respect to both the cosmetic and the speech consequences, are constantly being improved so that the parents can actually observe, once the initial shock has been dealt with, that much can be and is being done to ameliorate the child's disability.

One completely neglected area of research is that of the psychosocial problems of the adolescent and adult with cleft palate. While it may be argued that their problems are more intense than those of children with this defect, both because of the greater importance of cosmetic appearance at older ages and because of the greater independence from parental support and assistance, there is no evidence to support this point of view. Indeed, the informal observational impression suggests that the typical adult with cleft palate is happily married, gainfully employed, and a generally useful, contributing member of society.

REFERENCES

Backus, Ollie L. (1948). Speech defects. *Bull. Natl. Assoc. Secondary School Principals* **32**, No. *151*, 127–132.

Backus, Ollie L. (1950). Children with cleft palate and cleft lip. *In* "Speech Problems of Children." (W. Johnson, ed.) Grune & Stratton, New York.

Barker, Elizabeth I. (1951). A Study of Certain Aspects of Personality in Given Individuals Having Cleft Palate. M. S. Thesis, Univ. of Michigan, Ann Arbor, Michigan.

Barker, R. G., Wright, Beatrice A., Meyerson, L., and Gonick, Mollie R. (1953). "Adjustment to Physical Handicap and Illness. A Survey of the Social Psychology of Physique and Disability," rev. ed. Social Science Research Council, New York.

Billig, A. L. (1951). A psychological appraisal of cleft palate patients. *Proc. Penna. Acad. Sci.* **25**, 29–32.

Birch, J. (1952). Personality characteristics of individuals with cleft palate: research needs. *Cleft Palate Bull.* **2** (2), 7.

Bradley, Doris P. (1960). A study of parental counseling regarding cleft palate problems. *Cleft Palate Bull.* **10** (3), 71–72 (abstract).

Carr, Lela B. (1959). Problems confronting parents of children with handicaps. *Except. Children* **25**, 251–255.

Corah, N. L., and Corah, Patricia L. (1963). A study of body image in children with cleft palate and cleft lip. *J. Genet. Psychol.* **103**, 133–137.

Gluck, M. R., McWilliams, Betty Jane, Wylie, H. L., and Conkwright, Elizabeth Anne (1965). Comparison of clinical characteristics of children with cleft palates and children in a child guidance clinic. *Percept. Mot. Skills* **21**, 806.

Goodstein, L. D. (1958). Functional speech disorders and personality: methodological and theoretical consideration, *J. Speech Hearing Res.* **1**, 377–382.

Goodstein, L. D. (1960a). MMPI differences between parents of children with cleft palates and parents of physically normal children. *J. Speech Hearing Res.* **3**, 31–38.

Goodstein, L. D. (1960b). Personality test differences in parents of children with cleft palates. *J. Speech Hearing Res.* **3**, 39–43.

Goodstein, L. D. (1961). Intellectual impairment in children with cleft palates. *J. Speech Hearing Res.* **4**, 287–294.

Hackbush, Florentine (1951). Psychological studies of cleft palate children. *Cleft Palate Bull.* **1** (4), 7–8.

Haggard, E. A., Brekstad, A., and Skard, Ase G. (1960). On the reliability of the anamestic interview. *J. Abnorm. Soc. Psychol.* **61**, 311–318.

Harkins, C. S., and Nitsche, M. Maria (1950). The cleft palate child is crippled. *Crippled Child* **29**, 22–23.

Hill, M. J. (1956). An investigation of the attitude and information possessed by parents of children with clefts of the lip and palate. *Cleft Palate Bull.* **6** (1), 3–4.

Irwin, J. V., and Means, Beverly J. (1954). An analysis of certain measures of intelligence and hearing in a sample of the Wisconsin cleft palate population. *Cleft Palate Bull.* **4** (2), 4 (abstract).

Johnson, W., Brown, S. F., Curtis, J. F., Edney, C. W., and Keaster, Jacqueline (1967). "Speech Handicapped School Children." Harper, New York.

Kahn, J. P. (1956). Operations for hare lip and cleft palate: The emotional complications in children. *Calif. Med.* **84**, 334–338.

Kinnis, G. C. (1954). Emotional adjustment of the mother to the child with a cleft palate. *Med. Soc. Work* **3**, 67–71.

Lewis, Ruth (1961). A survey of the intelligence of cleft palate children in Ontario. *Cleft Palate Bull.* **11** (4), 83–85.

McDonald, E. T. (1962). "Understand Those Feelings." Stanwix House, Pittsburgh, Pennsylvania.

McGregor, Frances C., Abel, Theodora M., Bryt, A., Lauer, Edith, and Weissmann, Serena (1953). "Facial Deformities and Plastic Surgery: A Psychological Study." Thomas, Springfield, Illinois.

McWilliams, Betty J. (1956) Some observations of environmental factors in speech development of children with cleft palate. *Cleft Palate Bull.* **6** (1), 4–5.

May, Anna M., and Munson, S. E. (1955). Are cleft palate persons of subnormal intelligence? *J. Educ. Res.* **48**, 617–621.

Meyerson, L. (ed) (1948) Social psychology of physical disability. *J. Soc. Issues* **4** (4), 1–111.

Moffat, Helen M. (1951) Counseling parents of cleft palate children. *Cleft Palate Bull.* **1** (4), 8–9.

Morris, H. L. (1962). Communication skills of children with cleft lips and palates. *J. Speech Hearing Res.* **5**, 79–90.

Palmer, J. M., and Adams, M. R. (1962). The oral image of children with cleft lip and palate. *Cleft Palate Bull.* **12** (4), 72–76.

Palmer, M. F. (1960) Managing overprotective tendencies with speech-impaired children. *J. Speech Hearing Disorders* **25**, 405–408.

Prugh, D. G. (1956). Psychological and psychophysiological aspects of oral activities in childhood. *Pediat. Clin. N. Am.* **3**, 1049–1072.

Ruess, A. L. (1958). The clinical psychologist in the habilitation of the cleft palate child. *J. Speech Hearing Disorders* **23**, 561–578.

Ruess, A. L. (1965). A comparative study of cleft palate children and their siblings. *J. Clin. Psychol.* **21**, 354–360.

Sidney, Ruth A. (1951). An evaluation of the social adjustment of a group of children born with cleft palates. Ph. D. Thesis, Univ. of Pittsburgh, Pittsburgh, Pennsylvania.

Sidney, Ruth A., and Matthews, J. (1956). An evaluation of the social adjustment of a group of cleft palate children. *Cleft Palate Bull.* **6** (4), 10 (abstract).

Smith, R. M., and McWilliams, Betty Jane (1966). Creative thinking ability of cleft palate children. *Cleft Palate J.* **3**, 275–283.

Spriestersbach, D. C. (1961a). Counseling parents of children with cleft lips and palates *J. Chron. Diseases* **13**, 244–252.

Spriestersbach, D. C. (1961b). Evaluation of a technique for investigating the psychosocial aspects of the "cleft palate problem." *In* "Congential Anomalies of the Face and Associated Structures" (S. Pruzansky, ed.), pp. 345–366. Thomas, Springfield, Illinois.

Spriestersbach, D. C., Darley, F. L., and Rouse, Verna (1956). Articulation of a group of children with cleft lips and palates. *J. Speech Hearing Disorders* **21**, 436–445.

Spriestersbach, D. C., Darley, F. L., and Morris, H. L. (1958). Language skills in children with cleft palates. *J. Speech Hearing Res.* **1**, 279–285.

Spriestersbach, D. C., Moll, K. L., and Morris, H. L. (1961). Subject classification and articulation of speakers with cleft palates. *J. Speech Hearing Res.* **4**, 362–372.

Spriestersbach, D. C., Lierle, D. M., Moll, K. L., and Prather, W. F. (1962a). Hearing loss in children with cleft palates. *Plastic Reconstruc. Surg* **30**, 336–347.

Spriestersbach, D. C., Spriestersbach, Bette R., and Moll, K. L. (1962b). Incidence of clefts of the lip and palate in families with children with clefts and families with children without clefts. *Plastic Reconstruc. Surg.* **29**, 392–401.

Tisza, Veronica B., and Gumpertz, Elizabeth (1962) The parents' reaction to the birth and early care of children with cleft palates. *Pediatrics* **30**, 86–90.

Tisza, Veronica B., Silverstone, Betty, Rosenblum, G., and Hanlon, Nancy (1958). Psychiatric observations of children with cleft palate. *Am. J. Orthopsychiat.* **28**, 416–423.

Watson, C. G. (1964). Personality maladjustment in boys with cleft lip and palate. *Cleft Palate J.* **1**, 130–138.

Weachter, Eugenia H. (1959). Concerns of Parents Related to the Birth of a Child with a Cleft of the Lip and Palate with Implications for Nurses. M. A. Thesis, Univ. of Chicago, Chicago, Illinois.

Westlake, H. (1953). Understanding the child with a cleft palate. *Quart. J. Speech* **39**, 165–172.

Wolstad, D. M. (1932). The handicap of cleft palate speech. *Ment. Hyg. (N.Y.)* **16**, 281–288.

CHAPTER

VII

Diagnosis and Therapy

Ralph L. Shelton, Jr., Elise Hahn, and Hughlett L. Morris

PART ONE: DIAGNOSIS 226
   I. Velopharyngeal Competence 227
      A. Diagnostic Techniques 227
      B. Treatment Decision 236
  II. Speech Problems 237
      A. Diagnostic Techniques 237
      B. Treatment Decision 238
 III. Oral-Facial Structures 239
      A. Diagnostic Techniques 239
      B. Treatment Decision 241
  IV. Neural Function 241
      A. Diagnostic Techniques 241
      B. Treatment Decision 244
   V. Hearing Acuity and Auditory Perception 244
      A. Diagnostic Techniques 244
      B. Treatment Decision 245
  VI. Psychosocial Adjustment 245
      A. Diagnostic Techniques 245
      B. Treatment Decision 246
 VII. Language Maturity 246
      A. Diagnostic Techniques 246
      B. Treatment Decision 248
VIII. Concluding Statement 248

PART TWO: THERAPY 249
   I. Procedures for Articulation Therapy 251
  II. Therapeutic Exercise and Motor Learning 253
 III. Procedures for Voice Therapy 257
      A. Individuals with Normal Oral Structures 257
      B. Individuals with Inadequate Oral Structures 258
  IV. Procedures for Language Development and the Improvement of Com-
      munication 259
   V. Concluding Statement 261
      References 261

Part One: Diagnosis

Speech diagnosis for cleft palate problems includes investigation of the current status of the client, determination of the etiology of any problems that exist, prediction about future status, and development of a plan for the remediation of the problems identified. The activities of diagnosis involve sampling and measurement, and reliable and valid procedures and instruments must be employed.

Whenever possible the clinician makes use of standardized instruments for evaluation of the client's problems. However, he will often wish to investigate aspects of a client's behavior for which suitable tests or norms do not exist. In these instances he may be forced to generalize from his experience or to utilize nonstandardized check lists and rating scales developed from his experience; and, in any case, he must be prepared to change his initial impression of his client as well as to note changes in the client's behavior with time.

This chapter will emphasize problems arising from the relationship between articulation and the speech mechanism. For persons with defective palates, speech problems are frequently related to the condition of this mechanism, which, in many cases, can be modified by physical management in a way to facilitate speech learning. The speech clinician who works with persons with defective palates thus should cooperate closely with members of other professions, particularly those of medicine and dentistry. Since the speech clinician will often see the patient more frequently than will his professional colleagues, he must assume responsibility not only for habilitation of communication but also for referring him to other professional workers as indicated.

Most of the literature to be considered here is directly concerned with the problems of persons with defective palates. Some of it, although not specifically concerned with these problems, provides information useful for present purposes. The term "speech" as used in this chapter will refer to articulation, voice, and language. Disfluency will not be discussed because of its surprisingly infrequent occurrence in cleft palate persons (Takagi *et al.*, 1965). Certain matters of general importance in diagnosis of communication disorders, that is, those not central to problems related to cleft palate, will not be discussed in detail.

Procedures for taking case history material, both in general and with reference to cleft palate, are described elsewhere (Chapter 2 in Johnson *et al.*, 1963; Darley, 1964). Of particular value in the history of an individual with cleft palate is information about the treatment of the cleft palate problem, both physical and behavioral. The clinician should identify any physicians and dentists who are currently treating the patient, and for what purpose. This information will be vital in planning the speech training for the patient.

Of equal importance is the information in the history concerning the feelings and attitudes of the patient and his family about the status of treatment and, more specifically, the complaints which he now has. The patient's initial comments frequently reflect concerns which are uppermost in his mind and which the speech pathologist will need to cope with during the early stages of treatment. In working with the cleft palate patient, as with all patients with speech problems, a very good beginning is the question, simply put, "What can I do to help you?"

For organization of the material to be presented here, either the parameters to be evaluated or the instruments for their evaluation might be used. The former were chosen for consistency with the previous discussion of etiological factors (Chapter IV). The parameters to be evaluated are velopharyngeal competence, speech problems, oral-facial structures, neural function, hearing acuity and auditory perception, psychosocial adjustment, and language maturity.

I. Velopharyngeal Competence

A. DIAGNOSTIC TECHNIQUES

Defectiveness of the velopharyngeal port mechanism is the most important single factor contributing to the speech problems of persons with cleft palate. The task of diagnosing the adequacy of structure and the functions of this mechanism, then, is of central importance in this discussion.

1. *Examination of the Oral Cavity*

For examination of the oral cavity, the clinician may use a tongue blade and light source for evaluation of gross defects of structure while the structures are at rest and of structure and function during phonation. By such an examination he may observe whether there is an open cleft palate, whether the palate is intact but appears to be shortened, whether there is a fistula between the oral and nasal cavities, and whether there is movement of the palate and/or pharyngeal wall during phonation. If he has had experience in making such observations, he will be able to estimate the probable effect of the various observed factors on speech. As indicated by studies with lateral x-ray films, however, the port is hidden from view in the direct observation; it is behind and above the surface of the soft palate which is directly visualized. The addition of a laryngoscopic mirror may assist, but even by use of a mirror under optimal conditions, the clinician will still be able to visualize only the inferior aspects of the palatal and pharyngeal wall structures. In general, then, examining the oral cavity is not a satisfactory procedure for assessing the adequacy of the velopharyngeal mechanism for speech.

2. X-Ray films

A second technique which may be used to evaluate the relationship between structures involved in the velopharyngeal valve is that of x-ray films of the head. Lateral films have been helpful in viewing the relationship between the velum and the posterior pharyngeal wall. Frontal films, which give a coronal view of the head, have not been helpful, since the bony portions of the skull prevent delineation on the film of the soft tissues of the palate and of the lateral wall of the pharynx. Films taken from above or below the head have not been helpful for the same reasons.

Cinefluorographic, that is, motion-picture x-ray, films also have been used in studying velopharyngeal closure. Single-frame x-ray films are used to demonstrate structural relationships during rest or during a speech or nonspeech activity which can be sustained. In contrast, cinefluorographic x-ray films can be taken while the speaker is performing a variety of activities such as syllable repetition, connected speech, or swallowing. Information from the films can be obtained either by inspection, by comparative judgments, or by tracing the structures under consideration and measuring the distances between them. Various writers have discussed discrepancies between results obtained from the two types of films (Blackfield et al., 1961; Morris and Smith, 1962; Shelton et al., 1964). For study of speech movements, cinefluorographic films are preferred since a greater amount and variety of velopharyngeal activity can be sampled than in a single-view still film.

Measurement of the distance between the soft palate and the posterior pharyngeal wall of individual frames of a cinefluorographic film has demonstrated that many persons are inconsistent in the accomplishment of closure on the same task, depending on phonetic context, and that even the person who never achieves closure varies in the extent of opening depending on context (Moll, 1960; Bjork, 1961; Nylen, 1961). Shelton et al. (1964) found that some cleft palate speakers exhibit closure patterns judged to be normal and that others do not. It is not possible to say at present what closure pattern is essential for maximum speech learning. Undoubtedly some of the closure patterns described by Shelton et al. (1964) can be modified by articulation instruction (Nylen, 1961). Others require physical management.

In the above studies closure has been defined as contact between the soft palate and the posterior wall of the pharynx, and the distance between these structures has been studied. Neeley and Bradley (1964) were concerned about variability in extent of closure in persons who made contact between the palate and the posterior wall of the pharynx. In preparing a rating scale for study of cinefluorography recorded on video tape, they used terms such as "total blending," "partial blending," "touch but no blending," and "close approximation."

One problem with lateral x-ray films is that mesiolateral distances cannot be assessed. This limitation may be serious in assessing velopharyngeal area since, in certain individuals and under certain conditions, mesial movement of the lateral pharyngeal walls may contribute greatly to the reduction of the velopharyngeal space. In fact, consonant distortion by nasal escape of air has sometimes been observed in persons whose x-ray films show velopharyngeal closure. There is some evidence, however, that lateral films usually do provide a good index to velopharyngeal area. Bjork (1961) found that measurements of the distance between the soft palate and the posterior pharyngeal wall correlated highly with area measurements made from transverse laminagraphs of normal subjects.

Another method of assessing movement of the lateral walls of the pharynx (Cole and Campos-Giral, 1962) involves placement of a balloon containing radiopaque material in the pharynx and the use of radiography to show displacement of the balloon by the lateral pharyngeal walls. This procedure, however, is difficult to use for routine diagnostic purposes since the balloons must be positioned by individually fitted prosthodontic devices.

The use of radiographic techniques in the study of speech requires that the speech pathologist work closely with the radiologist. It is the radiologist who is legally responsible for the use of radiographic procedures and it is his responsibility to see that all equipment and techniques ensure maximum patient protection. He will assist the speech pathologist in reviewing the x-ray techniques available. The speech pathologist, however, will make final selection of the techniques to be used because he must decide whether they are suitable for the definition of structures important in speech production.

Since many of the structures to be considered are soft tissue and since definition of soft tissue by x-ray presents problems, evaluation by the speech pathologist of the radiographic technique to be used is important. Film contrast adequate for examination of soft tissue function during motion projection may not be adequate for identification of soft tissue borders during stop frame projection. Also, some speech tasks may be more appropriate than other tasks for demonstrating certain structural relationships. Thus, the speech pathologist is the one to specify the activity required of the subject during the film. Finally, the speech pathologist may wish to specify the conditions under which the films are to be taken. This may be the case particularly when the films are to be used for research and when great care needs to be used in maintaining appropriate angles, standard enlargement factors, and effort levels.

3. *Oral Manometers and Manometric Measures*

Various manometric devices for evaluation of velopharyngeal adequacy have been reported in the literature (Spriestersbach and Powers, 1959; Chase, 1960; Morris and Smith, 1962; Hanson, 1964; Hardy and Arkebauer, 1966). The majority of these assess air pressure either by using U-tube, water manometer devices, or mechanical pressure gauges. Each of the two types of evaluation has advantages and disadvantages (Dornette and Brechner, 1959; Hardy, 1965; Morris, 1966).

The U-tube water manometer, with readings usually made to the nearest half centimeter of water displacement, measures the pressure escaping through the nose (Buncke, 1959; Hess and McDonald, 1960; Shelton et al., 1961, 1965). This inexpensive device may be used to identify nasal escape of air and to provide a technique for visual feedback of nasal air escape to the client during training.[1] The normal speaker produces little or no displacement of the water except when he exhales nasally at the end of phonation. The technique has the disadvantage that only peak pressures can be read. More elaborate devices that permit write-out of nasal pressures over time are available. An additional use for a water manometer is in the calibration of an electrical manometer (Young, 1953).

A second manometric device is the Hunter oral manometer, which is available commercially.[2] It has been used clinically (Morris and Smith, 1962; Morris, 1966) and in research (Spriestersbach and Powers, 1959; Morris et al., 1961; Spriestersbach et al., 1961; Brooks et al., 1966). In general, two readings are obtained from the patient when it is used to assess velopharyngeal function. For the first reading he is asked simply to blow into the mouthpiece. The assumption is made that in his attempt to direct the airstream orally, his best attempt at velopharyngeal closure is demonstrated. For the second reading, he is again asked to blow into the mouthpiece but with his nostrils occluded by the examiner's fingertips to prevent a leak of oral pressure through the nasal cavities. This reading is usually referred to as the nostrils-occluded condition and provides an index of what reading might be expected if the patient could prevent nasal escape of air by closing the velopharyngeal port. The two readings are expressed as a ratio or quotient; ratios smaller than 1.00 demonstrate that the patient cannot prevent nasal escape by closing the velopharyngeal port and, thus, that he has a velopharyngeal problem.

[1] Hess, D. A., personal communications (1962).
[2] Hunter Manufacturing Company, Iowa City, Iowa.

Either positive or negative pressure readings can be used in computing a manometer ratio. There is no clear preference between the two types of readings if a bleed device is incorporated in the manometer to prevent the building up of oral pressure by contact between the tongue and palate rather than between the pharyngeal wall and palate (Morris, 1966).

A number of difficulties may be encountered in the clinical use of the manometric techniques. Hardy (1965) pointed out that use of oral manometer quotients is based on the assumption that the client produces maximum or at least equal respiratory effort on trials with the nares open and with them closed. He also pointed out that impounding pressure in the nasal cavities may result in inflation of the middle ears through the Eustachian tubes and that some speakers, especially children, may not produce maximum expiratory effort when this happens. Several writers have observed that subjects with poor palatopharyngeal closure sometimes, apparently as a result of tongue valving, are capable of producing large amounts of pressure during blowing. As discussed by Morris (1966) this problem can probably be prevented by use of a sufficiently large bleed valve. In general, the clinician is advised to familiarize himself with clients' responses to blowing tasks for purposes of general assessment but to base decisions on the outcome only when results are supported by other data. However, inadequate palatopharyngeal closure should be suspected when the oral pressure measures obtained with nares open divided by the measures obtained with the nares closed result in a ratio of less than 1.00.

4. *Intraoral Air Pressure*

The oral manometer is considered to be too gross an instrument for measuring amounts of intraoral air pressure. The device most commonly referred to in the literature for more precise measurements is the pressure-sensing tube, one end of which is placed in the mouth and the other end of which is attached to a pressure transducer. However, the instantaneous pressure readings which are obtained are not to be considered measurements of velopharyngeal competence. Nevertheless, there is a relationship between the two sets of events since, in the absence of velopharyngeal competence, little or no air pressure can be impounded in the oral cavity. In the present stage of development, then, the pressure-sensing tube cannot be considered to be a practical technique for diagnosing velopharyngeal competence, although it may possibly provide useful information in the future.

5. *Rate of Oral and Nasal Air Flow*

The pneumotachograph, described by Comroe (1950) and used by Isshiki and Ringel (1964), Kunze (1964), Lubker and Moll (1965), and Warren and Devereux (1966), was developed on the basis of a known relationship between a pressure drop across a grid and the rate of air flow through the grid. Various readings of air flow rate, taken either nasally or orally, or both, can be interpreted to indicate the efficiency of the velopharyngeal mechanism. The warm-wire anemoter, used by Quigley *et al.* (1964), operates by virtue of the cooling effect of the air flow from the mouth on a wire which is heated to a known temperature, and the measurement is of the amperage required to maintain that temperature in the presence of that cooling effect. Hardy (1965) has discussed problems in measuring rate of air flow and has specifically reviewed these two techniques. Subtelny *et al.* (1966) have developed instrumentation for studying oral and nasal pressure and flow. Certainly one advantage of all these devices is that measurements can be taken during continuous speech; another advantage is that the results are graphically recorded on paper for detailed study.

6. *Articulation Proficiency*

Important inferences regarding velopharyngeal competence can be made from tests of articulation proficiency when the speech clinician is careful to consider to what extent the level of proficiency may be due to learning and to what extent it is due to deficits in structure or function or both. Although the distinction is not always easy to make, a few generalizations are possible. Plosives, fricatives, and affricates are distorted and weakened by the escape of oral air pressure through the nasal cavity as a result of velopharyngeal incompetence. Recent work involving reduction of obturators worn by cleft palate speakers (Stick, 1966) and the relationship between speech therapy activities and articulation gain (Chisum, 1966) serves to make the definition of consonant distortion by nasal escape of air more specific. Stick's results suggest that the first effect when the posterior and lateral margins of the speech bulb are reduced in small decrements is an increase in nasal escape of air which, although inaudible to the listener, is measurable with a water manometer. The next effect is audible nasal escape of air until finally the available oral pressure is inadequate for the production of plosive and sibilant phonemes. Chisum reported that the audible nasal escape of air may range from unintelligible production of the phoneme because of emission of air through the nose to intelligible phoneme production accompanied by noises in the nasal passages generated by air escape. Similar distinctions have been used by Bzoch (1965). Frequent audible errors on plosives, fricatives, and affricates of the types described, then, can be interpreted as indicating a velopharyngeal problem. Another indication is the observation of nares constriction during the articulation of the so-called pressure consonants, which can be interpreted as an attempt by the speaker to prevent the nasal escape of oral air pressure from velopharyngeal incompetence.

Various types of observations of articulation proficiency are useful in evaluation of velopharyngeal competence. Word articulation tests are probably most conventionally employed because speech clinicians find it easier to evaluate the production of a speech sound in a single word than in connected speech. One such test specifically constructed for this purpose is the Iowa Pressure Articulation Test (Morris *et al.*, 1961), but others can be easily devised and indeed have been used in research and clinical reports (McWilliams, 1954; Greene, 1960; Shelton *et al.*, 1964; Brandt and Morris, 1965; Bzoch, 1965; Pitzner and Morris, 1966; Barnes and Morris, 1967).

The possibility of differences between a single word and connected speech in the ease of production of "pressure" consonants, particularly for those speakers with marginal or borderline competence, necessitates testing the production in connected speech. For this purpose Van Demark (1964, 1966) constructed a test with the score representing the number of plosives, fricatives, and affricates correctly produced in words elicited within sentences. In spite of methodological problems, which he describes in detail in his reports, the test provides useful and necessary diagnostic information.

Subtelny *et al.* (1961) measured intelligibility in terms of per cent of utterances intelligible to panels of listeners. Speech distorted by articulation errors may, however, be intelligible. An intelligibility score thus has a specific usefulness for measuring the degree to which the speakers may have difficulty in being understood by the listener; it cannot, of course, be used to identify specific speech sound errors resulting from poor palatopharyngeal closure.

For research purposes, psychological scale values derived from judges' responses to some aspect of speech, such as general defectiveness or severity of misarticulations, have often been useful. For clinical purposes, however, the techniques for obtaining such scale values are usually too cumbersome to be practical (see Chapter III for discussion of psychological scaling).

In summary, for evaluation of velopharyngeal competence from observations of connected speech, bias resulting from errors not related to adequacy of palatopharyngeal closure is to be avoided. Presumably nasals and glides are not affected by velopharyngeal incompetence; a speaker may learn, however, to substitute a glottal stop for a glide (Bzoch, 1965). The clinician must differentiate between such a learned response and similar errors that reflect physiological disability. Glottal stops may be used in any testing situation even after good physical repair because they are automatic responses to a set of stimuli. Comparison of articulatory responses made in connected speech with utterances made in test contexts will help the clinician to determine the consistency of error patterns and to differentiate between highly conscious performance and more automatic performance. To the extent that the examining speech pathologist wants to evaluate the "general effectiveness" of the individual as a speaker, however, he will want to include such observations in his diagnostic evaluations.

7. *Nasality*

Traditionally, assessment of the degree of nasality has been used as an index of velopharyngeal incompetence, particularly by individuals who are relatively naive about speech. It seems likely that many people, in using this term, have been referring both to voice quality and to control of the direction of the airstream during the production of consonants. Most appropriately, nasality refers to the degree of perceived nasal resonance during the production of vowels and the term will be so used in this discussion.

Many of the considerations for decisions about procedures to be used in assessing articulation proficiency are also relevant for assessing nasality. For example, judging the nasality demonstrated on isolated vowels may be considered an easier task than judging nasality during connected speech. Variability in degree of nasal resonance among vowels and among different contexts and speaking situations, however, makes construction of a testing instrument in the form of a standard speech sample difficult. Judgments of degrees of nasality on samples of connected speech also may reflect an irrelevant influence from defectiveness of articulation. In psychological scaling this problem can be managed by playing the tape-recorded speech samples backwards (Sherman, 1954), a procedure which eliminates any identification of articulation errors. Although scaling techniques for assessment of nasality have been useful in research, their use in diagnosis, with the scaling to be done by a single clinician, appears to lack adequate reliability (Shames *et al.*, 1960; Bradford *et al.*, 1964; Michel, 1965).

Development of techniques for reliable judging of degree of nasality in the clinical situation is needed. Carefully scaled tape-recorded speech samples to demonstrate varying degrees of nasality for use in training clinicians have not been made available commercially. Shames *et al.* (1960) have reported work of this kind, and scaled samples have been obtained (Sherman, 1954) and have been used for clinical training on a limited basis.

The problem of unreliability of judgments for clinical assessment of nasality has led many workers in the field to seek the development of instrumentation for obtaining measures which correlate highly with psychological scale values of severity of nasality. These could be used in evaluating severity for an individual patient and would eliminate the need for subjective judgments. Possibilities to consider are a measure of sound pressure level, a measure of phase shifting, and a measure obtained from evaluations of spectrograms. Techniques for obtaining such measures are discussed in Chapter III. Weiss (1954), Low (1955), Pierce (1962), Bryan (1963), and Shelton *et al.* (1967b) have studied the relationship between perceived nasality and measures of oral and nasal sound pressure level. Only the correlation coefficient reported by Weiss is high (.94). The coefficients reported by others are usually about .50 or lower. Although pressure measures may have merit in the evaluation of velopharyngeal closure, they are not satisfactory for the evaluation of degree of nasality.

Weatherly-White and his associates (1964, 1965, 1966) have described a nasality meter that is designed to differentiate between nasal and nonnasal voice in terms of the time relationships, or phase, of the frequencies in the speech sample. In the first publication (1964) the authors report being able to distinguish generally between cleft palate and normal speakers by examination of the readings obtained from the nasality meter. The findings of the most recent investigation (1966) indicate that direction of needle displacement is related to palatopharyngeal port opening. Further study is needed to establish the usefulness of this instrument in diagnosis.

Spectrograms or sonagrams of speech have been recommended for use as a diagnostic aid and for indicating changes which have resulted from therapy (Millard, 1957; Prins and Bloomer, 1965). Nylen (1961) reported that spectrography revealed changes in voice following surgery when those changes were relatively great, but, when differences in voice before and after surgery were perceptually less striking, spectrography was too gross a tool. As is suggested in Chapter III, spectrography does not provide a tool for the clinical evaluation of nasality at the present time for the reason that the interpretation of spectrograms for clinical purposes is confounded by the presence of multiple variables. Visual inspection of the spectrograph for study of nasality may indeed be a more difficult task than auditory inspection of a recording for the same purpose. The clinician who has access to a spectrograph is nevertheless advised to make spectrographs of nasal and nonnasal voice samples to extend his own experience.

In summary, none of the mechanical devices for assessing nasality seems satisfactory at this time. The works of Fant (1960) and Dickson (1962), which indicate that the relationships among measures relating to the physiology of nasality production, the acoustics of nasality transmission, and the perception of nasality are highly complex, support the idea that instrumentation cannot replace human judgments of severity of nasality. In fact, the development of an instrumental measure that correlates highly with nasality judgments should not be expected.

8. Stimulability

That speech observations can be useful in diagnosis of velopharyngeal competence has already been discussed. The clinician, of course, for this purpose, must distinguish between characteristics of speech which are related to velopharyngeal incompetence and those which are related to inappropriate learning of behavior patterns. Understandably, such a distinction is often very difficult to make. One way to distinguish between velopharyngeal problems and so-called functional problems is to observe whether the individual can be stimulated, by auditory and visual cues, to change his behavior (Morris and Smith, 1962; Barnes and Morris, 1967). This stimulability technique is important because success by the patient indicates that achievement of velopharyngeal competence is possible, and also that behavioral change is possible. Production of phonemes by conscious effort, however, does not guarantee that their use in automatic speech can be acquired. If repeated stimulation consistently results in consonant productions which are distorted by nasal emission and vowels which are unpleasantly nasal, the inference can be drawn, at least tentatively, that the individual is not able to change his speaking behavior because of velopharyngeal incompetence. Additional diagnostic observations are obviously needed before the final diagnosis is made.

B. Treatment Decision

Except when the physical defect is gross, none of the diagnostic procedures described above would, by itself, provide sufficient information upon which to base decisions. In general, diagnosis of the competence of the velopharyngeal mechanism leads to a choice of one of three possible decisions regarding treatment: physical management, behavioral therapy, or a deferment of diagnosis. Adequacy of velopharyngeal closure will range from gross insufficiency through possible sufficiency to competent closure. In some cases, it will be difficult to evaluate adequacy of palatopharyngeal closure and diagnosis will be deferred.

If the diagnostic techniques point conclusively to palatal insufficiency, then the treatment decision is referral for physical management. Typically, this referral will be made to the surgeon or dentist who has provided previous care. When the patient does not wish to return to the same surgeon or dentist, or when he cannot conveniently do so, the speech pathologist, by reviewing with the patient or his parents the facilities which are available, will help him or his parents to consider the possible options. Direct referral to a specific surgeon or dentist is to be avoided.

The parents should be given to understand that physical management alone may not alleviate the speech problems of the individual, that usually speech therapy also will be needed, and that further consultation with a speech pathologist may be indicated after physical management has been completed. To be emphasized is the fact that speech therapy in the absence of needed physical treatment is likely to be ineffective, and, as a matter of fact, attempts to teach a person speech responses that are beyond his physical capacity may result in the development of certain undesirable movements which treatment is designed to avoid or to eliminate.

If the diagnostic techniques indicate velopharyngeal competence, then the treatment decision is behavioral therapy, which will be discussed in the final portion of this chapter.

Diagnosis may be deferred because the speech clinician cannot make the relevant observations, usually because the child is too young to cooperate. It may also be deferred when the clinician is so unsure of what needs to be done that it seems best to continue making observations.

A word of caution seems indicated regarding the decision to defer diagnosis. Sometimes a speech clinician is hesitant to make a diagnosis of velopharyngeal incompetence. At the same time, he is aware that the patient is not responding to speech therapy and so, as an alternative, he simply defers treatment of any kind, hoping that the outlook for behavioral change will improve as the child grows older. In reality, however, the problem may be one of a structural deficit and, if this is true, probably the patient may be harmed by deferring treatment. The better choice, then, in case of doubt, is to make a referral for physical management. The decision to defer diagnosis always should be made with great care and with clear justification.

II. Speech Problems

A. DIAGNOSTIC TECHNIQUES

Observations of articulation and voice have been discussed with reference to their importance in the evaluation of the palatopharyngeal mechanism. Although useful in evaluating the mechanism, these observations do not provide sufficient information about speech to plan appropriate treatment. The child may have a good mechanism and yet have articulation errors. There is a need, then, for the traditional articulation tests in evaluating the cleft palate child's speech proficiency (Templin and Darley, 1960; Johnson et al., 1963; Darley, 1964; McDonald, 1964). Articulation testing is particularly useful for the assessment of general level of maturation of speech sound acquisition and of consistency of articulation error. The results permit comparison of the cleft palate child with normal children in terms of sound development. They provide information needed for conferring with the parents, the surgeon, or the dentist about the child's speech.

Mention should also be given to the use of articulation tests in the measurement of short-term change in articulation behavior in response to instruction. Remarkably little effort has been directed toward use of articulation tests to evaluate short-term change in articulation behavior. However, the work of Elbert (1966) and Elbert *et al.* (1967) indicates that short lists of phonemes, syllables, words, and sentences constructed to sample the learner's articulation of specific phonemes may be used to obtain reliable information about articulation and its change in response to therapy.

As indicated above, the problem of deciding whether a speech problem is "functional" or "organic" may be difficult. One index which can be obtained from results of articulation testing is a measure of inconsistency of misarticulation. If the individual misarticulates a speech sound only part of the time, he is obviously physically able to produce the sound correctly. In addition, whether speech problems are related to faulty learning may be indicated by the response given to auditory and visual stimulation. In one sense, the stimulation procedure is a very short period of trial therapy, designed to demonstrate whether the individual will be able to respond well and quickly to therapy. If the speaker can use auditory and visual cues and achieve correct articulation of a sound in the test situation, the assumption is that the error sound is the result of incorrect learning, not of a physical condition. It can also be assumed that the error can be corrected with appropriate retraining procedures.

The most frequently observed voice problem, as discussed previously, is nasality. In addition, however, the clinician should consider, in evaluating voice for a child with cleft palate, the possibility of deviant voice quality other than nasality. Brooks and Shelton (1963) found that 10% of a group of surgically or prosthetically managed children with cleft palate had voice problems other than, or in addition to, nasality. In two clinical studies involving several subgroups of cleft palate persons, Bzoch (1964a, b) has reported incidence of voice disorders other than nasality ranging from 17.5 to 52%. Since the voice disorders of harshness and hoarseness can result from vocal abuse, the possibility of vocal abuse from physical effort to use good speech in the absence of palatopharyngeal competence should be considered.

B. TREATMENT DECISION

Information regarding norms for maturation of articulation skills is helpful in deciding about treatment. The clinician may delay, for example, providing therapy for a child of age 6 who is having difficulty with /ɜ/ because many children at age 6 misarticulate /ɜ/ and because this sound is often corrected without therapy as the child grows older.

The decision of whether a speech problem is related to a physical condition or to patterns of learning is of major importance in diagnosis for the person with cleft palate. If indications are that the problem is related to patterns of learning, speech therapy is indicated. If the findings point to a relationship between the speech problem and physical conditions, then appropriate referral for a different kind of treatment other than speech therapy is usually indicated. In some cases, both speech therapy and other referrals may be indicated.

III. Oral-Facial Structures

A. DIAGNOSTIC TECHNIQUES

That deviations of several oral-facial structures can be important in contributing to the speech problems of an individual with cleft palate has been pointed out in Chapter IV, with the conclusion that in the majority of cases these deviations are not the major etiological factors. Their possible role in hampering speech production is, however, difficult to evaluate. Sometimes indirect measurements and sometimes ratings of the structures in question can be obtained with measurements of and with judgments of x-ray films or dental casts. The usual procedure is to depend upon clinical judgments of the structures made during an examination of the oral cavity. Reliability of such clinical observations can be questioned (Morris, 1965).

1. The Lips

Subjects with cleft lip only have essentially normal speech and thus the presence of a cleft lip, surgically repaired or not, is not expected to hinder the production of speech. Occasionally a surgically repaired cleft lip which seems very short and very immobile is seen, and, in some instances, the shortness and immobility might make production of the labial sounds difficult. A very practical criterion to employ in evaluating such a structure is to determine whether the individual can effect lip closure easily. If the upper lip is of sufficient length and mass for easy contact with the lower lip, structure and function can be judged adequate for speech production.

2. The Tongue

Although the tongue is important in speech production, it appears to be deviant in very few individuals. Diagnostic procedures, however, should include an evaluation of its adequacy for speech.

Tongue size is very difficult to assess, since it must be related to oral and pharyngeal volume, and no standardized measurement technique is available. Subjective evaluation is the basis for any diagnosis with reference to the adequacy of tongue size for good speech.

A retracted, elevated tongue position has been suggested as a possible cause of a speech problem for a person with a cleft palate (McDonald and Koepp-Baker, 1951). Recent work (Brooks *et al.*, 1965, 1966) indicates that the tongue may be excessively retracted during the articulation of certain sounds by those speakers with poor velopharyngeal closure. The relationship of tongue retraction to palatal adequacy makes reasonable an assumption that the articulators function as a unit and that the posture of one structure is dependent on the adequacy of other related structures.

Rates of tongue movements for persons with normal speech structures (Fairbanks and Spriestersbach, 1950; Sprague, 1961) and information about tongue motility for children with cleft palate (Matthews and Byrne, 1953) have been reported. The available information, however, does not permit easy distinction between normal and abnormal motility, nor does it establish that tongue motility is defective for speakers with cleft palate.

3. *Dentition*

Dental deviations, such as missing teeth or malocclusion, may be related to articulation errors. The relationship is not consistent, either for children with cleft palate or for those without cleft palate. Although many children with missing teeth articulate normally (Snow, 1961; Bankson and Byrne, 1962), the clinician in making a diagnosis and in planning therapy should consider whether dental deviations are an important factor. Orthodontic appliances sometimes temporarily hinder speech improvement; dental plates may be so thick in the area immediately behind the central incisors that there is little room for tongue placement necessary for acceptable articulation of certain sounds. Often however, the orthodontist or the prosthodontist can correct a problem of this kind if it is called to his attention. The clinician thus needs to be aware of dentition and possible effects of dental deviations upon articulation (Subtelny *et al.*, 1964).

4. *Nasal Cavities*

Obstruction of the nasal cavities may reduce the amount of nasal escape of air during speech to an extent which indicates better velopharyngeal function than is really possible when there is velopharyngeal incompetence. The cavities, typically, are inspected for obstruction with the aid of retractors (to enlarge the nares) and a light source. In addition, function is usually assessed by listening for possible auditory effects of the obstruction during expiration. While no single deviant oral-facial structure may have a detrimental effect on speech, the combination of subclinical deviations may have such an effect. Assessment of the combined effect of deviations of several oral-facial structures, however, is very difficult and, at best, conclusions should be tentative.

B. Treatment Decision

The criteria to be used in making decisions about treatment of deviant oral-facial structures are similar, to a large extent, to those considered for velopharyngeal incompetence. Since deviations of oral-facial structures are not amenable to behavioral therapy,[3] referrals to medical or dental specialists may be needed. However, some conditions such as abnormal tongue size are not treatable.

Since neural impairment, for the cleft palate population as a whole, has not been established, therapy for the improvement of motility of the lips or the tongue should be only for those who specifically need it and should not be routine for all. Although oral-facial deviations cannot be changed by behavioral therapy, sometimes the patient can learn to compensate for them. Behavioral therapy for this purpose is discussed later in this chapter.

IV. Neural Function

A. Diagnostic Techniques

Although motility of the oral structures, particularly of the soft palate, has been referred to throughout this section on diagnosis, neurological impairment has not been demonstrated to be a particular problem related to speech deviations of individuals with cleft palate. The diagnostician, however, should consider possible deviations in neural function resulting from cleft palate surgery (Nylen, 1961). He should also consider deviations in neural function which are related to congenital palatal insufficiency which has been described by Randall et al. (1960), Blackfield et al. (1963), and Crikelair et al. (1963). Techniques for assessing neural function are indicated in the following paragraphs.

Electromyography (EMG) is used to study both disorders and normal function of the lower motor neurone and muscle. In the study of the disorders, EMG readings help the medical clinician to locate the site of the neurological lesion. Electromyographic instrumentation has been described by Cooper (1965), Fromkin (1965), and Lubker (1968). The minimum equipment includes electrodes, a preamplifier and amplifier, a calibrator, and a recording apparatus. The electrical potential developed in the muscle is picked up by the electrodes, amplified, and then projected on an oscilloscope or through a speaker. It may also be recorded by tape recorder, camera, or pen writer. Simultaneous recordings from several different muscles by means of multiple

---

[3] Although they must be compatible with behavioral principles, physical therapy and myofunctional orthodontics are viewed here as physical treatment.

channel apparatus provide the best approach to the study of bodily movements or kinesiology (Rodriquez and Oester, 1961; Tavener, 1961). According to Fischer (1961), electromyography is the best, if not the only, tool for discovering minor dysfunction of the central nervous system and of the motor end plates.

The excitability characteristics of an isolated muscle or nerve fiber may be studied by means of a strength duration curve (Wynn-Parry, 1961a, b; Bauwens, 1961). The muscle or nerve is stimulated with an electronic stimulator, and the amount of current needed to produce a just perceptible contraction at each of a series of progressively shorter pulse durations is measured. The curve of strength duration is obtained when strength of current is plotted against duration of current. Such data indicate whether there is nerve damage and, if so, approximately how much. If repeated at intervals, the strength duration curve will indicate whether the condition of the lesion is improving, deteriorating, or remaining static.

Electrophysiological tests of motor function can be used in evaluation of motor disability in the individual with an articulation problem or palate malfunction. Some normative data regarding electromyographic measurement of levator veli palatini and pharyngeal constrictor action potentials during rest, sucking, and swallowing are available (Basmajian and Dutta, 1961; Fritzell, 1963), and EMG is being used increasingly in the study of distinctive phonetic features (MacNeilage, 1963; Harris et al., 1965; Fromkin, 1966).

Strength of muscular contraction, which may be related to neural function, has been measured by spring-balance methods, pressure systems, weight-lifting techniques, and strain gauge methods. Measurement of resistance that the palate muscles can overcome would require the attachment of some device to the superior surface of the palate. Such measurement is thus impractical for routine clinical procedure. Saltar (1958) described endurance as maintenance of a given level of contraction of a muscle or muscle group over a period of time or as maintenance of repeated exertions through a given range at a given rate over a period of time. She states that strength and endurance are not necessarily equally affected by exercise nor by disease.

She says that muscular coordination, which she defines as the ease and speed with which contractions can be made accurately, is difficult to measure and that it is not independent of strength. Poor articulation and also poor voice quality may indicate a lack of coordination of speech mechanism muscles, although this is not necessarily so.

Monitoring by means of oral sensation has been considered important to articulation behavior and in the correction of misarticulations (Van Riper and Irwin, 1958; McDonald, 1964). Presumably, defects in oral sensation can cause articulation problems (McCroskey, 1958; Ringel and Steer, 1963; Ringel and Ewanowski, 1965; Shelton et al., 1967a). Physiological and behavioral aspects of oral sensations and also test development are reported by Bosma (1967). Only those studies and topics of particular concern with reference to speech problems of persons with cleft palate will be reviewed here.

The possibility that no physiological mechanism is used for kinesthetic monitoring of movements of structures not associated with joints has been discussed by Shelton et al. (1967a). These structures include tongue, palate, lips, and facial muscles. Evidence indicates that receptors in muscles that were once thought to mediate kinesthesis actually transmit impulses to subcortical areas. No conscious sensation results from this transmission. Although this information does not contraindicate the point of view that oral sensation is important to speech, there is little reason to expect exercises directed toward creating conscious awareness of palate movement or position to be effective. There is less opportunity for touch cues from contact between the palate and other structures than from contact between the tongue or the lips and other structures; also, the palate may have fewer sensory receptors than the lips and tongue (Penfield and Rassmussen, 1950; Grossman, 1964; Ringel and Ewanowski, 1965). That impulses from receptors in oral muscles influence motor speech on an unconscious level appears to be a possible hypothesis. Under such a hypothesis, rehabilitation through motor practice would be a more practical approach than would perceptual training. The fact that on command the palate can be elevated to different heights without visual or auditory cues suggest the presence of kinesthetic function, especially when elevation short of contact with the posterior wall of the pharynx can be skillfully performed.

Assessment of oral sensory function in persons with speech defects with appropriate procedures might be useful in developing a better understanding of oral sensory physiology. Ringel and Ewanowski (1965) have suggested one such procedure by use of an oral esthesiometer for investigation of two-point discrimination capacity both extraorally and intraorally. This instrument permits control of stimulator force against the mucosa as well as separation of the stimulus points.

Several test-development projects are described in a reference edited by Bosma (1967), including a report by Rutherford and McCall (1967) on tactile acuity, two-point discrimination, tactile localization, tactile pattern recognition, and kinesthetic pattern recognition. In the same reference, McDonald and Aungst (1967) report work on the development and standardization of a test of oral stereognosis. Results of a factor analysis indicate that the test items are related to one common factor. Shelton et al. (1967a) report work in the same text on another test of oral stereognosis.

As in the McDonald and Aungst test, ability to identify small plastic forms by oral exploration is assessed. Eventually, with further development, these tools may be useful for clinical application. In the meantime, the clinician should recognize the possibility that sensory as well as motor factors may be etiological factors in any articulation disorder.

B. TREATMENT DECISION

Since the research on tests of neural function has provided only a meager basis for clinical implications, treatment decision with reference to neural deficit is difficult. During the past two decades, writings in speech pathology seem to indicate that, in the absence of adequate neural function, however defined, the expectations for success of retraining procedures are limited. For the patient with cleft palate who has velopharyngeal incompetence resulting from velar paresis the referral is for physical management as it is for the patient with velopharyngeal incompetence resulting from velar tissue insufficiency. For paralysis of the tongue or lips when no physical management procedures are available, the goals of treatment are usually lowered and behavioral therapy procedures are provided to help the patient compensate for the problem.

V. Hearing Acuity and Auditory Perception

A. DIAGNOSTIC TECHNIQUES

1. Standard Audiometric Techniques

For assessment of hearing acuity for individuals with cleft palate standard audiometric techniques are used (see Chapter V). Particular attention should be given to tests of middle ear function since hearing problems typical of individuals with cleft palate are those related to middle ear infections.

2. Tests of Auditory Perception

A number of tests of various aspects of auditory perception have been developed specifically for use in diagnosis of various speech pathologies. These include tests for assessment of the ability to identify phonemes when they are heard and to discriminate among phonetic units which are heard as somewhat similar. A review of the literature concerned with auditory perception, in general, is not appropriate here but is available from several sources (Karlin, 1942; Hanley, 1956; Templin, 1957; Wepman, 1958; Byrne, 1962).

Apparently no research on auditory perception factors, other than on hearing loss for pure tones and for speech, has been carried out for individuals with cleft palate speech problems. Liberman *et al.* (1957, 1961, 1962), however, have taken the position that the speaker learns to associate speech sounds with his articulation and that the articulatory movements and the corresponding neurological processes become part of the perceiving process: that is, the articulatory movements are important to speech perception. If this theory is correct, then speakers with cleft palate who have misarticulated speech sounds for long periods of time because of anatomical and physiological deficits might be expected to demonstrate disorders of auditory perception. It may be that such factors are particularly relevant in the case of an individual who now has the velopharyngeal competence requisite for normal speech but who persists in using speech which is comparable to that which he used when his problem was related to velopharyngeal incompetence. It is difficult to recommend testing instruments for assessing auditory perception. Tests of auditory discrimination and memory span have been devised by Templin (1957) and by Kirk and McCarthy (1961). Crary (1965) and Heck (1966) have discussed development of tests for evaluating sound synthesis ability and have presented test data obtained by administering such tests.

B. Treatment Decision

The criteria for the treatment decision for problems of hearing acuity for individuals with cleft palate are the same as for any individuals with such problems. Since the typical hearing problem associated with cleft palate is related to middle ear disease and is frequently responsive to medical care, medical referral is usually indicated. If the hearing loss appears to be irreversible, the possible value of methods for amplification and of auditory training should be considered.

Sometimes the treatment decision may include recommendations for ear training designed to develop the patient's ability to discriminate among speech sounds. The work of Prins (1963) and that of Aungst and Frick (1964) have indicated that discrimination ability of the patient should be considered in relation to his articulation errors. As in other therapy, the clinician should not use time developing skills that are already satisfactory.

VI. Psychosocial Adjustment

A. Diagnostic Techniques

In most aspects evaluation of the adequacy of psychosocial adjustment of individuals with cleft palate is very much like that of others, and, for this reason, the usual psychological testing instruments are employed.

Limitations on the usefulness of those instruments include lack of standardization and unavailability of an instrument suitable for evaluating adjustment of children.

That there apparently is in general no severe degree of psychological disturbance in parents of children with cleft palate has been reported (see Chapter VI). The possibility, however, that the amount of stress placed on the individual with the cleft and on his parents may vary from time to time seems reasonable. The parents, for example, may feel great stress immediately after the birth of the child and also at the time when decisions regarding physical management must be made. The same might be true for the time when the child starts school. The individual with the cleft may feel most stress when he first recognizes that he is different from other children in appearance or in speech proficiency, or when he first recognizes that he has a birth defect. He may also feel stress when he begins to seek attention from the opposite sex or when he begins his first job. The time at which appraisal is made of the psychosocial status of the patient and of his parents thus may influence an index of adjustment. The clinical speech pathologist, then, should be aware of the need to assess adjustment with reference to specific troublesome events or times.

B. TREATMENT DECISION

If the client is maladjusted to the extent that his psychological problems interfere with his ability to seek surgical or dental care or to benefit from speech therapy, then the speech pathologist should make an appropriate referral to a clinical psychologist, psychiatrist, or psychiatric social worker. If the adjustment problem seems relatively serious but is not interfering with routine treatment of problems associated with cleft palate, the speech pathologist may discuss the problem with the patient and make the appropriate referral and also may continue speech therapy, if indicated, at the same time.

VII. Language Maturity

A. DIAGNOSTIC TECHNIQUES

Children with cleft palate are on the average moderately retarded in the development of linguistic skill; also, it seems reasonable to assume that the language skills of adults with cleft palate would, in general, be somewhat below average. The clinical speech pathologist thus should include tests of linguistic function in the diagnostic procedures for the patient with cleft palate.

Templin (1957) described a set of measures designed for assessing language skills including response length, variability of response length, and structural complexity. These measures have been used by other investigators (Day, 1932; Davis, 1937; McCarthy, 1954; Winitz, 1959; Moll and Darley, 1960; Morris, 1960, 1962; Minifie *et al.*, 1963; Webster and Shelton, 1964). Comparison of these measures with available normative data can be useful clinically. They are time-consuming to use, however, and also the clinician should assure himself that his techniques are reliable and that the measures he uses are valid estimates of aspects of the child's language development. Recent research (Shriner and Sherman, 1967) has provided evidence that the best single measure in relation to observers' evaluations of language development among those mentioned is mean length in number of words for 50 responses. They developed, by means of a multiple-R procedure, an equation for prediction of observers' evaluations of degree of language development by using the above-mentioned measures obtained from analysis of samples of children's language consisting of 50 responses each. Results of a validity generalization procedure provided evidence that the measures most useful for this equation, as applied to language of children without speech problems, are useful also for predicting language development in samples from children with cleft palate accompanied by severe articulation problems. On the basis of their results clinical implications would seem to be that (1) the variability of response measure is not a useful one and (2) the mean length of response measure is the most useful single measure among those described in the references given at the beginning of this paragraph.

Clinicians often assess language development by the use of test items from tests which have been standardized for other purposes. An example of this is the use of selected items from verbal intelligence tests. The validity of the use of test items out of context and for purposes other than that for which they were standardized has been discussed by Anastasi (1961); she does not recommend this procedure.

Various tests designed for specific purposes other than assessing language development sometimes provide useful clinical information on the communication skills of a child with cleft palate. Tests of reading ability include the Metropolitan Readiness Tests (Hildreth and Griffiths, 1949), the Gates Primary Reading Tests (Gates, 1958), and the Wide Range Achievement Test (Jastak, 1946). The picture vocabulary intelligence tests (Ammons and Ammons, 1948; Dunn, 1959) provide a useful index for one aspect of language development. An interview scale constructed by Mecham (1958, 1960) may be especially useful in assessment of the language development of children who are not sufficiently mature to respond appropriately in a formal testing situation.

The Illinois Test of Psycholinguistic Abilities (Kirk and McCarthy, 1961; McCarthy and Kirk, 1961) was developed for use as a diagnostic language test. The authors have differentiated between diagnostic instruments and classification tests, and they have hypothesized that with their test therapeutic programs can be developed for specific profiles showing language deficits. The test was published as an experimental edition subject to revision depending upon additional clinical and theoretical work. Since publication, further study has been done on item analysis, reliability, and validity (McCarthy and Kirk, 1963; McCarthy and Olson, 1964), and a critical review has been published by Spradlin (1963).

Linguistic studies of normal and disordered language (Berko and Brown, 1960; Glanzer, 1962; Menyuk, 1964; Winitz, 1966) may eventually provide information useful for language assessment. Identification of persons with language disorders might be facilitated and language remediation might be programmed. Lee (1966) has compared developmental sentence types of a normal child with developmental sentence types of a child with delayed language and has reported that the child with delayed language is not only slower in language development but also does not produce certain types of syntactic structures.

The diversity of approaches to the study and the remediation of language disorders in children and the fact that these approaches are still taking form have been discussed in published monographs (Daley, 1962; Schiefelbusch, 1963).

B. TREATMENT DECISION

The major treatment decision to be considered for a language development problem is whether to provide behavioral therapy and, if so what kind. In general, the criteria to be used in making a decision for the patient with a cleft palate are the same as for any other individual.

VIII. Concluding Statement

With the exception of assessment of velopharyngeal competence, the diagnostic procedures for assessing speech problems presented by speakers with cleft palate are comparable to those to be used with the problems of other speech pathologies, and the same general procedures for therapy can be used. Assessment by the clinical speech pathologist of velopharyngeal problems is typically the most imperative diagnostic goal for the simple reason that the conclusions reached regarding velopharyngeal competence will determine whether physical management procedures are needed prior to behavioral treatment.

Part Two: Therapy

The therapeutic process is characterized by continued diagnosis in that there is periodic reevaluation of the predictions which were made about the outcome at the onset of retraining.

Considerations in planning speech therapy for an individual with cleft palate are, in general, the same as those for individuals with other speech pathologies and have been described in detail in various textbooks. There are several factors, however, that are unique to individuals with cleft palate and, more generally, to individuals with speech problems which are related to physical problems.

The individual with cleft palate is often being treated not only by the speech pathologist but also by other professional workers whose treatment may have a direct bearing on the effectiveness with which the individual can change his speech. For this reason the speech pathologist should maintain communication with the other workers in order that the various kinds of treatment may be coordinated. The speech pathologist will need to know the goals of other kinds of treatment and when they are expected to be reached; and, particularly with reference to velopharyngeal competence, he will need to provide information to the others about progress in speech.

The interdependence between speech training and certain other management procedures may be especially important. Speech training procedures for sibilant distortion related to dental deviations, for example, may depend on whether the dental deviations are to be treated. The scheduling of speech training and the choice of procedures for a child with a conductive-type hearing loss will be affected by decisions on otological treatment. Certainly speech training for an individual with velopharyngeal incompetence will be influenced by plans for management. If the only speech problems which the individual demonstrates are related to velopharyngeal incompetence for which there is to be physical management, then speech therapy should be deferred until after the management is completed. If physical management is not to be provided, then the speech clinician should consider whether speech therapy procedures which will help the individual to compensate for the physical problem are indicated.

At this point it is perhaps worth commenting upon the levels of knowledge and skill possessed by those professional persons trained to provide physical care for persons with cleft lip and palate. The view is taken here that these levels are such that most individuals with clefts can be given the anatomical and physiological requisites for satisfactory speech. That being the case, the speech pathologist should exert every effort to develop relationships with these professional colleagues, particularly the surgeons and dentists, and to achieve levels of understanding and trust with the patient and his parents, which will enable him to make referrals freely when he feels that the patient's present physical status is limiting the level of the goals which would be possible under relatively ideal conditions of physical intactness and function. In any event, the speech pathologist is responsible for informing other professional workers, the patient, and the parents of the goals of speech therapy, this responsibility being particularly important when the prediction is for only a limited amount of improvement. The patient, for example, may have speech problems related not only to velopharyngeal incompetence but also to inappropriate learning, in which case the decision might be to do speech therapy only for the latter, at least until physical management had been completed; the speech clinician, then, obviously should be responsible for providing realistic information on the goals of speech therapy to all concerned. Unrealistic goals on the part of anyone concerned can result in great harm to the patient.

Changes in speech behavior in some cases can occur relatively quickly because of changes in status of the physiological and anatomical bases for speech. The patient and clinician, for example, may be experiencing considerable success in therapy until the patient has an adenoidectomy. After recovery, because of the loss of adenoid tissue in the anteroposterior dimension of the nasopharynx, velopharyngeal competence may be deficient, and, for this reason, the rationale, objectives, and procedures for speech therapy have to be changed in a rather abrupt fashion. Changes which result from physical management, in the opposite direction, from incompetence to competence, may also come about just as abruptly. Goals for therapy thus must be defined somewhat tentatively, with the knowledge that, if physical status changes, their revision may be needed.

Whether parents can assist effectively in therapy for young children, particularly when therapy with the clinician cannot be scheduled at sufficiently frequent intervals, is often a consideration. That therapy can be more effective, in general, with help from parents who have been trained to assist than without such help has been demonstrated (Sommers, 1962; Sommers et al., 1964). The speech clinician should approach such delegation with care, perhaps with even more care than for children with other speech pathologies. If, however, the mother evidences any rejection of the child, if her level of anxiety about the problem indicates guilt feelings, or if she appears to be overprotective of the child, she cannot be expected to assume successfully the role of a teacher. The clinician also must be careful in estimating the mother's intelligence and her ability to understand the child. The mother may, if she lacks the needed intelligence and understanding to conduct therapy, pursue speech practice relentlessly and with no flexibility in a way that will be harmful to the child. Particular caution, then, is to be observed in making a decision on whether the mother of a child with cleft palate should be requested to help with therapy.

I. Procedures for Articulation Therapy

For the individual who has had a cleft palate but who now has essentially normal oral structures, articulation therapy will be very much like that designed for the person with a so-called functional articulation problem. The procedures are planned, first of all, to provide speech sound discrimination training if needed; second, to teach appropriate phonetic placement of the articulators if indicated; and, third, to accomplish automatic use of the newly acquired speech acts.

Specific generalizations about procedures for individuals with inadequate oral structures are difficult to make for the reason that much depends on which oral structures are inadequate. Therapy goals for the individual with inadequate oral structures must be specific, detailed, and will need to be made very clear, both to the client and the clinician. The goals may in reality be the achievement of compensatory behavior and may require experimental procedures.

An individual with velopharyngeal incompetence, for example, cannot be expected to have the oral air flow necessary for acceptable production of plosives and fricatives. Therapy stressing the accomplishment of sudden oral explosion of plosives or the accomplishment of fricatives is unrealistic. However, if physical management of the velopharyngeal incompetence is postponed or if for some reason it cannot be improved, a program may be planned to teach as nearly acceptable articulation as possible. Speech is more intelligible when characterized by acceptable phonetic placement for consonant articulation, even though it is characterized by nasality, omissions, general distortions, and glottal stops, than is speech with the same types of errors accompanied by unacceptable placement. In the latter instance, the substitution of pharyngeal fricatives and the presence of more deviant articulatory distortions may be expected to compound the problems of intelligibility brought about by generally inaccurate placement of the articulators.

Typical of therapy for the purpose discussed above is the teaching of light, quick, and appropriate articulation contacts for the plosives. Sustained tense contacts may cause enough breath to escape through the nasal passages that the result is an undesirable facial grimace which comes about from an attempt to prevent the nasal escape of air. The admonition to "try harder" thus will often increase the conspicuousness of the speech deviations.

For the /p/ and /b/ the client may practice the clicking sound which results when fairly relaxed, moistened lips are tapped together lightly as the mandible is elevated and lowered, a procedure sometimes referred to by the children as "fish talk." The /p/ and /b/ should be combined with open vowels to increase the amount of jaw action. At first they are whispered, with the client attempting to lessen the degree of facial grimace, if this is a problem, as he watches himself in the mirror. Words and short phrases can be introduced with attention concentrated on the tactile sensations of lip closure and on acoustic effect. Such practice will aid children with relaxed, everted lower lips.

Procedures similar to those given in the above paragraph can be used for /t/ and /d/. The mandible should be held in a depressed position as the tongue tip taps the gum ridge. If /k/ and /g/ are substituted for /t/ and /d/, with strong backward elevation of the tongue, therapy should include emphasis on ear training and mirror work with the jaw held down while the tongue tip rises for /t/, /d/, /n/, /l/ and /r/. Light contacts should be stressed.

For the /k/ and /g/ the individual may have learned to impound the breath by closing the glottis and increasing the pressure to obtain a sudden explosive release when he expels the breath with a resulting sound which is like a quick cough. One way to eliminate this glottal substitution is to teach a forward placement of the tongue and palatal contact with the tongue in such syllables as /iki/ and /igi/. This may be difficult when the maxillary arch is very narrow. Appropriate tongue placement may be so difficult for the patient that the clinician should give specific attention to raising the level of tongue carriage. He may, for example, instruct the patient to hold the tongue tip lightly against the back of the lower incisors while the body of the tongue is pressed upward against the palatal arch. It will be easier at first for the patient to maintain a high level of tongue carriage if the chin is held down. When contact between body of the tongue and the palate is achieved without excessive effort, the clinician can indicate with a tongue blade that only the posterior portion of the tongue contacts the palate for /k/ and /g/. The act of raising instead of lowering the back of the tongue is thus emphasized.

Fricatives can sometimes be taught by emphasis on light quick constriction with oral breath flow of brief duration. Prolongation of a fricative often only increases nasal emission. The /s/ and /z/ usually present great difficulty. In the effort to produce friction, the speaker with cleft palate frequently leaves the upper and lower teeth slightly apart and achieves the friction sound by moving the tongue back toward the pharyngeal wall. With a light closure between the teeth and stress upon correct placement for /s/ and /z/ a short oral air flow can be sufficient to make the sounds intelligible.

Teaching an individual to compensate for structural deviations other than velopharyngeal incompetence, such as collapsed maxillary arch or severe malocclusion, may be needed. Structural deviations, however, occur in such variety that detailed description of the procedures to be used is not feasible. Suffice it to say that the objective is to assist the patient to do the best he can in the presence of structural deviations, always remembering that the goal of such therapy is intelligible, rather than skilled, speech.

In summary, careful definition of the criteria to be used is needed before any decision on whether speech therapy should be initiated for the individual with inadequate oral structures. Any possibility of successful reduction of structural problems should be interpreted as indicating a need for careful consideration of whether it is best to defer speech training until after the physical management has been completed. Only when the speech clinician believes that physical management would not help or when parents are opposed to such management, should compensatory movements be taught.

Indirect articulation therapy may sometimes be used with very young children. The first procedure is to create a play situation for the child to observe (Hahn, 1960). The clinician arranges toys, describing his activities as he works. The child usually becomes interested and, as he imitates or participates in the play activity, he is likely to imitate also in a verbal way. As verbal interchange between the clinician and the child becomes more frequent in occurrence, the clinician may explain how he makes a speech sound in a word and later may make comments about the way the child articulates the sound. The aim is to interest the child to the extent that direct therapy will become appropriate. Age is not the criterion for deciding between indirect and direct methods of therapy. The introduction of direct methods should always be as early as feasible and depends on the intelligence, maturation, and physical capabilities of the child.

II. Therapeutic Exercise and Motor Learning

Strengthening and training of the muscles of the velopharyngeal mechanism have often been recommended and used as techniques for improving the speech of individuals with cleft palate. For example, Berry and Eisenson (1956) have recommended development of palatopharyngeal closure by exercise. They appear to have abandoned their earlier consideration (Berry and Eisenson, 1942) of physiotherapy and electrotherapy guided by the physician for the accomplishment of the closure. Nor did they reiterate in the later work their earlier suggestion that Passavant's ridge may be developed by tapping the back wall of the pharynx. In 1956 they emphasized development of flexible articulators to bring the mechanism into balance for speech. Van Riper (1947) presented a procedural outline for working with the speech problems of persons with cleft palate which included strengthening the muscles of the soft palate. Recently (1963) he has continued to place emphasis on physical therapy techniques but has not provided either rationale or evidence for support of this recommendation.

Various references (Moser, 1942; Ecklemann and Baldridge, 1945; Wells, 1945, 1948; Buck and Harrington, 1949) published during the 1940's have included, along with statements about goals and teaching techniques, recommendations for specific physical exercises. Some have advocated exercising specific muscles of the speech mechanism before teaching speech; some have placed emphasis on development of voluntary control of muscle; and some have discussed the importance of exercises directed toward gaining flexibility of muscles. Advice in general was to start with simple movements before working with more complex movements which would later be used in speech.

One of the better known discussions of blowing exercises was written by Kantner (1947). He maintained that the assumption that blowing exercises help the patient to learn better voluntary control of the palate muscles is "well founded clinically by virtue of the improvement often noted following a regime of such exercises." In his view, however, blowing exercises are relatively unimportant in the program of speech training for the person with cleft palate and he did not consider the possibility of administering these exercises as isolated drills apart from speech teaching. In his opinion, blowing exercises strengthen palate muscles, but he stated that such a relationship is difficult to prove. He was more certain that blowing exercises strengthen the breathing muscles but did not state whether strengthening breathing muscles might help in speech training. If persons with cleft palate are, in general, deficient in respiratory function, however, the nature of the deficit has not been defined and most practicing speech clinicians lack the means to identify it. Kanter questioned whether increased palatal efficiency for blowing is spontaneously carried over into speech. He mentioned that strenuous blowing encourages the development of undesirable movements of the nostrils and lips. This statement is in agreement with the report by Morris and Smith (1962) with reference to the association of facial grimaces with extreme palatopharyngeal deficiency. Kanter thought that blowing might increase pharyngeal wall movement but stated that he could give no evidence to support this idea. He recommended blowing exercises only for the client whose mechanism approximates adequacy.

Blowing exercises have been recommended by Morley (1951). She has written about these exercises as follows:

In some cases blowing practice quickly and automatically produces the desired result, but in others it is necessary to devise some means which will make the patient conscious of the movement of the soft palate and of closure of the sphincter. Where some anatomical deficiency exists, exercises should be directed towards the development of the muscles, both pharyngeal and palatal, in order that nasopharyngeal closure may be obtained where possible. Much can be done in this way, though the result may not always be permanent. Two cases in my experience obtained complete nasopharyngeal closure after much exercise. In one case the speech was normal, but in the other the soft palate was immobile, and some nasal tone persisted without nasal escape of air. Both were discharged but when seen again after an interval of twelve months, both had nasal escape. Apparently, in relaxing their efforts, this extra development of muscle had disappeared, everyday speech being insufficient to maintain it. Though still good, their speech could not be classed as normal.

Use of blowing exercises has been criticized by McDonald and Koepp-Baker (1951) who observed that speech therapy for cleft palate persons can be effective even though blowing exercises are omitted. They wrote, "Clinical experience with over 200 patients has demonstrated that cleft palate patients can develop intelligible and, in many cases, near-normal speech without recourse to blowing exercises." They also have maintained that blowing exercises often result in failure and frustration, thus creating psychological problems. In addition, in their opinion, the cleft palate speaker typically seems to use too much air pressure, and blowing exercises result in his using even more.

In summary, these reports of clinical impressions do indicate that greater movement of the articulators of persons with cleft palate has in some cases been developed by exercise of the articulators. No information, however, is available about the physical or psychological characteristics of persons who might be expected to make physical gains through exercise, about whether these gains would influence speech, or about whether the gains would be maintained.

Exercises for speech musculature are devised to develop strength, endurance, extent of movement, and new skills of the articulators. While certain of these goals seem useful for therapy procedures, others do not (Shelton, 1963). The assumption that increase in the strength with which the soft palate approximates the posterior pharyngeal wall results in an improvement of speech is untested and seems unwarranted. The speech clinician is concerned with whether palatal length and mobility are adequate for approximation needed for speech, not with the amount of pressure which is exerted against the posterior pharyngeal wall by the soft palate. He is usually not concerned with whether an increase in endurance is needed for better speech, with the possible exception of the infrequent case of inconsistent velopharyngeal competence when more nasal emission of oral air pressure under conditions of apparent fatigue is observed. Very often, extended range of motion, particularly of the palate, is a goal of therapy, and a successful procedure to accomplish this goal could be useful. No palatal exercises, however, have been demonstrated to result in range of motion greater than the range of motion for speech. Such exercises, in addition to speech work, thus appear to have no value beyond that to be expected from speech drill.

The question of whether motor exercise of the articulators is important in speech training for the person with cleft palate should be considered with reference to the role of motor learning in the acquisition of motor skill. Upon several points there appears to be agreement among several authors (Paillard, 1960; Fitts, 1965; Fleichman, 1965) who have reviewed the literature. Fitts has discussed the learning of complex skills in terms of three phases: cognitive, fixation, and autonomous. Training for the purpose of accomplishing the first of these phases emphasizes what to do and what to expect. The fixation phase involves practice. The automation phase involves (1) gradual increase in speed of performance, and (2) resistance to the effects of stress and interference from other concurrent activities. Paillard discusses the acquisition and automatization of the skilled act. Both Paillard and Fitts refer to the theory that, with acquisition of motor skill, control of the act is gradually switched from cortical to lower centers. This may be compatible with the idea that unconscious proprioceptive cues are important to articulation skill. The difficulty of differentiating learned aspects of skill from autonomous modulations in the neuromuscular response has been discussed by Hellebrandt et al. (1961). They say that:

> So much which transpires is automatic that it is difficult to determine what, specifically, constitutes the learned aspect of the skill under study. The primary set for jumping appears to be present at birth, only awaiting central nervous system maturation to unfold in primitive stereotyped form.
>
> It remains for us to determine what aspects of the neuro-muscular patterning associated with the excecution of so-called willed or purposive movement are amenable to modification other than the autonomous modulation induced by gradation in the severity of the effort. Until we know the answer to these questions we cannot do rational programming for the motor re-education of the disabled.

The conclusion that motor learning is influenced by the physical capacity of the learner, by practice with knowledge of results, and by other variables which affect learning, such as reinforcement, appears reasonable.

The question of whether motor exercises of the articulators for teaching new speech skills is of value must be considered in relation to the question of whether nonspeech exercises have as much value as exercises accompanied by speech. Nonspeech exercises have often been recommended, primarily for children with neuropathologies of speech. Shelton et al. (1966) reviewed literature and reported data which indicate that some persons with articulation errors and no obvious physiological etiology are deficient in the execution of nonspeech oral movements. The differences between children with articulation errors and those without are, on the average, small. For an individual child, however, a deficit in motor skill may be clinically significant. The premise that learning is facilitated by starting with simple tasks and gradually progressing to more complex tasks, and that nonspeech tasks are simple while speech tasks are more complex, has been the apparent basis for recommending motor exercises of the articulators. Hixon and Hardy (1964), however, have suggested that the central nervous system may organize speech emission through a series of neural patterns or networks which are unique for that particular automatic type of motor response. They have reported that, for cerebral palsy subjects, measures of oral activity involving phoneme production correlate more highly with ratings of speech defectiveness than do measures of nonspeech oral activity. A possible inference is that motor tasks as a part of the speech act are of more value than are motor tasks for the same structures but which are practiced without speech.

The speech clinician, if he is to be effective with all patients, probably needs to understand the principles of motor learning. If motor exercises are needed to prepare a patient for working directly on speech, the preparatory work might best be accomplished by a physical therapist in cooperation with the speech clinician. At present, however, no specific evidence can be cited to indicate (1) that motor exercises are of value for increasing velopharyngeal competence, or (2) that exercises of palatal structures are of value for accomplishing good, automatic articulation under conditions of stress.

III. Procedures for Voice Therapy

A. INDIVIDUALS WITH NORMAL ORAL STRUCTURES

Much consideration has been given to the clinical problem of functional nasality, that is, hypernasality which has no structural basis (Van Riper and Irwin, 1958). Much of the reported research and the hypothesizing took place before reliable diagnostic techniques for assessing velopharyngeal competence were available. Present knowledge of the relationship between velopharyngeal competence and nasal voice quality, particularly for those with marginal or borderline competence, gives rise to the question of whether a diagnosis of functional nasality is justified as often as formerly supposed. Although level of tongue carriage apparently may be a factor in the production of nasal voice quality, lack of velopharyngeal competence should also be considered as a possible cause of the tongue carriage problem.

B. Individuals with Inadequate Oral Structures

The decision to initiate voice training when the voice problem is the result, at least in part, of inadequate oral structures, is made according to the same criteria as the decision to provide speech training for an articulation disorder when the deviations are the result of inadequate oral structures. The typical voice problem is nasality resulting from velopharyngeal incompetence. In these cases referrral for physical management is indicated. Only if physical management is impractical should compensatory therapy be considered. If the decision is made to attempt compensatory therapy, the goals, which of necessity will be limited in nature, should be made clear to the patient and to all other professional workers concerned. The clinician should be particularly alert to any signs of defeatism or frustration on the part of the patient and if they occur should either terminate or modify the therapy program.

For purposes of compensatory therapy the clinician often should try out various techniques on an experimental basis. He may observe, for example, that the patient appears to channel more than is necessary of the energy and airstream through the incompetent velopharyngeal port because of a relatively small oral port. An obvious experimental technique, then, is to instruct the patient to increase the size of mouth opening and to lower the elevation of tongue carriage. Speech drill during which the patient is required to observe articulation of /a/ in contrast to that of /i/ and /u/ can sometimes be quite helpful to his understanding of therapy goals. This is true for two reasons: (1) The mouth opening is greater and the tongue position is lower for /a/ than it is for /i/ and /u/; and (2) /a/ on the average is perceived as less nasal than are /i/ and /u/ (Lintz and Sherman, 1961). The influence of adjacent consonants is known to affect degree of nasality perceived on vowels (Lintz and Sherman, 1961). Vowels in combination with voiceless plosives, for example, are on the average perceived as less nasal than the same vowels in combination with voiced plosives. Information of this kind can be used to build drill materials to help the patient to hear differences among degrees of nasality, to understand what he needs to change, and to listen to himself critically.

The clinician should consider, particularly for the patient with borderline or marginal velopharyngeal competence, whether fatigue affects the ability to maintain the best level of voice quality the patient is able to achieve. Although their reports have not been well documented by research findings, clinicians and patients have both frequently observed that the degree of nasality increases with fatigue. Changes in degree of nasality which accompany changes in degree of fatigue are perhaps more noticeable and more frequently to be observed in those whose velopharyngeal competence, although good enough under optimal conditions, is lacking under certain adverse conditions, most particularly the condition of fatigue. If the patient can learn to predict the situations in which he will have difficulty in maintaining voice quality free from unpleasant nasality, he may be able by conscious effort to achieve better voice quality in these situations than he otherwise would. To maintain for all speech tasks in all circumstances the best quality achieved under the best of conditions is probably an unrealistic goal for many patients, most definitely for those who have a serious lack of velopharyngeal competence.

Denasality which is the result of atresia of the velopharyngeal port by a pharyngeal flap or an obturator is sometimes a problem for the speaker with cleft palate. This problem usually is not amenable to behavioral therapy. Physical management, that is, trimming of the obturator bulb or of the pharyngeal flap, may establish an airway sufficient for breathing through the nose and for the production of acceptable nasal consonants.

IV. Procedures for Language Development and the Improvement of Communication

Children with cleft palate are reported to show delay in language development (Bzoch, 1956; Morris, 1960, 1962). The reasons for this delay have been discussed in Chapter IV. For the young child who shows a considerable amount of delay, the speech pathologist may plan therapy procedures which are specifically for the purpose of language development.

Although descriptions of language acquisition are available to the clinician (McCarthy, 1954), a comment on clinical training seems relevant here. In the very early stages of training, the goal may be simply to encourage the young child to make noises which reinforce actions. He may be encouraged in parallel play with the clinician to vocalize during such activities as walking an animal, pushing a car, or flying an airplane. When he gives evidence of being at this noise-reinforcement level, formal language building can begin.

In a second stage, the child is led to imitate verbally the noise-reinforcement tasks. The clinician also repeats short phrases which are related to the activity at hand and uses meaningful language units. No external reward is needed since the child probably still is not communicating but is now using language to structure his behavior. During this stage the clinician does not attempt to lead the child to initiate vocalization.

In the third and fourth stages, monologue and dramatic play, the child continues by describing and by giving directions to the objects being used in play. He may further assume the role of the object, extending himself, as it were. In the last stage, the child begins to perceive more clearly the use of language as a tool of communication with other people and, without being pressured to respond in any situation, uses the tool more freely and with greater facility.

It seems evident that the clinician, in inducing use of language forms, is often teaching correct articulation placement by model and is also displaying the use of vocal changes to express feeling (Hahn, 1960); and, if the oral structures are adequate for normal speech, such language stimulation procedures can lead to direct articulation therapy.

Consideration also must be given to the possibility that adults with cleft palate may need assistance. This is obviously true in spite of the fact that research reports on their communication behavior are not available. Such may be the case particularly for the individual who by preference or otherwise must adapt to the condition of velopharyngeal incompetence and to the various problems in speech production which result. Therapy designed for the purpose of improving the general ability to communicate in the presence of such problems as velopharyngeal incompetence must take into account aspects of communication which can be improved. Several of these aspects have been referred to before. One aspect is the expressive use of voice. Within the limitations of his mechanism, the patient can learn to modify pitch, loudness, and quality to convey meaning. A second aspect is the expressive use of the body. Gestures of the face and body can be helpful in communication. Exaggerations are to be avoided, of course. A third aspect is the possibility of adaptations to the response of the listener. The act of communication is not complete until the listener's response occurs. Many persons with speech handicaps are taught to concentrate so strongly on monitoring their own speech behaviors that they neglect the continual adaptation which a skilled speaker-listener must make to variations in the overt response to his message. The maintenance of eye contact is important, in that it serves to provide information to the speaker about when he needs to modify his speaking behavior. Individuals with cleft palate can be taught such adaptations. The fourth aspect is that of evidence of the speaker's self-acceptance. Many intangible factors can contribute to his feeling of self-esteem or self-confidence. One is probably the speaker's belief in himself as a valued person rather than as a handicapped individual. Probably the most important contribution the clinician can make toward the fostering of this feeling is the respect that he gives the patient with whom he is working.

V. Concluding Statement

The recommended procedures in speech therapy for the individual with cleft palate obviously will vary greatly from person to person, depending upon the present functional adequacy of the speech mechanism, the patterns of behavior associated with past physical deviations, and also such factors as age, intelligence, health, family and school environments, and emotional factors which contribute to motivation for self-improvement.

In most situations, therapeutic procedures used with individuals with the functional articulation and voice problems will be useful. Therapy certainly should be planned with due consideration of the physical changes brought about by physical management of cleft and associated problems, and by growth. Also considered must be changes in the individual's capacity to learn. In summary, many techniques of therapy are useful for various purposes depending on the particular factors important for individual cases.

REFERENCES

Ammons, R. B., and Ammons, Helen S. (1948). "The Full-Range Picture Vocabulary Test." Psychological Test Specialists, Missoula, Montana.

Anastasi, Anne (1961). "Psychological Testing," 2nd ed. Macmillian, New York.

Aungst, L. F., and Frick, J. V. (1964). Auditory discrimination ability and consistency of articulation of /r/. *J. Speech Hearing Disorders* **29**, 76–85.

Bankson, N. W., and Byrne, Margaret C. (1962). The relationship between missing teeth and selected consonant sounds. *J. Speech Hearing Disorders* **27**, 341–348.

Barnes, Ida J., and Morris, H. L. (1967). Interrelationships among oral breath pressure ratios and articulation skills for individuals with cleft palate. *J. Speech Hearing Res.* **10**, 506–514.

Basmajian, J. V., and Dutta, C. R. (1961). Electromyography of the pharyngeal constrictors and levator palati in man. *Anat. Record* **139**, 561–563.

Bauwens, P. (1961). *In* "Electrodiagnosis and Electromyography" (S. Licht, ed.), 2nd ed., pp. 171–200. Elizabeth Licht, New Haven, Connecticut.

Berko, Jean and Brown, R. (1960). *In* "Handbook of Research Methods in Child Development" (P. H. Mussen, ed.), pp. 517–557. Wiley, New York.

Berry, Mildred F., and Eisenson, J. (1942). "The Defective in Speech," Chapter 13. Appleton, New York.

Berry, Mildred F., and Eisenson, J. (1956). "Speech Disorders," Chapter 14. Appleton, New York.

Bjork, L. (1961). Velopharyngeal function in connected speech. *Acta Radiol. Suppl.* **202**.

Blackfield, H. M., Miller, E. R., Owsley, J. Q., Jr., and Lawson, Lucie I. (1961). Comparative evaluation of diagnostic techniques in patients with cleft palate speech. *Cleft Palate Bull.* **11**, No. 3, 64–66.

Blackfield, H. M., Miller, E. R., Lawson, Lucie I., and Owsley, J. G., Jr. (1963). Cinefluorographic evaluation of velopharyngeal incompetence in individuals with no overt cleft of the palate. *Cleft Palate Bull.* **13**, No. 3, 68 (abstract).

Bosma, J. F., ed. (1967). "Symposium on Oral Sensation and Perception." Thomas, Springfield, Illinois.

Bradford, L. F., Brooks, Alta R., and Shelton, R. L., Jr. (1964). Clinical judgment of hypernasality in cleft palate children. *Cleft Palate J.* **1**, 329–335.

Brandt, Sara D., and Morris, H. L. (1965). The linearity of the relationships between articulation errors and velopharyngeal incompetence. *Cleft Palate J.* **2**, 176–183.

Brooks, Alta R., and Shelton, R. L., Jr. (1963). Incidence of voice disorders other than nasality in cleft palate children. *Cleft Palate Bull.* **13**, 63–64.

Brooks, Alta R., Shelton, R. L., Jr., and Youngstrom, K. A. (1965). Compensatory tongue-palate-posterior pharyngeal wall relationship in cleft palate. *J. Speech Hearing Disorders* **30**, 166–173.

Brooks, Alta R., Shelton, R. L., Jr., and Youngstrom, K. A. (1966). Tongue-palate contact in persons with palate defects. *J. Speech Hearing Disorders* **31**, 14–25.

Bryan, G. A. (1963). Relationship Among Nasal and "Oral" Sound Pressures and Ratings of Nasality in Cleft Palate Speech. Ph. D. Thesis, Univ. of Oklahoma, Norman, Oklahoma.

Buck, M., and Harrington, R. (1949). Organized speech therapy for cleft palate rehabilitation. *J. Speech Hearing Disorders* **14**, 43-52.

Buncke, H. J., Jr. (1959). Manometric evaluation of palatal function in cleft palate patients. *Plastic Reconstruc. Surg.* **23**, 148–158.

Byrne, Margaret C. (1962). Development and evaluation of a speech improvement program for kindergarten and first grade children. *Rept. Coop. Res. Proj. No. 620* (8255). U. S. Office of Educ. Dept. of Health, Educ. Welfare, Washington, D.C.

Bzoch, K. R. (1956). An Investigation of the Speech of Pre-school Cleft Palate Children. Ph. D. Thesis, Northwestern Univ., Evanston, Illinois.

Bzoch, K. R. (1964a). The effects of a specific pharyngeal flap operation upon the speech of forty cleft-palate persons. *J. Speech Hearing Disorders* **29**, 111–120.

Bzoch, K. R. (1964b). Clinical studies of the efficacy of speech appliances compared to pharyngeal flap surgery. *Cleft Palate J.* **1**, 275–286.

Bzoch, K. R. (1965). Articulation proficiency and error patterns of pre-school cleft palate and normal children. *Cleft Palate J.* **2**, 340–349.

Chase, R. A. (1960). An objective evaluation of palatopharyngeal competence. *Plast. Reconstruc. Surg.* **26**, 23–29.

Chisum, Linda (1966). Relationship Between Remedial Speech Instruction Activities and Articulation. M. A. Thesis, Univ. of Kansas, Lawrence, Kansas.

Cole, R. M., and Campos-Giral, R. (1962). A method of evaluating the degree of mesial movement of the latter pharyngeal walls. *Asha* **4**, 409 (abstract).

Comroe, J. H., Jr., ed. (1950). *Methods Med. Res.* **2**.

Cooper, F. S. (1965). Research techniques and instrumentation: EMG. *In* "Proceedings of the Conference: Communicative Problems in Cleft Palate." *ASHA Rept.* **1**, 153–168.

Crary, Delores F. (1965). Sound Synthesis Ability of Kindergarten Children. M. A. Thesis, Univ. of Kansas, Lawrence, Kansas.

Crikelair, G. F., Kastein, Shulamith, and Fowler, E. P., Jr. (1963). Velar dysfunctions in absence of cleft palate. *Cleft Palate Bull.* **13**, 8–9.

Daley, W. T. (1962). "Speech and Language Therapy with the Brain-Damaged Child." Catholic Univ. of Am. Press, Washington, D. C.

Darley, F. L. (1964). "Diagnosis and Appraisal of Communication Disorders." Prentice-Hall, Englewood Cliffs, New Jersey.

Davis, Edith A. (1937). The development of linguistic skill in twins, singletons with siblings, and only children from age five to ten years. *Inst. Child Welfare Monogr. Ser. No. 14.* Univ. of Minnesota Press, Minneapolis, Minnesota.

Day, Elizabeth J. (1932). The development of language in twins. I. A comparison of twins and single children. *Child Develop.* **3**, 179–199.

Dickson, D. R. (1962). An acoustic study of nasality. *J. Speech Hearing Res.* **5**, 103–111.

Dornette, W. H. L., and Brechner, V. L. (1959). "Instrumentation in Anesthesiology." Lea & Febiger, Philadelphia, Pennsylvania.

Dunn, L. M. (1959). "Manual for the Peabody Picture Vocabulary Test." American Guidance Service, Inc., Minneapolis, Minnesota.

Eckelmann, Dorathy and Baldridge, Patricianne (1945). Speech training for the child with a cleft palate. *J. Speech Hearing Disorders* **10**, 137–147.

Elbert, Mary (1966). Evaluation of Articulation Change During Remedial Speech Instruction. M. A. Thesis, Univ. of Kansas, Lawrence, Kansas.

Elbert, Mary, Shelton, R. L., Jr. and Arndt, W. B., Jr. (1967). A task for evaluation of articulation change: 1. Development of methodology. *J. Speech Hearing Res.* **10**, 281–288.

Fairbanks, G. T., and Spriestersbach, D. C. (1950). A study of minor organic deviations in "functional" disorders of articulation. 1. Rate of movement of oral structures. *J. Speech Hearing Disorders* **15**, 60–69.

Fant, G. (1960). "Acoustic Theory of Sound Production." Mouton, The Hague, The Netherlands.

Fischer, E. (1961). *In* "Electrodiagnosis and Electromyography" (S. Licht, ed.), 2nd ed., pp. 66–112. Elizabeth Licht, New Haven, Connecticot.

Fitts, P. M. (1965). *In* "Training Research and Education" (R. Glaser, ed.), pp. 177–197. Wiley, New York.

Fleichman, E. A. (1965). *In* "Training Research and Education" (R. Glaser, ed.), pp. 137–175. Wiley, New York.

Fritzell, B. (1963). An electromyographic study of the movements of the soft palate in speech. *Folio Phoniat.* **15**, 307–311.

Fromkin, Victoria A. (1965). Some phonetic specifications of linguistic units: an electromyographic investigation. *Working Papers in Phonetics No. 3.* Univ. of California at Los Angeles, Los Angeles, California.

Gates, A. I. (1958). "Manual for the Gates Primary Reading Tests." Bureau of Publications, Teachers College, Columbia Univ., New York.

Glanzer, M. (1962). Toward a psychology of language structure. *J. Speech Hearing Res.* **5**, 303–314.

Greene, Margaret C. L. (1960). Speech analysis of 263 cleft palate cases. *J. Speech Hearing Disorders* **25**, 43–48.

Grossman, R. C. (1964). Methods for evaluating oral surface sensation. *J. Dental Res.* **43**, 301 (abstract).

Hahn, Elise (1960). Speech therapy for the pre-school cleft palate child. *J. Speech Hearing Disorders* **23**, 605–609.

Hanley, C. N. (1956). Factorial analysis of speech perception. *J. Speech Hearing Disorders* **21**, 76–87.

Hanson, M. L. (1964). A study of velopharyngeal competence in children with repaired cleft palates. *Cleft Palate J.* **1**, 217–231.

Hardy, J. C. (1965). Air flow and air pressure studies. *ASHA Rept.* **1**, 141–152.

Hardy, J. C., and Arkebauer, H. J. (1966). Development of a test for velopharyngeal competence during speech. *Cleft Palate J.* **3**, 6–21.

Harris, Katherine S., Lysaught, Gloria F., and Schvey, M. M. (1965). Some aspects of the production of oral and nasal labial stops. *Lang. Speech* **8**, 135–147.

Heck, Frances (1966). Measurement of Sound Synthesis Ability in Kindergarten, First, and Second Grade Children. M. A. Thesis, Univ. of Kansas Lawrence, Kansas.

Hellebrandt, F. A., Rarick, G. L., Glassow, Ruth, and Carns, Marie L, (1961). Physiological analysis of basic motor skills. I. Growth and development of jumping. *Am. J. Phys. Med.* **40**, 14–25.

Hess, D. A., and McDonald, E. T. (1960). Consonantal nasal pressure in cleft palate speakers. *J. Speech Hearing Res.* **3**, 201–211.

Hildreth, Gertrude H., and Griffiths, Nellie L. (1949). "Metropolitan Readiness Tests." Harcourt, New York.

Hixon, T. J., and Hardy, J. C. (1964). Restricted motility of the speech articulators in cerebral palsy. *J. Speech Hearing Disorders* **29**, 293–306.

Isshiki, N., and Ringel, R. L. (1964). Air flow during the production of selected consonants. *J. Speech Hearing Res.* **7**, 233–244.

Jastak, J. (1946). "Wide Range Achievement Test." C. L. Storey, Wilmington, Delaware.

Johnson, W., Darley, F. L., and Spriestersbach, D. C. (1963). "Diagnostic Methods in Speech Pathology." Harper, New York.

Kantner, C. E. (1947). The rationale of blowing exercises for patients with repaired cleft palates. *J. Speech Hearing Disorders* **12**, 281–286.

Karlin, J. E. (1942). A factorial study of auditory function. *Psychometrika* **7**, 251–279.

Kirk, S. A., and McCarthy, J. J. (1961). The Illinois Test of Psycholinguistic Abilities—an approach to differential diagnosis. *Am. J. Mental Deficiency* **66**, 399–412.

Kunze, L. H. (1964). Evaluations of methods of estimating sub-glottic air pressure. *J. Speech Hearing Res.* **7**, 151–164.

Lee, Laura L. (1966). Developmental sentence types: A method for comparing normal and deviant syntatic development. *J. Speech Hearing Disorders* **31**, 311–330.

Liberman, A. M., Harris, Katherine S., Hoffman, H. S., and Griffith, B. C. (1957). The discrimination of speech sounds within the across phoneme boundaries. *J. Exptl. Psychol.* **54**, 358–368.

Liberman, A. M., Harris, Katherine S., Eimas, P., Lisker, L., and Bastian, J. (1961). An effect of learning on speech perception: The discrimination of durations of silence with and without phonemic significance. *Lang. Speech* **4**, 175–195.

Liberman, A. M., Cooper, F. S., Harris, Katherine S., and MacNeilage, P. F. (1962). A Motor Theory of Speech Perception. Paper presented at the Speech Communication Seminar, Speech Transmission Laboratory, Royal Institute of Technology, Stockholm.

Lintz, Lois B., and Sherman, Dorothy (1961). Phonetic elements and perception of nasality. *J. Speech Hearing Res.* **4**, 381–390.

Low, G. M. (1955). An Objective Index of Nasality. Ph. D. Thesis, Univ. of Minnesota, Minneapolis, Minnesota.

Lubker, J. F. (1968). An electromyographic-cinefluorographic investigation of velar function during speech production. *Cleft Palate J.* In press.

Lubker, J. F., and Moll, K. L. (1965). Simultaneous oral-nasal air flow measurements and cinefluorographic observations during speech production. *Cleft Palate J.* **2**, 257–272.

McCarthy, Dorothea (1954). *In* "Manual of Child Psychology" (L. Carmichael, ed.), rev. ed., pp. 492–630. Wiley, New York.

McCarthy, J. J., and Kirk, S. A. (1961). "Examiners Manual, Illinois Test of Psycholinguistic Abilities," Institute for Research on Exceptional Children. Univ. of Illinois, Urbana, Illinois.

McCarthy, J. J., and Kirk, S. A. (1963). "The Construction, Standardization, and Statistical Characteristics of the Illinois Test of Psycholinguistic Abilities," Institute for Research on Exceptional Children. Univ. of Illinois, Urbana, Illinois.

McCarthy, J. J., and Olson, J. L. (1964). "Validity Studies on the Illinois Test of Psycholinguistic Abilities," Institute for Research on Exceptional Children. Univ. of Illinois, Urbana, Illinois.

McCroskey, R. (1958). The relative contributions of auditory and tactile cues to certain aspects of speech. *Southern Speech J.* **24**, 84–90.

McDonald, E. T. (1964). "Articulation Testing and Treatment: A Sensory-Motor Approach." Stanwix House, Pittsburgh, Pennsylvania.

McDonald, E. T. and Aungst, L. F. (1967). *In* "Symposium on Oral Sensation and Perception" (J. F. Bosma, ed.). Thomas, Springfield, Illinois.

McDonald, E. T., and Koepp-Baker, H. (1951). Cleft palate speech: an integration of research and clinical observation. *J. Speech Hearing Disorders* **16**, 9-20.

MacNeilage, P. F. (1963). Electromyographic and acoustic study of the production of certain final cluster. *J. Acoust. Soc. Am.* **35**, 461–463.

McWilliams, Betty J. (1954). Some factors in the intelligibility of cleft palate speech. *J. Speech Hearing Disorders* **19**, 524–527.

Matthews, J., and Byrne, Margaret, C. (1953). An experimental study of tongue flexibility in children with cleft palate. *J. Speech Hearing Disorders* **18**, 43–47.

Mecham, M. J. (1958). "Verbal Language Development Scale." Educational Test Bureau, Minneapolis, Minnesota.

Mecham, M. J. (1960). Measurement of verbal language development in cerebral palsy. *Cerebral Palsy Rev.* **21**, 3–4.

Menyuk, Paula (1964). Comparison of grammar of children with functionally deviant and normal speech. *J. Speech Hearing Res.* **7**, 109–121.

Michel, J. F. (1965). Reliability of phonational quality classification. *Asha* **7**, 426–427 (abstract).

Millard, R. T. (1957). The role of the sound spectrographic tracing in cleft palate patients. *Cleft Palate Bull.* **7**, 7–8.

Minifie, F. D., Darley, F. L., and Sherman, Dorothy (1963). Temporal reliability of seven language measures. *J. Speech Hearing Res.* **6**, 139–148.

Moll, K. L. (1960). Cinefluorographic techniques in speech research. *J. Speech Hearing Res.* **3**, 227–241.

Moll, K. L., and Darley, F. L. (1960). Attitudes of mothers of articulatory-impaired and speech-retarded children. *J. Speech Hearing Disorders* **25**, 277–384.

Morley, Muriel E. (1951). "Cleft Palate Speech," 5th ed. Livingstone, Edinburgh and London.

Morris, H. L. (1960). Communication Skills of Children With Cleft Lips and Palates. Ph. D. Thesis, Univ. of Iowa, Iowa City, Iowa.

Morris, H. L. (1962). Communication skills of children with cleft lips and palates. *J. Speech Hearing Res.* **5**, 79–90.

Morris, H. L., ed. (1965). "Cleft Lip and Palate: Criteria for Physical Management." Univ. of Iowa, Iowa City, Iowa.

Morris, H. L. (1966). The oral manometer as a diagnostic tool in clinical speech pathology. *J. Speech Hearing Disorders* **31**, 362–369.

Morris, H. L., and Smith, Jeanne K. (1962). A multiple approach for evaluating velopharyngeal competency. *J. Speech Hearing Disorders* **27**, 218–226.

Morris, H. L., Spriestersbach, D. C., and Darley, F. L. (1961). An articulation test for assessing competency of velopharyngeal closure. *J. Speech Hearing Res.* **4**, 48–55.

Moser, H. M. (1942). Diagnostic and clinical procedures in rhinolalia. *J. Speech Hearing Disorders* **7**, 1–4.

Neely, Betty J. M., and Bradley, Doris P. (1964). A rating scale for evaluation of video tape recorded x-ray studies. *Cleft Palate J.* **1**, 88–94.

Nylen, B. O. (1961). Cleft palate and speech. *Acta Radiol. Suppl.* **203**.

Paillard, J. (1960). *In* "Handbook of Physiology—Neurophysiology" (J. Field *et al.*, eds.), Vol. 3, pp. 1679–1709. Am. Physiol. Soc., Washington, D. C.

Penfield, W., and Rasmussen, T. (1950). "The Cerebral Cortex of Man." Macmillan, New York.

Pierce, B. R. (1962). Nasal Resonance Differences Resulting from Speech Appliance Modifications in Cleft Palate Adults. Ph. D. Thesis, North-western Univ., Evanston, Illinois.

Pitzner, Joan H., and Morris, H. L. (1966). Articulation skills and adequacy of breath pressure ratios of children with cleft palates. *J. Speech Hearing Disorders* **31**, 26–40.

Prins, T. D. (1963). Relations among specific articulatory deviations and responses to a clinical measure of sound discrimination ability. *J. Speech Hearing Disorders* **28**, 382–388.

Prins, T. D., and Bloomer, H. H. (1965). A word intelligibility approach to the study of speech change in oral cleft patients. *Cleft Palate J.* **2**, 357–368.

Quigley, L. F., Jr., Shiere, F. R., Webster, R. C., and Cobb, C. M. (1964). Measuring palatopharyngeal competence with the nasal anemometer. *Cleft Palate J.* **1**, 304–313.

Randall, P., Bakes, F. P., and Kennedy, C. (1960). Cleft palate-type speech in the absence of cleft palate. *Plastic Reconstruc. Surg.* **25**, 484–495.

Ringel, R. L., and Ewanowski, S. J. (1965). Oral perception. 1. Two-point discrimination. *J. Speech Hearing Res.* **8**, 389–398.

Ringel, R. L., and Steer, M. D. (1963). Some effects of tactile and auditory alterations on speech output. *J. Speech Hearing Res.* **6**, 369–378.

Rodriquez, A. A., and Oester, Y. T. (1961). *In* "Electrodiagnosis and Electromyography" (S. Licht, ed.), 2nd ed. pp. 286–341. Elizabeth Licht, New Haven, Connecticut.

Rutherford, D., and McCall, G. (1967). *In* "Symposium on Oral Sensation and Perception" (J. Bosma, ed.). Thomas, Springfield, Illinois.

Saltar, Nancy (1958). *In* "Therapeutic Exercises" (S. Licht, ed.), pp. 127–158. Elizabeth Licht, New Haven, Connecticut.

Schiefelbusch, R. L. (1963). Language studies of mentally retarded children. *J. Speech Hearing Disorders, Monogr., Suppl. No.* **10**, 3–7.

Shames, G. H., Matthews, J., and Lutz, K. R. (1960). Audible Scales for Measuring Voice Quality in Adults. Report of a project of the University of Pittsburgh Speech Department and of the Office of Vocational Rehabilitation, U. S. Dept. Health, Educ. Welfare, Washington, D. C.

Shelton, R. L., Jr. (1963). Therapeutic exercise and speech pathology. *Asha* **5**, 855–859.

Shelton, R. L., Jr., Bankson, N. W., and Brooks, R. S. (1961). Nasal pressure in first grade non-cleft palate children. *J. Kansas Speech Hearing Assoc.* **2**, 2–8.

Shelton, R. L., Jr., Brooks, Alta R., and Youngstrom K. A. (1964). Articulation and patterns of palatopharyngeal closure. *J. Speech Hearing Disorders* **29**, 390–408.

Shelton, R. L., Jr., Brooks, Alta R., and Youngstrom, K. A. (1965). Clinical assessment of palatopharyngeal closure. *J. Speech Hearing Disorders* **30**, 37–43.

Shelton, R. L., Jr., Arndt, W. B., Jr., Krueger, A. L., and Huffman, Evelyn (1966). Identification of persons with articulation errors from observation of nonspeech movements. *Am. J. Physical Med.* **45**, 143–150.

Shelton, R. L., Jr., Arndt, W. B., Jr., and Hetherington, J. J. (1967a). *In* "Symposium on Oral Sensation and Perception" (J. F. Bosma, ed.). Thomas, Springfield, Illinois.

Shelton, R. L., Jr., Knox, A. W., Arndt, W. B., Jr., and Elbert, Mary (1967b). The relationship between nasality scale values and oral and nasal sound pressure level. *J. Speech Hearing Res.* **10**, 549–557.

Sherman, Dorothy (1954). The merits of backward playing of connected speech in the scaling of voice quality disorders. *J. Speech Hearing Disorders* 19, 312–321.

Shriner, T. H., and Sherman, Dorothy (1967). An equation for assessing language development. *J. Speech Hearing Res.* 10, 41–48.

Snow, Katherine (1961). Articulation proficiency in relation to certain dental abnormalities. *J. Speech Hearing Disorders* 26, 209–212.

Sommers, R. K. (1962). Factors in the effectiveness of mothers trained to aid in speech correction. *J. Speech Hearing Disorders* 27, 178–186.

Sommers, R. K., Furlong, Ann K., Rhodes, F. E., Fichter, G. R., Bowser, D. C., Copetos, Florence G., and Saunders, Zane G. (1964). Effects of maternal attitude upon improvement in articulation when mothers are trained to assist in speech correction. *J. Speech Hearing Disorders* 29, 126–132.

Spradlin, J. E. (1963). *In* "Handbook of Mental Deficiency" (N. R. Ellis, ed.), pp. 512–555. McGraw-Hill, New York.

Sprague, Ann L. (1961). The Relationship Between Selected Measures of Expressive Language and Motor Skill in Eight-Year-Old Boys. Ph. D. Thesis, Univ. Of Iowa Iowa City, Iowa.

Spriestersbach, D. C., and Powers, G. R. (1959). Articulation skills, velopharyngeal closure, and oral breath pressure of children with cleft palate. *J. Speech Hearing Res.* 2, 318–325.

Spriestersbach, D. C., Moll, K. L., and Morris, H. L. (1961). Subject classification and articulation of speakers with cleft palates. *J. Speech Hearing Res.* 4, 362–372.

Stick, S. L. (1966). A Description of the Procedures Used to Fit and Reduce a Prosthetic Speech Appliance and Their Effect on Articulation. M. A. Thesis, Univ. of Kansas, Lawrence, Kansas.

Subtelny, Joanne D., Koepp-Baker, H., and Subtelny, J. D. (1961). Palatal function and cleft palate speech. *J. Speech Hearing Disorders* 26, 213–224.

Subtelny, Joanne D., Mestre, J. D., and Subtelny, J. D. (1964). Comparative study of normal and defective articulation of /s/ as related to malocclusion and deglutition. *J. Speech Hearing Disorders* 29, 269–285.

Subtelny, Joanne D., Worth, J. H., and Sakuda, M. (1966). Intraoral pressure and rate of flow during speech. *J. Speech Hearing Res.* 9, 489–518.

Takagi, Y., McGlone, R. E., and Millard, R. (1965). A survey of speech disorders of persons with clefts. *Cleft Palate J.* 2, 28–31.

Taverner, D. (1961). *In* "Electrodiagnosis and Electromyography" (S. Licht, ed.), 2nd ed., pp. 342–384. Elizabeth Licht, New Haven, Connecticut.

Templin, Mildred C. (1957). "Certain Language Skills in Children." Univ. of Minnesota Press, Minneapolis, Minnesota.

Templin, Mildred C., and Darley, F. L. (1960). "The Templin-Darley Tests of Articulation." Bureau of Education Research and Service, Extension Division, Univ. of Iowa, Iowa City, Iowa.

Van Demark, D. R. (1964). Misarticulations and listener judgments of the speech of individuals with cleft palates. *Cleft Palate J.* 1, 232–245.

Van Demark, D. R. (1966). A factor analysis of the speech of children with cleft palate. *Cleft Palate J.* 3, 159–170.

Van Riper, C. G. (1947). *In* "Speech Correction," 2nd ed., Chapter 12. Prentice-Hall, Englewood Cliffs, New Jersey.

Van Riper, C. G. (1963). "Speech Correction: Principles and Methods," 4th ed. Prentice-Hall, Englewood Cliffs, New Jersey.

Van Riper, C. G., and Irwin, J. V. (1958). "Voice and Articulation." Prentice-Hall, Englewood Cliffs, New Jersey.

Warren, D. W., and Devereux, J. L. (1966). An analog study of cleft palate speech. *Cleft Palate J.* **4**, 103–114.

Weatherley-White, R. C. A., Dersch, W. C., and Anderson, Ruth M. (1964). Objective measurement of nasality in cleft palate patients: a preliminary report. *Cleft Palate J.* **1**, 120–124.

Weatherley-White, R. C. A., Stark, R. B., and DeHaan, C. R. (1965). The objective measurement of nasality in cleft palate patients. *Plastic Reconstruc Surg.* **35**, 588–598.

Weatherley-White, R. C. A., Stark, R. B., and DeHaan, C. R. (1966). Acoustic analysis of speech: validation studies. *Cleft Palate J.* **3**, 291–300.

Webster, Martha J., and Shelton, R. L., Jr. (1964). Estimation of mean length of response in children of normal and below average intellectual capacity. *J. Speech Hearing Res.* **7**, 101–102.

Weiss, A. I. (1954). Oral and Nasal Sound Pressure Levels as Related to Judged Severity of Nasality. Ph. D. Thesis, Purdue Univ., Lafayette, Indiana.

Wells, Charlotte G. (1945). Improving the speech of the cleft palate child. *J. Speech Hearing Disorders* **10**, 162–168.

Wells, Charlotte G. (1948). Practical techniques in speech training for cleft palate cases. *J. Speech Hearing Disorders* **13**, 71–73.

Wepman, J. W. (1958). "Auditory Discrimination Test." J. W. Wepman, Chicago, Illinois.

Winitz, H. (1959). Language skills of male and female kindergarten children. *J. Speech Hearing Res.* **4**, 377–386.

Winitz, H. (1966). *In* "Speech Pathology" (R. W. Rieger and R. S. Brubaker, eds.), pp. 42–76. North-Holland Publ., Amsterdam.

Wynn Parry, C. B. (1961a). Electrodiagnosis. *J. Bone Joint Surg.* **43B**, 222–236.

Wynn Parry, C. B. (1961b). *In* "Electrodiagnosis and Electromyography" (S. Licht, ed.), pp. 241–271. Elizabeth Licht, New Haven, Connecticut.

Young, N. B. (1953). An Investigation of Intranasal Pressure during the Phonation of Consonant-Vowel Combinations and Sentences. M. A. Thesis, Univ. of Washington, Seattle, Washington.

CHAPTER
VIII

Some Professional Implications

D. C. Spriestersbach

I. "Professions" 269
II. The Team 273
III. The Speech Pathologist 275
    A. His Training and Orientation 275
    B. His Roles 276
IV. Summary 278
    References 279

I. "Professions"

Preceding chapters have included discussion not only of various aspects of the work of speech pathologists in the management of the problems of individuals with cleft lip and palate but also of the work of others who have "professional" interests in and concerns with the management of these problems. Although we routinely describe specialties and accompanying activities and concerns as "professional," this description is, in fact, often poorly understood. Consequently, a discussion of its general implications should be helpful not only to speech pathologists, to whom this book is particularly addressed, but also to all other specialists who are interested in cleft palate. This general discussion will be followed by an examination of some of the specific professional issues directly related to problems often associated with cleft palate.

In the immediately following discussion we are not talking about any one particular specialty, nor are we assuming that there are professionals who are competent to deal equally well with all of the problems of the person with a cleft lip or palate. On the contrary, we are talking about speech pathologists, dentists, surgeons, psychologists, pediatricians, social workers, nurses, obstetricians, classroom teachers, vocational counselors, and any others who have an interest in the problems of cleft palate. The general issues important for any one of these professions should be relevant also for any one of the others. The particular examples which have been chosen for discussion here thus have no significance specific only to certain ones of the specialties or professions. Equally relevant examples could have been presented from the fields of specialists other than the one used for illustration.

If one belongs to a "profession," it is assumed that he has something to profess. In this context we are usually talking about ways in which knowledge is given practical expression—the content of the expression, the techniques for its effective expression, and the uses to be made of the knowledge expressed in what types of settings. Some 50 years ago Abraham Flexner (1915) presented what is now recognized as a classic address entitled "Is Social Work a Profession?" He said

> ... to make a profession in the genuine sense something more than a mere claim or an academic degree is needed. There are certain objective standards that can be formulated...

Then he proceeded to develop six criteria which he summarized as follows:

> ... professions involve essentially intellectual operations with large individual responsibility; they derive their raw material from science and learning; this material they work up to a practical and definite end; they possess an educationally communicable technique; they tend to self-organization; they are becoming increasingly altruistic in motivation.

He discussed some of these criteria:

> ... the real character of the activity is the thinking process; a free, resourceful and unhampered intelligence applied to problems and seeking to understand and master them—that is in the first instance characteristic of a profession... the responsibility of the practitioner is at once large and personal.... He is not under orders; though he be cooperating with others, though the work be team work rather than individual work, his responsibility is not less complete and personal... it is the steady stream of ideas... which keeps professions from degenerating into mere routine, from losing their intellectual and responsible character... members of a given profession are pretty well agreed as to the specific objects that the profession seeks to fulfill, and the specific kinds of skill that the practitioner of the profession must master in order to attain the object in question.

Perhaps Flexner's one criterion which is passed over most frequently, undoubtedly because of its assumed obviousness, is that of "an educationally communicable technique." In this connection it is interesting to note one of the concluding impressions in the report, edited by Morris (1965), of a conference on the criteria for physical management of individuals with cleft lip and palate:

> The participants found it difficult to identify many of the diagnostic criteria which they use in making management decisions. They tended to describe specific manage-

ment techniques and criteria which they use in evaluating the results of management rather than describing their personal diagnostic criteria. Furthermore, even when the diagnostic criteria were identified, the participants had difficulty in describing, in operational terms, the nature of observations which they make or the relationship of these observations to the criteria and to the consequent management decisions.

One possible inference which can be made from this observation is that the training and experience of the participants have led them to adopt, by-and-large, highly standardized procedures which they employ to accomplish certain objectives for a specific patient group without regard to differences within that patient group. Another possible inference which can be made, perhaps with more validity than the first one, is that the training and experience of the participants have led them to evaluate differences within a patient group, but in a relatively nonverbal way. Because the evaluations may be nonverbal, the participants had difficulty in expressing them...

An example of the difficulty which the participants experienced in identifying diagnostic criteria is revealed by the use (particularly by the surgeons) of the phrase "in my hands." This phrase was repeatedly interjected into the discussions, most frequently with regard to discussion about techniques used for management. Two interpretations of this comment can be made. The first is that the participant is aware of differences between surgeons (or between dentists, etc.) in the criteria selected, in the observations made and the interpretation of those observations, and in the management techniques employed. Consequently, he is trying very hard not to generalize to other operators from his own experiences. A second interpretation, not necessarily exclusive of the first, is that the participant is indicating by such terminology that frequently he really does not understand the mechanism by which certain results are achieved, but that he has become convinced that when he performs a specific procedure, certain results will be obtained. To the extent that the second interpretation is valid, the implications are that identification of diagnostic criteria during this conference was difficult because the participants in reality did not know what the criteria are.

These comments were made following a two and one-half day conference of 42 persons chosen because of their national and international reputations in dealing with individuals with cleft lip and palate. They had spent the entire time in intense discussions, trying to identify the criteria used in management of the problem. Their difficulties in accomplishing this task point up, if we are willing to accept Flexner's criterion of an "educationally communicable technique," how far we have to go before we have arrived at the point when we have described adequately the professional skills important for dealing with the problem of cleft lip and palate. Another implication of the criterion of "an educationally communicable technique" is that every aspect of clinical work with patients, including those with cleft lip and palate, is subject to scientific study. There are at least two ways to view the clinician (adapted from Baldwin, 1963). In the first view he can be conceived of primarily as a classifier. In this instance his main function is to identify and to classify a problem properly. Having done so, he treats the problem according to general recommendations which he has learned from some "authority." He makes minimal use of variations in treatment which have resulted from experience and intellectual inquiry. In the extreme he is a technician. He tends to emphasize the similarities among, rather than the differences between, his patients.

In the second view the clinician can be conceived of as an investigator. Such a person attempts to understand the complex processes of the problem as it exists in the individual at a particular time. He expects to theorize about the problem, to observe the problem systematically, and, following his observations, to arrive at a diagnosis and treatment plan. He recognizes the limitations of his understanding of the problem and approaches each assessment with humility and an eagerness to learn more. To meet most effectively the needs of the individual he tends to emphasize the importance of those differences between his patients which demand modification and adaptation of his approach. In short, he is a scientist, using the methods of science in a laboratory environment. He has great potential for intellectual growth and for increasing his own social effectiveness. Any professional person who deserves the respect of his peers must acquire an understanding in depth of the problems of his concern and he must constantly up-date this understanding through a continual program of study and systematic observation.

A great many persons fail to appreciate that the methods of science can be applied to their work as clinicians or as clinical researchers. They fail to state the problem in the form of an answerable question or to formulate an hypothesis which can be tested by appropriate observations. This is the first step in the scientific method, but its accomplishment is anything but simple. If the question is to have relevance and timeliness, the researcher (clinician) must have a deep understanding of all facets of the problem. The time of stating the problem is one of uneasiness for even the most sophisticated and experienced investigator. Less experienced investigators have a tendency to want to pass quickly over the step or ignore it completely to "get on with the show," implying that it is an unnecessary step anyway, or that this step is perhaps less deserving of the amount of time and care that other later steps may warrant. It seems expedient to move quickly to the observational step and to decide later how best to make use of the data that are accumulated. But the question which is asked establishes the limits of the issue to be studied and it also determines the type of observations to be made and the nature of the data which are to be accumulated. The wise researcher (clinician) knows that there is no shortcut for this vital step.

The material presented in the preceding chapters makes abundantly clear that a large and distinctive body of information relating to the cleft palate problem has been derived from "science and learning" (Flexner,

1915) by a host of persons from many professional disciplines. But this is no time for resting on our laurels. There are still large gaps in our knowledge which limit the clarity of our understanding and the effectiveness of the habilitative programs which we are able to provide. On the other hand, we should take heart in our accomplishments to date. Each of the interested professional groups can point with pride to its unique contribution and to the extensiveness of the body of material which it alone can draw upon in dealing with the problem. As a consequence, there is little justification for the professional defensiveness that one might expect to find in less developed fields in which professional workers are attempting prematurely to achieve status and recognition because they have not first taken the time to demonstrate that they have something significant to profess.

II. The Team

Now in order are a few comments about teamwork, the arrangement under which much of the clinical and research work in cleft palate is done. The need for and the success of the arrangement needs no documentation here. In fact, all of the preceding chapters in this book have pointed up the complexity of the problem and the consequent overlap of interests and concerns of the professional persons involved. The results are obvious to all who have dealt with the problem. But this is not to say that there are no problems in the team approach.

There is the tendency to make ourselves the focus of attention instead of the clinical problem. We manifest this tendency in several ways. Most commonly we are apt to exhibit a kind of professional defensiveness which makes it difficult for us to admit that other professions have knowledge and skills that we do not have. It is devastating to our egos and to the images we have of our professions to admit that we can profit from the advice of persons in other professions about problems which we had previously assumed, or had been taught, that we were quite competent to handle. In this circumstance we tend to be poor listeners; we tend to assume that our role is to inform others rather than to be informed. During our nonverbal moments in professional conferences, we marshall our thoughts so that we can expound our ideas during the next opportunity that we have to speak. We tend to worry and fret about our "proper role" and to demand "our professional rights" even before we have demonstrated that we have any skills that deserve recognition. When we do these things, we usually fail to take the pediatric view; in fact, we tend to forget the patient by allowing our needs to obscure his (Spriestersbach, 1962). Koepp-Baker (Morris, 1965) has this to say about the team:

... the team is not a panacea nor is it in every way the best and only way a cleft palate child may be habilitated. The team is merely a device for maximizing information and effort. Often there is a prodigious waste of time in the processes of the team. There can be mere mechanism without content. There may be a tendency to manipulate the least essential as if it were the most essential. There may be a tendency to substitute mere talk for true information of an objective sort...

There is the problem of effective communication between the members of the various professions represented on the team. This problem is related to the one of the focus of attention which has just been discussed. When we are concerned about our professional status we tend to use a vocabulary designed to demonstrate the learned character of our understanding, the sophistication of our approach, and the "scientific" bases for our observations. We assume this posture apparently because we are afraid that our teammates will not listen to us if we do not. Those of us who are the listeners appear to accept the assumptions made by the speaker. As a consequence, teams may spend their time going through stylized verbal rituals that have little relation to the real world and contribute little to the development of the team's understanding of the needs of the patient. Again to quote Koepp-Baker (Morris, 1965):

The value of group interaction is derived principally from free and open communication. This channel must be unimpeded. The disquiet and restiveness produced by the specialistic jargon and vocabulary is reduced as the members of the group are required to communicate with others engaged in the same quest. The group is a strong check on vacuous, obfuscating talk and unsupported ideas.

Effective teams must take the time, formally or informally, to learn, at least in a general way, about those aspects of the problem of interest and concern to the other team members. Only in this way can the team establish effective communication which enables each member to understand how his management plan should be modified or to suggest how others' plans should be modified.

Cooperative effort is much more time-consuming than unilateral action. Cooperative effort involves consulting, sharing, convincing, motivating, checking, and coordinating. Because of the complexities of the problem and our personal needs as team members, there is an inertial aspect to cooperative endeavor. It is manifested by comments such as "Why bother? The family won't appreciate what we are trying to do anyway" and "Things are good enough as they are." Teams will prosper only if they recognize the time-consuming character of their enterprise and justify it out of a conviction that the best interests of the patient are being served as a result.

There is the need for the systematic restimulation of teams. Usually they are involved in the evaluation of large groups of patients over considerable periods of time. Observations on a given Tuesday can become very tiresome and mundane. Perhaps one of the best ways to counter the flagging spirit is through the systematic study of selected aspects of the problem in an attempt to describe the problem more completely and objectively, and to document the changes which take place through management and with the passage of time. The formulation, challenging, and reformulation of hypotheses that go on as a result of this investigative process can help the team view each patient with a freshness which can make each clinic day an exciting and stimulating affair.

Finally there is the problem of designating the leader, for all groups must have one. It is obvious that the personality of the leader and the role that he plays will have a great effect upon the way in which the team functions. In most medical settings the leader is a physician since he has the ultimate responsibility for the well-being of the patient. In other habilitation settings the person with the greatest responsibility for the management being provided in that setting may be the leader. But, whoever the leader, if he is to be effective, he will seek to understand the potential contribution of each of the other members and will manage the team in such a way as to maximize those contributions.

III. The Speech Pathologist

A. His Training and Orientation

The material in this book has dealt primarily with the communication aspects of the "cleft palate problem." Even so, it dramatizes the breadth of training which the speech pathologist must have to cope effectively with that aspect of the problem. And then there are issues related to growth and development; to medical, dental, and psychological management; to educational programs; to vocational planning; and to the development of satisfying interpersonal relations. "The cleft palate problem" is no field for the speech pathologist who is a professional neophyte or who has only cursory training. Rather, it is a field requiring extended study of anatomy, physiology, psychology, acoustics, electronics, and speech and hearing science as well as the identification and treatment of the pathological processes of verbal communication.

In addition, the speech pathologist must have an orientation to the problem which encourages continual growth of understanding and professional skill. A review of the changes which have taken place in the management of cleft lip and palate in the last 10 years reveals how imperative it is to keep abreast of the times and to maintain the ability to adopt new techniques and new perspectives. The secret to success here, of course, is the outlook which comes from the application of the scientific method to the problem— from question to observation, to evaluation, to revision, to further questions, etc., in a never-ending, though certainly not monotonous, cycle. This point of view needs no further expansion here since Moll (Morris, 1965, pp. 10–19) has expanded on its implications as they apply specifically to some of the problems in cleft palate management.

Finally, the speech pathologist, as does any other serious professional, affiliates with other members of his profession in those organizations that are designed to help him maintain an effective interchange with others who have similar training, interests, and standards of integrity and ethical principles. For the speech pathologist interested in cleft lip and palate, the two primary organizations are the American Speech and Hearing Association and the American Cleft Palate Association.

B. His Roles

In the early years of the evolution of his professional role, the speech pathologist's interest in the problems of the person with a cleft lip or palate were derived primarily from his role as a clinician. During those years he accepted the speaker as he found him and did his valiant best to help the speaker achieve satisfactory speech. Frequently it was a frustrating experience for both. Emphasis was placed upon strengthening the muscles of the lips, tongue, and pharyngeal walls; upon tongue carriage and its precision of movement and placement; upon orality; and upon the production of nasal-free vowels. The results typically were far from satisfactory. Extended periods of therapy with poor results were the rule, a state of affairs hardly designed to establish the speech pathologist as an effective member of the cleft palate team. In many respects it was a period that need not have been, for the speech pathologist already understood the essentials of speech production. Apparently he failed to apply his knowledge to the problems of the speaker with a cleft lip and palate because of his view of his role and his relationships with the members of other professions interested in the problem. It is no mere coincidence that the improvements which have been made in the postmanagement adequacy of the speech mechanisms of persons with cleft palate have resulted in great measure from the change in the role of the speech pathologist from clinician to diagnostician.

It is trite to observe that one of the paramount reasons for the physical management of the cleft lip and palate is to provide the anatomical and physiological requisites for satisfactory speech. It is obvious, then, that one of the primary criteria for evaluating the effectiveness of the physical management is the end product of the effort, that is, speech. But the speech pathologist has been reluctant to accept his role as the expert in the evaluation of the end product. More specifically, he frequently has been too timid, or perhaps unable, to specify the physical requisites for satisfactory speech and to identify those instances when the physical management has fallen short in meeting the requirements. Whitehouse (1965) has discussed in some detail the significant part that this type of feedback can play in a team effort.

Unquestionably the most significant role of the speech pathologist in dealing with cleft lip and palate is that of diagnostician. The physicians and the dentists now have amazing skill in dealing with the physical habilitation aspects of the problem. But they need a feedback of relevant commentary. They need to know not only when the speech mechanism is inadequate following management but also in what ways it is inadequate. Surely this is the proper role for the speech pathologist.

The feedback must be provided in terms of the structural relationships and functions which are adequate or inadequate. It does not include instructions concerning the physical management procedures to be used or the techniques for accomplishing the physical management. But this role as diagnostician need not create problems of professional relationships with the physician and the dentist. On the contrary, if the speech pathologist does his work competently, the relevance of his observations in assisting the experts in physical management to modify their procedures will be quickly recognized by them and his place in the team will be secure.

A special aspect of the diagnostic role of the speech pathologist concerns his evaluation of radiographic data. These data should be obtained only under the direct supervision of a radiologist. However, few radiologists have had training which qualifies them as experts in the production of speech. Consequently, they must be advised concerning the radiographic observations that are relevant in evaluating the adequacy of the speech mechanism. Once relevant films of satisfactory quality have been obtained, only persons who understand the anatomical and physiological requisites for satisfactory speech are competent to evaluate them. It is to be hoped that the speech pathologist will be such a person; a radiologist may or may not be.

Of course, the speech pathologist plays a significant role as a clinician, that is, as one who attempts to change verbal behavior. Explanation of this role has been developed in detail in Chapter VII. It is sufficient here to emphasize his role only as it is important in the continual appraisal of the changes that are being made in behavior. In this role, the speech pathologist continues to function as a diagnostician, reporting to other members of the team when he is confronted with problems which are not within his sphere of competence or when he feels that other changes must be effected in the speaker before he can continue with his work.

In some instances the speech pathologist serves as coordinator of the cleft palate team. Such a role is probably justified only in those situations in which are seen patients whose physical management is handled in several hospitals or medical centers. In these instances the speech pathologist, or some other nonmedical member of the team, may be called upon to serve as a "neutral" coordinator.

Finally, there is the role of the speech pathologist as counselor. There are many aspects of the cleft palate problem which call for counseling. Among them are matters concerning speech production, the etiology of clefts, the typical program of physical management, the utilization of community resources, school adjustment, peer relationships, and vocational planning. Spriestersbach (1961) has discussed some of these needs in some detail. The least that can be expected of the speech pathologist is that he should do what he can to ensure that competent persons are made available to do the indicated counseling. Further, he can be expected to recognize, through his contacts with parents and patients, when professionals other than himself should be consulted. Finally, he should be expected to establish the kind of rapport with parents and patients, as a result of his interest and concern for them, which will give them enough security to reveal their needs for counseling to him. He, in turn, must be secure enough to meet those needs which are in the area of his competence and to be willing to make the necessary referrals when those needs are not in the area of his competence.

IV. Summary

In summary, one cannot help but be impressed, even awed, by the complexity of the cleft palate problem. To work on it, the professional must have a broad and exacting training and a high degree of professional skill. To be effective in this work, he must also have concern for the persons with the problem and must feel secure in his relationships with the professionals from other fields of specialization who share his concern. And most of all, he must not be caught in the possible trap to which the expression "cleft palate speaker" can lead him. He must not view these speakers as persons who can be understood only by the application of a special set of psychological principles. On the contrary, he must realize that he is dealing with a person with feelings, frustrations, and dreams much like his own and that his role, as speech pathologist, includes assisting his client to express those feelings, frustrations, and dreams effectively through speech.

REFERENCES

Baldwin, R. D. (1963). Impediments to the acquisition and use of medical knowledge. *Science* **141**, 1237–1238.

Flexner, A. (1915). Is social work a profession? *School Soc.* **1**, 901–911.

Morris, H. L., ed. (1965). "Cleft Lip and Palate: Criteria for Physical Management." The Univ. of Iowa, Iowa City, Iowa.

Spriestersbach, D. C. (1961). Counseling parents of children with cleft lips and palates. *J. Chron. Diseases* **13**, 244–252.

Spriestersbach, D. C. (1962). Professional survival groups. *Cleft Palate Bull.* **12**, 63–66.

Whitehouse, F. A. (1965). Teamwork as a dynamic system. *Cleft Palate J.* **2**, 16–27.

Author Index

Numbers in italics refer to the pages on which references are listed in bibliographies at end of each article.

A

Abd-el-Malek, S., 12, *22*
Abel, Theodora M., 202, 216, *223*
Abramson, A., 9, 16, *22*
Adams, M. R., 141, *167*, 215, *223*
Alexander, M. H., 184, *198*
Ammons, Helen D., 247, *261*
Ammons, R. B., 247, *261*
Anastasi, Anne 247, *261*
Anderson, Ruth M., 99, *118*, 235, *268*
Ansberry, M., 120, 131, *168*
Arkebauer, H. J., 121, 130, *165*, 230, *263*
Arndt, W. B., Jr., 234, 238, 243, 257, *263*, *266*
Aungst, L. F., 243, 245, *261*, *265*

B

Backus, Ollie L., 202, 213, *222*
Bakes, F. P., 241, *266*
Baldridge, Patricianne, 68, 95, *114*, 254, *263*
Baldwin, R. D., 271, *279*
Ballenger, J. J., 172, 176, 180, 181, 185, 187, 188, 190, 191, 193, 197, *199*
Bankson, N. W., 230, 240, *261*, *266*
Barker, Elizabeth J., 215, *222*
Barker, J. O., 70, *113*
Barker, R. G., 201, 202, *222*
Barnes, Ida J., 127, 129, *165*, 233, 236, *261*
Basmajian, J. V., 242, *261*
Bastian, J., 245, *264*
Battle, R. J. V., 64, *113*

Bauwens, P., 242, *261*
Belt, L. A., 21, *23*
Bensen, J. F., 97, 98, *113*
Bentley, F. H., 64, 66, *113*
Berko, Jean, 248, *261*
Berry, Mildred F., 85, 93, 110, 111, 112, *114*, 120, 132, *165*, 172, *198*, 253, *261*
Bevans, C., 16, *24*
Billig, A. L., 210, *222*
Bingham, H. G., 175, 176, 177, 178, 179, 181, 185, 193, *199*
Birch, J., 214, 217, *222*
Björk, L., 9, 11, *23*, 228, 229, *261*
Black, J. W., 19, *23*, 121, *165*
Blackfield, H. M., 228, 241, *261*
Blakeway, H., 63, *114*
Bloomer, H. H., 136, *165*, 235, *266*
Boky, H., 191, *199*
Borel-Maisonny, S., 64, 66, 67, *118*
Bosma, J. F., 7, 9, *23*, 243, *261*
Bowser, D. C., 250, *267*
Bradford, L. F., 234, *262*
Bradley, Doris P., 207, *222*, 229, *265*
Brandt, Sara D., 129, 143, 157, *165*, 233, *262*
Breckner, V. L., 230, *263*
Brekstad, A., 220, *223*
Brooks, Alta R., 9, *24*. 127, 157, *167*, 228, 230, 233, 234, 238, 240, *262*, *266*
Brooks, R. S., 9, *24*, 175, 177, 192, *199*, 230, *266*
Brown, R., 248, *261*
Brown, S. F., 120, 132, 134, *166*, 202, *223*

281

Brown, S. J., 108, *115*
Bryan, G. A., 234, *262*
Bryt, A., 202, 216, *223*
Buck, M., 254, *262*
Buck, M. W., 152, *166*
Buncke, H. J., Jr., 122, *166*, 230, *262*
Burgi, E. J., 72, 73, *114*
Byrne, Margaret C., 69, 72, 74, 76, 77, 79, 85, 86, *114*, 132, *167*, 240, 244, *261*, *262*, *264*
Bzoch, K. R., 69, 73, 74, 76, 77, 78, 80, 81, 82, 83, 84, 85, 86, 87, 89, 90, 91, 92, 93, 96, 101, 108, 110, *114*, 134, 136, 137, *166*, 232, 233, 238, 259, *262*

C

Calnan, J. S., 64, *114*
Campbell, E. J. M., 3, *23*
Campos-Giral, R., 229, *262*
Carmody, F. J., 8, *23*
Carns, Marie L., 256, *264*
Carr, Anna., 120, 131
Carr, Lela B., 208, *222*
Casteel, R. L., 172, 175, 176, 190, *198*
Chalet, N. J., 188, *198*
Chase, R. A., 230, *262*
Chiba, T., 22, *23*
Chisum, Linda 232, *262*
Christiansen, R. L., 21, *24*
Christovich, L. A., 21, 22, *23*
Cobb, C. M., 232, *266*
Cobb, Lois H., 87, 101, 108, 110, *114*
Coffey, R. J., 97, *115*
Cole, R. M., 229, *262*
Comroe, J. H., Jr., 231, *262*
Conkwright, Elizabeth Anne, 214, *222*
Conway, H., 65, *114*
Cooker, H. S., 69, *114*
Cooper, F. S., 5, 9, 16, 17, 21, *22*, *24*, 241, 245, *262*, *264*
Copetos, Florence G., 250, *267*
Corah, N. L., 215, *222*
Corah, Patricia L., 215, *222*
Counihan, D. T., 69, 73, 74, 76, 77, 79, 80, 82, 83, 85, 86, 87, 89, 90, 91, 92, 96, 101, 106, 107, *114*, 124, 134, 151, *166*, 172, *198*
Crary, Delores F., 245, *262*

Crikelair, G. F., 241, *262*
Crosby, C. A., 72, 81, 102, *114*
Curtis, J. F., 5, *23*, *46*, *60*, 88, 95, 105, 108, 111, *114*, *115*, *117*, 120, 149, 153, *166*, 202, *223*

D

Darley, F. L., 69, 71, 74, 81, 82, 83, 84, 85, 86, 87, 88, 89, 90, 91, 94, 107, 109, *115*, *116*, *117*, 126, 142, *167*, 209, 210, *224*, 226, 227, 230, 233, 237, 247, *262*, *264*, *265*, 267
Davis, Edith, A., 247, *262*
Davis, H., 139, *166*, 171, *198*
Day, Elizabeth J., 247, *263*
De Haan, C. R., 99, *118*, 235, *268*
Dersch, W. C., 99, *118*, 235, *268*
Devereux, J. L., 57, *60*, 129, *168*, 231, *268*
Dickinson, D. G., 3, *24*
Dickson, D. R., 46, *60*, 99, *114*, 235, *263*
Diedrich, W. M., 9, *24*, 69, 72, 74, 76, 77, 79, 85, 86, *114*
Dietze, H., 69, *114*
Doerfler, L. G., 171, 193, 195, *198*
Donaldson, J. A., 187, *198*
Dornette, W. H., L., 230, *263*
Doubek, F., 65, 98, *114*, *118*
Drettner, B., 173, 175, 176, 188, 190, 191, *198*
DuBois, A. B., 129, *168*
Dunn, H. K., 38, *60*
Dunn, L. M., 247, *263*
Dutta, C. R., 242, *261*

E

Eagles, E. L., 171, 193, 195, *198*
Eckelmann, Dorathy, 68, 95, *114*, 254, *263*
Eckstein, A., 64, *114*
Edney, C. W., 108, *115*, 120, *166*, 202, *223*
Egbert, J., H., 142, *166*
Eguchi, B. Y., 68, 74, 80, 106, *114*
Eimas, P., 245, *264*
Eisenson, J., 110, 111, 112, *114*, 120, *165*, 172, *198*, 253, *261*
Elbert, Mary, 234, 238, *263*, *266*
Embrey, J. E., 175, 177, 192, *199*

Ersner, M. S., 184, *198*
Ewanowski, S. J., 243, *266*

F

Falck, Vilma T., 68, 69, 71, 72, 96, 106, 107, *114*
Fant, G., 35, 37, 38, 44, 45, 46, 48, *60*, 97, 99, *114*, 235, *263*
Farmer, A. W., 64, 66, 67, *115*
Farnsworth, D. W., 4, *23*
Fichter, G. R., 250, *267*
Fischer, E., 242, *263*
Fitts, P. M., 256, *263*
Flanagan, J. L., 54, 55, *60*
Fleichman, E. A., 256, *263*
Fletcher, S. G., 7, 9, *23*, 186, *198*
Flexner, A., 270, 272, 273, *279*
Foster, T. D., 64, *114*, 134, *166*
Fowler, E. P., Jr., 241, *262*
Fraser, M., 171, 186, 188, 195, *199*
Frick, J. V., 245, *261*
Fritzell, B., 22, *23*, 69, 70, *115*, 242, *263*
Fromkin, Victoria A., 22, *23*, 241, 242, *263*
Fujimura, O., 22, *23*, 46, 48, *60*
Furlong, Ann K., 250, *267*

G

Gaines, F. P., 171, *198*
Gannon, J., 171, 176, 180, 181, 193, *198*
Gates, A. J., 247, *263*
Glanzer, M., 248, *263*
Glassow, Ruth, 256, *264*
Glover, D. M., 64, 66, 78, *115*, 186, 188, *198*
Gluck, M. R., 214, *222*
Goetzinger, C. P., 175, 177, 192, *199*
Gonick, Mollie R., 201, 202, *222*
Goodstein, L. D., 142, 147, *166*, 207, 208, 210, 212, 217, 218, 219, *223*
Goodwin, F., 104, *117*
Graham, M. D., 139, *166*, 173, 175, 180, 188, 192, 195, *199*
Gray, G. H., 65, *115*
Greene, Margaret C. L., 64, 66, 68, 78, 93, *114*, *115*, 134, *166*, 233, *263*
Griffith, B. C., 245, *264*
Griffiths, Nellie, L., 247, *264*
Grossman, R. C., 243, *263*
Gumpertz, Elizabeth 204, *224*

H

Hackbusch, Florentine, 214, *223*
Hagerty, R. F., 10, *23*, 124, 150, *166*
Haggard, E. A., 220, *223*
Hahn, Elise, 253, 260, *263*
Halfond, M. M., 172, 176, 180, 181, 185, 187, 188, 190, 191, 193, 197, *199*
Halle, M., 44, *60*
Hamlen, M., 65, 66, 67, *115*
Hanley, C. N., 244, *263*
Hanley, T. D., 111, *117*
Hanlon, Nancy, 202, 214, *224*
Hanson, M. L., 99, *115*, 230, *263*
Hardy, J. C., 230, 231, 232, 257, *263*, *264*
Harkins, C. S., 213, *223*
Harrington, R., 254, *262*
Harris, Katherine S., 5, 17, 20, 21, 22, *23*, *24*, 242, 245, *263*, *264*
Hattori, S., 46, 48, *60*
Hayes, C. S., 197, *199*
Heck, Frances, 245, *263*
Heffner, R.-M. S., 12, 16, 22, *23*
Heinz, J. M., 44, *60*
Hellebrandt, F. A., 256, *264*
Hess, D. A., 96, 97, 101, 103, 104, 105, 111, *115*, *264*
Hetherington, J. J., 243, *266*
Hildreth, Gertrude H., 247, *264*
Hill, M. J., 10, *23*, 207, *223*
Hixon, T. J., 57, *60*, 257, *264*
Hoffman, H. S., 245, *264*
Hoffmeister, F. S., 124, 150, *166*
Holborow, C. A., 179, 181, 183, 185, 186, 188, *199*
Holbrook, R. T., 8, *23*
Holdsworth, W. G., 64, 67, *115*, 184, *199*
Hollien, H., 5, *23*
Holmes, E. M., 172, 176, 180, 181, 184, 187, 193, *199*
Holmes, F. L. D., 104, *115*
Holt, D. L., 122, 151, *166*
House, A. S., 38, 41, 42, 45, 48, 50, 51, 52, *60*, 97, 99, 105, 111, *115*
Hudgins, C. V., 8, 19, *23*, *24*, 121, *166*, *168*
Huffman, Evelyn, 257, *266*
Huffman, W. C., 65, 66, 67, *117*
Hughes, G. W., 44, *60*

I

Irwin, J. V., 12, 22, *25*, 68, 95, 112, *118*, 120, *168*, 171, 174, *199*, 210, *223*, 242, 257, *267*
Isshiki, N., 55, *60*, 121, *166*, 231, *264*

J

Jastak, J., 247, *264*
Johnson, W., 107, 108, *115*, 120, *166*, 202, *223*, 226, 227, 237, *264*
Jolleys, A., 64, 67, *115*, 145, *166*
Jones, H. W., 65, *115*
Jordan, E. P., 72, *115*

K

Kahn, J. P., 202, 205, *223*
Kajiyama, M., 22, *23*
Kaltenborn, A., 158, *166*
Kane, J. J., 10, *23*
Kantner, C. E., 95, 100, *115*, 254, *264*
Karlin, J. E., 244, *264*
Kastein, Shulamith, 241, *262*
Keaster, Jacqueline, 108, *115*, 120, *166*, 191, *199*, 202, *223*
Kelleher, R. E., 97, *115*
Kennedy, C., 241, *266*
Kenyon, J. S., 13, *23*
Kinnis, G. C., 203, *223*
Kirk, S. A., 245, 248, *264*
Klinger, H., 69, 74, 81, *115*
Knott, T. A., 13, *23*
Knox, A. W., 234, *266*
Kobes, H. R., 172, *199*
Kodman, F., 150, *166*
Koepke, G. H., 3, *24*
Koepp-Baker, H., 69, 98, 106, 107, 111, *116*, *118*, 125, 128, 131, 133, 151, 152, 153, 158, *166*, *167*, *168*, 172, 186, 188, 189, 193, *199*, 233, 240, 255, *265*, *267*
Kos, C. M., 189, *199*
Kozhevnikov, V. A., 21, 22, *23*
Krueger, A. L., 257, *266*
Kunze, L. H., 55, *60*, 231, *264*
Kydd, W. L., 21, *23*

L

Ladefoged, P., 3, 16, 22, *23*, *24*
Lauer, Edith, 202, 216, *223*

Lawson, Lucie J., 228, 241, *261*
Leach, E. A., 69, 72, 73
Lee, Laura L., 248, *264*
LeMesurier, A. B., 64, 66, 67, *115*
Levine, H. S., 171, 193, 195, *198*
Lewis, Ruth, 210, 211, 212, *223*
Liberman, A. M., 17, *24*, 245, *264*
Lieberman, P., 5, *24*
Lierle, D. M., 65, 66, 67, 87, 101, 108, 110, *114*, *116*, *117*, 139, *168*, 173, 175, 176, 177, 179, 180, 181, 182, 186, 188, 189, 192, 194, *199*, *200*, 209, *224*
Lindsay, W. K., 64, 66, 67, *115*
Linthicum, F. H., 191, *199*
Lintz, Lois B., 101, 102, 103, *115*, 163, *166*, 258, *264*
Lis, E. F., 172, *199*
Lisker, L., 245, *264*
Loeb, W. J., 180, 188, *199*
Low, G. M., 98, *115*, 234, *264*
Lubker, J. F., 97, *115*, 231, 241, *264*
Lutz, K. R., 106, *117*, 234, *266*
Lysaught, G. F., 21, 22, *23*, 242, *263*

M

McCall, G., 243, *266*
McCarthy, Dorothea, 108, *116*, 141, 154, 155, *166*, *167*, 247, 248, 259, *264*
McCarthy, J. J., 245, 248, *264*
MacCollum, D. W., 64, 101, *116*
McCroskey, R., 243, *265*
McDermott, R. P., 69, 72, 81, 88, 89, 94, *116*, 127, 135, 136, *167*
McDonald, E. T., 97, 98, 111, *115*, *116*, 152, 153, 158, *167*, 207, *223*, 230, 237, 240, 242, 243, 255, *264*, *265*
McGlone, R. E., 21, *24*, 226, *267*
McGregor, Frances C., 202, 216, *223*
McIntosh, C. W., Jr., 101, 102, *116*
MacNeilage, P. F., 5, 12, 17, 22, *24*, 242, 245, *264*, *265*
McWilliams, Betty J., 69, 71, 72, 74, 86, 87, 89, 90, 94, 96, 106, 107, 108, *116* 208, 211, 214, *222*, *223*, *224*, 233, *265*
Malecot, A., 19, *24*
Masters, F. W., 175, 176, 177, 178, 179, 181, 185, 193, *199*
Matthews, J., 72, 73, 106, *114*, *117*, 132, 141, *167*, 215, *224*, 234, 240, *264*, *266*

May, Anna M., 210, *223*
Means, Beverly J., 171, 174, *199*, 210, *223*
Mecham, M. J., 247, *264*
Melnik, W., 171, 193, 195, *198*
Melrose, J., 195, *200*
Menyuk, Paula, 248, *264*
Merrill, Maud A., 148, *168*
Mestre, J. D., 240, *267*
Meyerson, L., 201, 202, *222, 223*
Michel, J. F., 234, *264*
Milisen, R. L., 90, *116*
Millard, R. T., 99, *116*, 224, *267*, 235, *264*
Miller, E. R., 228, 241, *261*
Miller, G. F., 187, *199*
Miller, M. H., 172, 185, 188, 193, *199*
Minifie, F. D., 247, *265*
Moffat, Helen M., 208, *223*
Moll, K. L., 9, 11, 22, *24*, 65, 66, 67, 69, 74, 75, 76, 77, 82, 83, 86, 87, 91, 92, 97, 99, *115, 116, 117*, 126, 128, 131, 139, 140, 142, 147, 156, 157, *167, 168*, 173, 175, 176, 177, 179, 181, 182, 186, 189, 192, 194, *200*, 203, 209, 219, *224*, 228, 230, 231, 247, *264, 265, 267*
Moore, P., 4, 5, *25*
Moran, R. E., 65, 67, *116*
Morley, M. E., 64, 66, 68, 92, 112, *116*, 120, 132, 144, 145, *167*, 254, *265*
Morris, H. L., 69, 72, 74, 75, 76, 77, 82, 83, 86, 87, 88, 91, 92, 108, *116, 117*, 126, 127, 128, 129, 131, 140, 142, 143, 146, 148, 153, 154, 156, 157, 164, *165, 167, 168*, 195, *200*, 209, 210, 219, 223, *224*, 228, 230, 231, 233, 236, 239, 247, 254, 259, *261, 262, 265, 266, 267*, 270, 273, 274, 276, *279*
Morrison, Sheila, 72, *116*
Moser, H. M., 254, *265*
Moses, E. R., Jr., 22, *24*
Munson, S. E., 210, *223*
Murphy, A. J., 3, *24*

N

Neely, Betty J. M., 229, *265*
Nitsche, M. Maria, 213, *223*
Noll, J. D., 91, 92, *117*
Nylen, B. O., 228, 235, 241, *266*

O

Obregon, G., 65, *116*
O'Brien, L. W., 69, *118*
Oester, Y. T., 242, *266*
Oldfield, M. C., 64, *116*
Olin, W. H., 180, *199*
Oliver, Dorothy, 132, 134, *166*
Olson, J. L., 248, *264*
Owsley, J. Q., Jr., 228, 241, *261*

P

Paillard, J., 256, *266*
Palmer, J. M., 141, *167*, 215, *223*
Palmer, M. F., 206, 213, *223*
Parmenter, C., 16, *24*
Penfield, W., 243, *266*
Perlman, H. B., 183, *199*
Perrin, E. H., 72, *116*
Pettit, H. S., 10, *23*
Phillips, Betty R. 72, 73, *116*
Pierce, B. R., 234, *266*
Pike, K. L., 16, 19, *24*
Pinson, A. B., 68, 82, 87, 88, *116*, 124, *167*
Pitzner, Joan H., 84, *116*, 128, 142, 146, *167*, 233, *266*
Podvinec, S., 183, *199*
Powers, G. R., 76, 77, 79, 96, 97, 101, 102, 106, *117*, 123, 125, 135, 138, 142, 151, 156, 162, 164, *167, 168*, 186, *200*, 230, *267*
Prather, Elizabeth M., 72, *117*
Prather, W. F., 139, *168*, 173, 175, 176, 177, 179, 181, 182, 186, 189, 192, 194, *200*, 209, *224*
Prins, T. D., 235, 245, *266*
Proffitt, W. R., 21, *24*
Proud, G. O., 175, 177, 192, *199*
Prugh, D. G., 214, *223*
Pruzansky, S., 172, *199*

Q

Quigley, L. F., Jr., 97, *115*, 232, *266*

R

Radley, J. P., 44, *60*
Randall, P., 191, 195, *200*, 241, *266*
Rarick, G. L., 256, *264*

Rasmussen, T., 243, *266*
Reed, G. F., 172, 176, 180, 181, 184, 187, 193, *199*
Reidy, J. P., 64, 66, *117*
Renfrew, Catherine E., 92, 93, *117*
Rhodes, F. E., 250, *267*
Rich, A. R., 183, *199*
Richardson, Sylvia O., 64, 101, *116*
Riello, A., 148, *167*
Ringel, R. L., 121, *166*, 231, 243, *264*, *266*
Ritchie, W., 64, 110, *117*
Robinson, D. W., 175, 176, 177, 178, 179, 181, 185, 193, *199*
Rodriguez, A. A., 242, *266*
Rosenblum, G., 202, 214, *224*
Rosov, R., 21, *23*
Rouse, Verna, 69, 71, 74, 81, 82, 83, 84, 85, 86, 87, 88, 89, 90, 91, 94, *117*, 209, *224*
Rubin, H. J., 4, *24*
Ruess, A. L., 211, 214, 215, *223*, *224*
Rutherford, D., 120, 134, *168*, 243, *266*

S

Sakuda, M., 121, 130, *168*, 232, *267*
Saltar, Nancy, 242, *266*
Sataloff, J., 171, 186, 188, 195, *199*
Saunders, Zane G., 250, *267*
Schiefelbusch, R. L., 248, *266*
Schvey, M. M., 22, *23*, 242, *263*
Schweiger, J. W., 180, *199*
Shames, G. H., 106, *117*, 234, *266*
Shelton, R. L., Jr., 9, *24*, 69, 72, 74, 76, 77, 79, 85, 86, *114*, 127, 157, *167*, 228, 230, 233, 234, 238, 240, 243, 247, 255, 257, *262*, *263*, *266*, *268*
Sherman, Dorothy, 71, 91, 92, 96, 97, 101, 102, 103, 104, *115*, *117*, 163, *166*, 234, 247, 258, 264, *265*, *267*
Shiere, F. R., 232, *266*
Sholes, G. N., 12, 22, *24*
Shriner, T. H., 247, *267*
Shuchardt, K., 64, *114*
Sidney, Ruth A., 141, *167*, 215, 217, *224*
Siegel, G. M., 72, *117*
Silverman, S. R., 139, *166*, 171, *198*
Silverstone, Betty, 202, 214, *224*
Simmons, J. R., 103, *117*
Skard, Ase, G., 220, *223*
Skolnik, E. M., 171, 173, 175, 176, 177,

180, 181, 182, 184, 185, 186, 188, 190 191, 197, *200*
Smith, E. M., 3, *24*
Smith, Jeanne K., 65, 66, 67, *116*, *117*, 131, *167*, 228, 230, 236, 254, *265*
Smith, R. M., 211, *224*
Smith, S., 6, *24*, 97, 99, *117*
Snodgrass, R. M., 181, *200*
Snow, Katherine, 136, *167*, 240, *267*
Sommers, R. K., 250, *267*
Sonesson, B., 5, *24*
Sonninen, A. A., 8, *24*
Spradlin, J. E., 248, *267*
Sprague, Ann L., 240, *267*
Spriestersbach, Bette R., 203, 209, *224*
Spriestersbach, D. C., 69, 71, 74, 75, 76, 77, 79, 81, 82, 83, 84, 85, 86, 87, 88, 89, 90, 91, 92, 94, 95, 96, 97, 101, 102, 103, 106, 107, 109, *115*, *116*, *117*, 123, 125, 126, 128, 131, 136, 139, 140, 142, 147, 151, 156, 157, 162, 164, *167*, *168*, 173, 175, 176, 177, 179, 181, 182, 186, 189, 192, 194, *200*, 203, 204, 205, 209, 210, 219, *224*, 226, 227, 230, 233, 237, 240, *263*, *264*, *265*, *267*, 273, 278, *279*
Stark, R. B., 99, *118*, 235, *268*
Starr, C. D., 69, 74, 76, 77, 79, 82, 83, 84, 85, 86, 89, 90, 91, 92, 93, 101, *117*
Steer, M. D., 111, *117*, 243, *266*
Stetson, R. H., 8, 19, 22, *23*, *24*, 89, *117*, 121, *166*, *168*
Stevens, K. N., 38, 41, 42, 44, 48, 50, 51, 52, *60*, 97, 99, 105, 111, *115*
Stick, S. L., 232, *267*
Stool, S. E., 191, 195, *200*
Strong, L. H., 12, 22, *24*
Subtelny, J. D., 9, 22, *24*, 69, 106, 107, *117*, *118*, 121, 125, 128, 130, 134, 151, 156, *168*, 232, 233, 240, *267*
Subtelny, Joanne, D., 9, 22, *24*, 69, 106, 107, *117*, *118*, 121, 125, 128, 130, 134, 151, 156, *168*, 233, 240, *267*
Swanson, L. T., 64, 101, *116*
Sweitzer, R. S., 195, *200*

T

Takagi, Y., 226, *267*
Tangen, G. V., 173, 185, 186, 187, 188, 191, 193, *200*

Tavener, D., 242, *267*
Templin, Mildred C., 71, 74, 76, 77, 84, 87, 108, 109, *118*, 143, *168*, 237, 244, 245, 247, *267*
Terman, L. M., 148, *168*
Timcke, R., 4, 5, *25*
Tisza, Veronica B., 202, 204, 214, *224*
Trauner, R., 65, *118*
Travis, L. E., 120, *168*
Truby, H. M., 8, 9, 12, 21, 22, *25*

V

Van Demark, Ann A., 84, 90, 92, *118*
Van Demark, D. R., 69, 71, 74, 84, 90, 92, 93, 96, 97, 106, *118*, 161, *168*, 233, *267*
van den Berg, Jw., 4, 6, *25*, 55, *60*
Van Hattum, R. J., 72, 96, 97, 101, 106, *118*
Van Riper, C. G., 12, 22, *25*, 68, 95, 112, *118*, 120, *168*, 242, 254, 257, *267*
Veau, V., 64, 66, 67, *118*
Velander, E., 64, 66, *118*
von Leden, H., 4, 5, *25*

W

Wagner, J. A., 171, 184, *200*
Wardill, W. E. M., 64, *118*, 145, *168*
Warren, D. W., 57, *60*, 129, *168*, 231, *268*
Watkins, J., 64, 66, *113*
Watson, C. G., 141, *168*, 216, 218, *224*
Weachter, Eugenia H., 204, *224*

Weatherley-White, R. C. A., 99, *118*, 235, *268*
Webster, Martha J., 247, *268*
Webster, R. C., 97, *115*, 232, *266*
Wechsler, D., 148, *168*
Weiss, A. J., 96, 98, 105, *118*, 234, *268*
Weissmann, Serena, 202, 216, *223*
Wells, Charlotte G., 254, *268*
Wepman, J. W., 244, *268*
West, R., 120, 131, *168*
Westlake, H., 120, 134, *168*, 203, 204, 216, *224*
Whaley, J. B., 172, 188, *200*
Whitehouse, F. A., 277, *279*
Wildman, A. J., 122, *168*
Williams, H. B., 65, *118*
Williamson, A. B., 105, *118*
Wilson, D. K., 69, *118*
Winitz, H., 149, *168*, 247, 248, *268*
Wishik, S. M., 171, 193, 195, *198*
Wolstad, D. M., 210, *224*
Wood, K. S., 141, *168*
Woodhouse, F. M., 65, *118*
Worth, J. H., 121, 130, *168*, 232, *267*
Wright, Beatrice A., 201, 202, *222*
Wright, H. N., 72, *118*
Wylie, H. L., 214, *222*
Wynn Parry, C. B., 242, *268*

Y

Yamanoto, K., 46, 48, *60*
Young, N. B., 97, *118*, 230, *268*
Youngstrom, K. A., 9, *24*, 127, 157, *167*, 228, 230, 233, 240, *262*, *266*

Subject Index

A

Acoustic signals of speech, 28–30
  amplitude, 29
  duration, 28–29
  periodicity vs. aperiodicity, 28
  spectral composition, 29–30
Acoustic theory, 30–45
Acoustics of nasalization, 45–52
Adenoids, tonsils, and hearing loss, 187–189
Age and hearing loss, 191–193
Age at surgery and hearing loss, 171–181
Air flow measurement, 6
Allergy and hearing loss, 191
Amplitude, speech signal, 29
Articulation in cleft palate speech, 68–95
  articulation status, 74–80
    age differences, 75–76
    age of physical management, 79–80
    sex differences, 78–79
    type of cleft differences, 76–78
    type of physical management, 79
  measurement procedures, 69–73
    reliability of, 70–72
    selection of, 73
    subjectivity of, 70
    validity of, 70–72
  misarticulation patterns, 80–95
    consistency of articulation, 94–95
    consonant articulation, place of, 84–86
    consonant production, manner of, 82–84
    consonant, voicing, 86–87
    phonetic context, 87–89
    types of misarticulation, 89–94
    vowel-consonant differences, 81–82
Articulation disorders, etiology, 121–149,
  156–162

anatomical and physiological bases,
  121–140
  cleft lip, 131–132
  combination of factors, 136–137
  dentition, 134–136
  hearing acuity, 138–140
  nasal cavities, 137–138
  tongue motility and carriage, 132–134
  velopharyngeal incompetence, 121–131
behavioral bases, 140–149
  learning factors, 142–147
  mental retardation and brain injury,
    147–149
  psychosocial factors, 140–142
discussion of, 156–162
Articulation in normal speech, 6–22
  adjustments for speech sounds, 13–22
    consonants, 13–14, 16–19
    recording of articulatory data, methods
      of, 21–22
    vowels, 13–16
  configurations, methods of studying, 6–7
  pharyngeal configurations, 7–9
    radiological study, 8–9
  upper vocal tract couplings and configu-
    rations, 9–13
Articulation therapy, 249–257
  exercise and motor learning, 253–257
  procedures, 251–253

C

Cleft lip and articulation, 131–132
Cleft type and hearing loss, 175–176
Congenital anomalies and hearing loss,
  181–182

D

Degree of cleft and hearing loss, 176–177
Dentition and articulation, 134–136
Diagnosis, speech, 226-248
  hearing acuity and auditory perception, 244–245
  language maturity, 246–248
  neural function, 241–244
  oral-facial structures, 239–241
  psychosocial adjustment, 245–246
  speech problems, 237–239
  velopharyngeal competence, 227–237
Duration, speech signal, 28–29

E

Eustachian tube and palatal muscle function, 182–187
  dysfunction and hearing loss, 184–187
  normal function, 182–184

H

Hearing acuity and articulation, 138–140
Hearing acuity and auditory perception, evaluation of, 244–245
  standard audiometric techniques, 244
  tests of auditory perception, 244–245
  treatment decision, 245
Hearing loss and aural pathology, incidence, 170–194
  cleft palate population, 171–174
  general school age population, 170–171
  related variables, 174–194
    adenoids and tonsils, 187–189
    age, 191–193
    age at surgery, 171–181
    allergy, 191
    cleft type, 175–176
    congenital anomalies, 181–182
    degree of cleft, 176–177
    eustachian tube and palatal muscle function, 182–187, 196
    nasal obstruction, swollen turbinates, and sinuses, 189–191
    physical management type, 171–181
    reflux of food, 193
    respiratory infections, upper, 193–194
    sex, 177

Hearing loss, criterion, 194, 195
Hearing loss, implications of research for management, 194–198

L

Language development, 108–110, 153–156, 164–165, 246–248, 259–260
  characteristics of, in the cleft palate population, 108–110
  diagnostic techniques, 246–248
  etiology of problems, 153–156, 164–165
  therapy procedures, 259–260
  treatment decision, 248
Larynx, 53–58

M

Mannerisms, 112, 137–138
Measures of degree of nasality, 96–100
  of the acoustic spectrum, 99–100
  of air flow or pressure, 97–98
  by listener-judgment procedures, 96–97
  of nasal sound pressure, 98–99
Mental retardation, brain injury, and articulation, 147–149

N

Nares constriction, 137
Nasal cavity deviations and articulation, 137–138
Nasal coupling with pharyngeal-oral tract, 45–51
Nasal obstruction, swollen turbinates, sinuses, and hearing loss, 189–191
Nasality, 81–82, 95–107, 150–153
  in individuals with cleft palates, 101–107
    articulation and intelligibility, 105–107
    phonetic factors, 101–103
    vocal intensity, 104–105
    vocal pitch, 103–104
    voice quality disorder, 150–153
    and vowel articulation, 81–82
  measurement techniques for, 96–100
    listener-judgment procedures, 96–97
    "objective" measures, 97–100
Neural function, 241–244
  diagnostic techniques, 241–244
  treatment decision, 244

O

Oral-facial structures, diagnosis of deviations, 239–241
   dentition, 240
   lips, 239
   nasal cavities, 240
   tongue, 239–240
   treatment decision, 241

P

Parents, 203–208, 219
   immediate concerns, 203–207
   learning about the defect, 203
   psychological adjustment, 207–208
   socioeconomic differences, 219
Periodicity vs. aperiodicity of speech signal, 28
Personality, and adjustment of the child, 213–217
Physical management type, 171–181
Professional considerations, 269–278
   other "professions," 269–273
   speech pathologist, 275–278
      roles, 276–278
      training and orientation, 275–276
   teamwork, 273–275
Psychological adjustment, 245–246
   diagnostic techniques, 245–246
   treatment decision, 246
Psychosocial aspects, problems of studying, 218–220
   heterogenity of samples, 218–219
   representativeness of samples, 219–220
   retrospective reports, 220
Psychosocial development of the child, 209–213
   intelligence, 209–212
   social competence, 212–213
Psychosocial factors and etiology of articulation problems, 140–142
Psychosocial problems, 217–218

R

Reflux of food and hearing loss, 193
Respiration and cleft palate speech, 52, 59–60, 254
Respiration in normal speech, 2–4, 58–60

Respiratory infections, upper, and hearing loss, 193–194

S

Sex and hearing loss, 177
Spectral composition, nasalized speech signal, 44–50
   antiresonances and zeros, 46–47
   bandwidth, 44–45, 47
   damping, 47, 50
   vowels, 47–49
Spectral composition, normal speech signal, 29–30, 33–44
   antiresonance and zeros, 36–38
   bandwidth, 35–36, 43
   damping, 36
   formants, 43–44
   resonance, 35–38, 43
   source spectrum, 33–38
   vowels, 40–42
Speech characteristics, problems in the study of, 69–109
   measurement procedures, 69–70, 73–74, 80, 96–97, 103, 106–107
   sampling errors, 75, 76, 79, 88
   validity, 70–72, 96–100
   variability of findings, 63–66, 78, 80, 83–84, 89–91, 101, 109
Speech problems, diagnosis of, 237–239
   techniques of diagnosis, 237–238
   treatment decision, 238–239
Speech problems, and subgroup differences, incidence of, 63–68
   age of management, 67
   cleft type, 66
   other subgroups, 67–68
Speech sounds, excitation of vocal cavities, 53–58
   vocal cavity constriction, 57–58
   vocal fold vibration, 53–57

T

Teamwork, 273–275
Therapy, speech, 249–261
   articulation, 251–253
   exercise and motor learning, 253–257
   language development and communication, 259–260

voice, 257–259
Tongue motility and carriage, effects on articulation, 132–134

V

Velopharyngeal closure, normal speech, 10–11
Velopharyngeal competence, evaluation of, 227–237
  articulation proficiency, 232–234
  examination of the oral cavity, 227–228
  intraoral air pressure, 231
  nasality, 234–235
  oral manometers and manometric measures, 230–231
  rate of oral and nasal air flow, 231–232
  stimulability, 235–236
  treatment decision, 236–237
  x-ray films, 228–230
Velopharyngeal incompetence, 51–52, 84, 121–131
Vocal cavity constriction and speech sounds, 57–58
Vocal fold vibration, 4–6, 53–57
  and subglottic effects, 5–6, 55–57
    on intensity, 5, 55–56
    on pitch, 5, 56–57
Voice disorders, 110–112, 149–153, 162–164
  intensity, 110–111
  loudness, 149–150
  pitch, 110–111, 149
  quality, 111–112, 150–153
Voice therapy, 257–259